Law and Ethics for Health Practitioners

Law and Ethics for Health Practitioners

SONIA ALLAN, OAM CF

LLB (Hons), BA(Hons), MPH (Merit), LLM (Dist), PhD, GDLP GCHE
Associate Professor (Health Law)
Deakin Law School, Deakin University, Victoria, Australia

ELSEVIER

Sydney   Edinburgh   London   New York   Philadelphia   St Louis   Toronto

Elsevier Australia. ACN 001 002 357
(a division of Reed International Books Australia Pty Ltd)
Tower 1, 475 Victoria Avenue, Chatswood, NSW 2067

ISBN: 978-0-7295-4303-3

Notice

Practitioners and researchers must always rely on their own experience and knowledge in evaluating and using any information, methods, compounds or experiments described herein. Because of rapid advances in the medical sciences, in particular, independent verification of diagnoses and drug dosages should be made. To the fullest extent of the law, no responsibility is assumed by Elsevier, authors, editors or contributors for any injury and/or damage to persons or property as a matter of products liability, negligence or otherwise, or from any use or operation of any methods, products, instructions, or ideas contained in the material herein.

National Library of Australia Cataloguing-in-Publication Data

 A catalogue record for this book is available from the National Library of Australia

Senior Content Strategist: Melinda McEvoy
Content Project Manager: Shubham Dixit
Edited by Matt Davies
Proofread by Annabel Adair
Cover by Georgette Hall
Internal design: Standard
Index by Innodata Indexing
Typeset by Toppan Best-set Premedia Limited
Printed in China by RR Donnelley Asia

Last digit is the print number: 9 8 7 6 5 4 3 2 1

CONTENTS

Foreword viii

Preface.. x

About the Author xii

Acknowledgements xii

Contributors and Reviewers xiii

Section 1 INTRODUCTION TO LAW AND ETHICS FOR HEALTH PRACTITIONERS 1

1   INTRODUCTION TO THE AUSTRALIAN LEGAL SYSTEM.....................2

2   INTRODUCTION TO THE AUSTRALIAN HEALTH SYSTEM..............16

3   INTRODUCTION TO ETHICS AND ETHICAL DECISION MAKING 24

Section 2 PROFESSIONAL REGULATION AND KEY CONCEPTS RELEVANT TO HEALTHCARE DELIVERY 31

4   PROFESSIONAL REGULATION OF HEALTH PRACTITIONERS 32

5   MANAGEMENT OF HEALTH INFORMATION 48

6   NEGLIGENCE 63

7   INTENTIONAL TORTS 79

8   CRIMINAL LAW AND ISSUES RELATED TO HEALTH CARE 92

Section 3 MATTERS OF LIFE AND DEATH... 107

9   REGISTRATION OF BIRTHS AND DEATHS AND THE CORONERS COURT..108

10   ABORTION, WRONGFUL BIRTH, WRONGFUL LIFE AND PRENATAL INJURY 116

11   ASSISTED REPRODUCTION AND SURROGACY 124

12   ADVANCE CARE PLANNING AND THE WITHHOLDING AND WITHDRAWAL OF TREATMENT...........132

Section 4 FURTHER PRACTICE CONSIDERATIONS 145

13   THE REMOVAL AND DONATION OF HUMAN BLOOD, TISSUE AND ORGANS 146

14   THE REGULATION OF DRUGS AND POISONS...152

15   MENTAL HEALTH LEGISLATION 162

16   CHILD AND ELDER ABUSE 174

Section 5 LAW AND ETHICS IN ACTION 183

17 WORKING WITH LEGAL REPRESENTATIVES 184

18 CASE STUDIES: GUIDED APPLICATION OF LEGAL AND ETHICAL PRINCIPLES 196

INDEX 249

This book is dedicated to my father, Alberto Magri

FOREWORD

What is health law? Thirty years ago, when I was an undergraduate in law school, there were no health law electives available to study. In that time, only pioneers such as Prof. Loane Skene (The University of Melbourne), the dearly departed John McPhee (The University of Newcastle) and Prof. Colin Thomson (University of Wollongong) were starting to teach health law as a distinct subject, rather than as a component of private laws such as torts. It was work like theirs that created a foundation for a new subdiscipline, and they built it from the basic blocks of contract, tort and crime. Those efforts were later joined with the applied philosophy of Prof. Tom Campbell (Australian National University), the expert advocacy experience of Prof. Ian Freckelton (now The University of Melbourne), the concern over the legal dimensions of the HIV/AIDS epidemic in the work of Prof. Roger Magnusson (The University of Sydney) and the joint disciplinary knowledge of law and medicine in the late, great Prof. Tom Faunce (Australian National University). The power of this combined scholarship was soon noticed by others in Australia and overseas – Australian health law had been born.

It is dangerous to generalise about those wonderful years of scholarship, but it was marked by great collegiality and support for younger colleagues. Very quickly a second generation of scholarship started to emerge. The author of this text, Assoc. Prof. Sonia Allan, is part of that generation, and her work on the laws of reproductive technologies are internationally renowned. While the first-generation scholars had been busy creating a new legal subdiscipline, the second-generation scholars were very much engaged with getting the health professions to understand the impact of law and regulation on their practices and to encourage the health professions to incorporate legal thinking into their everyday experience. Law is not just something that 'happens' to a health practitioner when they do something wrong – it is an embedded part of the normative framework of everyday professional life. It is essential for health practitioners to understand and incorporate the law into their day-to-day working lives and to see it as something that can facilitate best practice.

Sonia has had a career devoted to this message, and this book is a testament to her dedication. This book is aimed at helping health professionals (and lawyers new to health law) to understand how law (and the related ethical principles) work in every aspect of health practice. Sonia's task has been to make clear the normative frameworks of Australian health law and, in the lucid chapters of this book, she has succeeded. It is hard to imagine how difficult this task is in our frenetic little federation. With six states, two territories and a federal jurisdiction, there is much law to discuss, but Sonia does this with such ease that it makes one underestimate the enormity of the undertaking.

I am very honoured to have been asked to write this foreword and I do so as Sonia's colleague and fellow member of the second generation of Australian health lawyers. I congratulate her on this achievement, and I look forward to seeing how the book is received by the next generation – the third generation – of Australian health law. What will be their contribution? It is hard to say, but whatever their mission becomes, it will have been made much easier because of the hard work of Sonia contained in this text.

Let me return to the original question: what is health law? It began as the principles of contract, tort and crime that relate to health professionals. Over time, the growth of regulation has meant that those common law principles, while still important, no longer dominate discussion, and equal time has been devoted to specific regulation of health care in different contexts. In the future, these growth patterns will continue and health law will grow further in size and independence. Those of you seeking to become part of the next generation will do well to start here.

PROF. CAMERON STEWART
Sydney Law School
July 2019

PREFACE

*L*aw and Ethics for Health Practitioners contains extensively researched information on the professional and practice obligations of healthcare practitioners when providing health services. Critical examination of the law and ethics is presented on a wide array of health law matters, relevant to individual as well as population health.

Detailed discussion of the law illustrates that much of health law regulation falls to the states and territories and differs across the country in a variety of ways. The Commonwealth's integral role in relation to healthcare law and policy is also detailed. In addition, examination of the role of ethics, professional codes of practice, and guidelines, is integrated into the book to provide health practitioners with a robust understanding of the regulatory environment within which they work. Practical guidance is also provided to demonstrate a process for reasoned decision making when faced with challenging healthcare issues. Such a process exemplifies how health practitioners may move beyond intuitive responses to such issues to consider the ethical and legal dimensions of a problem, options for resolution, and the justification for the decision made.

The book is structured in five sections:

- Section 1 provides an *Introduction to Law and Ethics for Health Practitioners* examining the Australian legal system, the Australian healthcare system, and providing an introduction to ethics and ethical decision making.
- Section 2 examines *Professional Regulation and Key Concepts Relevant to Healthcare Delivery*.

This section includes consideration of health practitioner registration and accreditation schemes, healthcare complaints systems, management of patient information, and civil and criminal areas of law relevant to healthcare practice standards and delivery.

- Section 3 focuses on *Matters of Life and Death*, including detailed consideration of the registration of births and deaths, and the Coroners Court. Regarding the beginning of life, Section 3 also examines ethically and legally challenging matters such as abortion, wrongful birth and wrongful life claims, pre-natal injury, assisted reproduction and surrogacy. Regarding the end of life, Section 3 considers advance care planning, and the withholding and withdrawal of treatment.
- Section 4 moves to examine the law regarding blood, tissue and organ donation; the regulation of drugs and poisons; mental health legislation; and child and elder abuse. These matters all reflect individual as well as population health concerns.
- Section 5 draws the discussion throughout the book together, providing further insights into *Law and Ethics in Action*. It contains practical information about working with legal representatives, as well as providing an extensive array of case studies illustrative of legal and ethical dilemmas that practitioners may face. The book benefits from the case studies having been drafted by a wide variety of healthcare practitioners drawn from

medicine, midwifery, nursing, paramedicine, pharmacy, physiotherapy, podiatry, and speech pathology. Their contributions and experience enable modelling of an applied approach to reasoned decision making and the translation of law and ethics into practice.

SONIA ALLAN OAM CF BA (Psych)(Hons), LLB (Hons), LLM (Global Health Law) (Dist), MPH(Merit), PhD
May 2019

ABOUT THE AUTHOR

Associate Professor Sonia Allan OAM CF trained as a psychologist prior to coming to the law. Her experience in working with adults and children in a variety of healthcare settings led to significant interest in the interplay between ethics, law, regulation and health. It also led to the desire to impact health regulation in positive ways for those who work in the health sector, those who access health services, and the wider community. She has for more than 25 years focused her study, research and work on health and law.

ACKNOWLEDGEMENT

Sonia thanks Deakin University, School of Law, where she is employed as an Associate Professor of Health Law. Sonia is also very grateful to the members of the Elsevier concept, editorial and publishing team, and Matt Davies for his editing. She especially thanks her children, Mahalia Rose and Gabriel Jackson, who continually share with her such endeavours and are full of wonder, curiosity and joy.

Elsevier Australia and Sonia Allan would like to acknowledge the contribution of Kim Forrester and Debra Griffiths who authored *Essentials of Law for Health Professionals* 4e, which was originally published in 2001, on which this publication is based. We also wish to thank the contributors and the reviewers of this book, whose work and feedback has been tremendous.

CONTRIBUTORS AND REVIEWERS

CONTRIBUTORS

Prof. Clare Delany, BAppScPhysio, MPhysio(Manip), LLM, PhD
Department of Medical Education, The University of Melbourne, Clinical Ethicist, Children's Bioethics Centre, The Royal Children's Hospital

Jackie Dempsey, RN, GDLP, LLB
Campus Course Advisor Parramatta, Associate Lecturer, School of Nursing and Midwifery, Western Sydney University

Dr Sally de-Vitry Smith, PhD
National Program Manager, Australian Nurse-Family Partnership, Abt Associates

Trish Johnson, BAppSc(SpPath), MMgt, MSPA
Manager, Ethics and Professional Issues, Speech Pathology Australia

Dr Suze Leitão, PhD, CPSP, FSPA
Life Member of SPA, Associate Professor, School of Occupational Therapy, Social Work and Speech Pathology, Faculty of Health Sciences, Curtin University, Honorary Research Associate, Telethon Kids Institute, Associate Investigator, ARC Centre of Excellence in Cognition and its Disorders, Macquarie University

Dr Dominique Martin, MBBS, BA(Hons), PhD
Associate Professor in Bioethics and Professionalism, School of Medicine, Deakin University

Nikolaos Nikolopoulos, BPod(Hons), LLM(LP), MBusSys, PDLP
Podiatry Department, La Trobe University

Dr Maree Donna Simpson, GradCert (UnivTeach&Learn), BPharm, BSc(Hons), PhD, MPS, SFHEA
Associate Professor, Pharmacy & Health Studies Group Discipline Leader, Head of Pharmacy, Charles Sturt University

Dr Ruth Townsend, DipParaSc, GDLP, LLB, LLM, PhD
Senior Lecturer, Paramedic Law, Ethics and Professionalism, Charles Sturt University

Brett Vaughan, BSc, MHlthSc, GradCertTertEd
Lecturer, Department of Medical Education, The University of Melbourne

REVIEWERS

Dr Judith Anderson, PhD
General Manager, Opal Specialist Aged Care, Adjunct Senior Lecturer, Charles Sturt University

Dr Georgia Clarkson, DipEd, DipAmbPara, BA, MEd, PhD
Senior Lecturer, Paramedicine, Australian Catholic University

Jaci Mason, RN, RMN, BSc(Hons), PGCHPE, FHEA, DipNLP, MSc, PhD Candidate
Lecturer, School of Nursing, Midwifery and Paramedicine, Curtin University

Dr Rebekkah Middleton, DipAppSc(Nursing), BN, MNRes, PhD, GCEN, GCCM
Senior Lecturer, BN Academic Program Director, L&T Scholar, School of Nursing, University of Wollongong

Andrea Miller, BN(Hons), MEd, MClinNurs, GDHS, GCULT, GCST
(Acting) Director of Undergraduate Studies (Curriculum), School of Nursing, College of Health and Medicine, University of Tasmania

Section 1

INTRODUCTION TO LAW AND ETHICS FOR HEALTH PRACTITIONERS

1

INTRODUCTION TO THE AUSTRALIAN LEGAL SYSTEM

LEARNING OBJECTIVES

Upon completing this chapter you should be able to:

- explain why the study of health law is an essential aspect of your professional practice
- discuss the features of the Australian legal system
- identify the sources of law and explain the different types of law
- discuss the hierarchy of the courts and understand the concept of jurisdiction
- explain the distinction between criminal and civil law
- describe the doctrine of precedent, natural justice and the presumption of innocence
- demonstrate the ability to locate and read a case and an Act of Parliament.

INTRODUCTION

In Australia the law plays a fundamental role in the provision of health care. It, to a significant degree, determines the structure and operation of the Australian health system, regulates the delivery of healthcare services, and establishes the rights and obligations of health practitioners and recipients of care. Understanding the law in relation to health, health care and the delivery of healthcare services, however, is complex. It requires an understanding of the Australian federal system of governance, as well as of the primary sources of law – legislation and the common law decisions of judges. One must also understand the general features of the Australian legal system and how the law operates. The obligations and responsibilities arising from the

federal government's commitment to international treaties and declarations also impact significantly on the provision of healthcare services within the Australian context. This chapter therefore introduces the reader to key concepts and elements of the Australian system of governance, the legal system and sources of law.

AUSTRALIA AS A FEDERATION

Australia is a fully independent democratic nation, with historical links to Britain as a colonial power. On 1 January 1901 the Australian Constitution[1] established a federal system of government. Various powers were distributed between a national government (the Commonwealth) and the six former colonies (now states) of New South Wales, Victoria, Queensland, South Australia, Western Australia and Tasmania. Within the Commonwealth there is also now the self-governing Australian Capital Territory and the Northern Territory plus the external territories of Norfolk Island, Christmas Island and the Cocos (Keeling) Islands.

DISTRIBUTION OF POWER BETWEEN THE STATES AND THE COMMONWEALTH

The federal structure of government and distribution of power between the states and the Commonwealth is fundamental to Australia's governance and its legal system. The legislative (law-making) powers of the Commonwealth Parliament are primarily found in sections 51 and 52 of the Australian Constitution. Section 51 lists 40 areas over which the Commonwealth Parliament has law-making power, including powers to regulate international and interstate trade and commerce (s 51(1); the corporations power (s 51(xx)); the external affairs power (s 51(xxix)); the taxation power (s 51(ii)); the quarantine power (s 51(xxxii)); power relevant to insurance other than state insurance (s 51(xiv)); and power regarding the provision of allowances and benefits (s 51(xxxiiiA)) (see further Chapter 2).

State parliaments can also refer matters to the Commonwealth Parliament under section 51(xxxvii) of the Constitution. This means that states can ask the Commonwealth to make laws about an issue that is usually a state responsibility. Any resultant federal law only applies in the state(s) that referred the matter or that decide to adopt the law.

The Commonwealth Parliament has exclusive power to make laws in areas such as defence and communication (s 52). Matters not listed in sections 51 or 52 of the Constitution, where federal powers are defined, are state responsibilities. These areas where states have law-making powers include roads, schools, ambulance services, hospitals, police, prisons.[2]

The government power to make laws can be categorised as:

- **exclusive**, when only the government is able to exercise power to legislate – for example, the federal government has exclusive power to legislate in relation to foreign affairs
- **concurrent**, when both levels of government are able to legislate on the matter – for example, regarding industrial relations, roads and health
- **residual**, when the states continue to be able to legislate on any issue provided it is in relation to peace, order and good government, and without the need for authority from the Commonwealth government or any other authority – for example, legislation relating to the control of drugs and poisons.

When the Commonwealth and state parliaments both may make laws on the same matter, sometimes there may be conflict. Such conflict is resolved by reference to section 109 of the Constitution, which provides that when there is an inconsistency between a state law and a Commonwealth law, the Commonwealth law applies. The state law is said to be invalid to the extent of the inconsistency.

In recent decades, decisions of the High Court regarding constitutional disputes, including issues relating to section 51 of the Constitution, have led to an expanding of the power and influence of the Commonwealth government while simultaneously reducing state powers. For example, section 51(xxix) of the Constitution confers on the Commonwealth Parliament the power to legislate with respect to 'external affairs'. This has been interpreted by the High Court to mean that the Commonwealth Parliament may legislate to implement an international treaty, which then binds the states to that treaty. Some examples of international declarations and conventions of particular relevance to the health professions include the following:

- The *Universal Declaration of Human Rights* sets out basic rights and fundamental freedoms to which all human beings are entitled. This includes Article 25, which provides that 'everyone has the right to a standard of living adequate for the health and well-being of himself and his family, including food, clothing, housing, medical care, and necessary social services'.[3]
- The *International Covenant on Economic, Social and Cultural Rights*, and the associated General Comment 14, support individual rights in attaining the highest attainable standard of physical and mental health.[4]
- The *Convention on the Elimination of all Forms of Discrimination against Women*, in particular Article 11(1), protects women's rights in relation to work and protects against dismissal in relation to pregnancy or maternity. Article 12 ensures equitable access to healthcare services, including in relation to family planning, pregnancy and the postnatal period, and Article 14 protects the right of rural women to access healthcare services (among other things).
- The 1989 *Convention on the Rights of the Child* requires states to recognise the right of children to enjoy the highest attainable standard of health and to facilities that treat illness and provide rehabilitation services.[5]
- The *Convention on the Rights of Persons with Disabilities* protects the rights and dignity of people

with disabilities. It requires parties to the Convention to promote, protect and ensure the full enjoyment of human rights of people with disabilities and to ensure they enjoy full equality under the law.[6]

THE SEPARATION OF POWERS

To prevent abuse of power and to provide for a fair and just system of government that includes 'checks and balances', there is an enshrined 'separation of powers' between the three branches of government: the executive, legislative and judiciary.

Members of the executive are elected via popular vote. They are tasked with putting the laws passed by the legislature into operation.

Members of the legislature represent both the ruling and opposing political parties and are drawn from different geographical constituencies. The legislative branch of government in each state (except Queensland) and the federal government has two houses of parliament (referred to as 'bicameral') consisting of a lower house of representatives and an upper house of review. Queensland and the territories each have 'unicameral' legislatures, in which there is no upper house. The legislature is responsible for making laws.

Judges are appointed by the executive with the approval of the legislature. The separation between the executive and the judiciary at the federal, state and territory levels means judges are prevented from being part of the executive or the legislature. The judiciary interprets law and can also determine constitutional issues regarding whether the government is acting within its power. Courts exercising their jurisdiction must be free from legislative or executive interference.

The two primary sources of law in Australia – legislation and case law – emanate from the legislative and judicial branches of government (see Box 1.1).

LEGISLATION

In Australia each parliament has the power to make laws and amend or repeal existing laws. The laws enacted by the federal and state/territory governments are written down within Acts of Parliament and are commonly referred to as 'legislation' or 'statutes'. An Act passed by parliament is considered a primary source of the law

---

BOX 1.1
SOURCES OF LAW

JUDGE-MADE OR COMMON LAW
- Judges decide on cases brought before the courts.
- Court proceedings are initiated by litigants who have a dispute needing a legal remedy.
- Judges develop the common law principles known as precedents.
- Cases are decided on the evidence presented and also within the parameters of established precedent or prior judgments.
- Judges apply legal remedies to actual disputes between people or about points of law including equitable principles.
- The *ratio decidendi* is the 'reason for deciding' or the principle of law upon which the case was decided.
- The judgment may contain comments that clarify a situation but do not make new law (*obiter dicta*). Comments made in *obiter* are not regarded as new law.

LEGISLATION OR STATUTORY LAW
- Legislation passed by parliament on a matter is known as a statute or Act (primary legislation).
- Statutory bodies and ministers have the power to make regulations and rules (delegated legislation).

---

because the government has the mandate to enact laws on behalf of the people who have elected it to power. Legislation has priority over judge-made law (case law) to the extent of any inconsistency because judges are not popularly elected.

Some states and territories also have codes on particular areas of law, which are a type of legislation that purports to cover a complete area of law because it existed at the time the code was enacted. For example, refer to Chapter 8 for the criminal law codes.

The Passage of Legislation

While a law is progressing through parliament, it is referred to as a 'Bill'. Once passed by parliament and assented to by the Governor-General (federal legislation) or Governor (state legislation), it becomes an Act of Parliament. The process involved in passing an Act entails following certain procedures in a prescribed sequence as shown in Fig. 1.1.

Most Bills introduced in parliament are government Bills initiated by the minister with portfolio responsibility for the area the Bill addresses. For example, the

The need is established for a new law or changes to an old law

↓

Members of parliament are made aware of the need for change

↓

Notice is given to the lower house that a Bill will be introduced at the next sitting

↓

First reading

↓

Second reading and debate

↓

Committee stage

↓

Third reading

↓

Upper house follows a similar process as that in the lower house

↓

The Bill is presented to the Governor-General or Governor for Royal Assent

↓

The Act of Parliament is proclaimed

Fig. 1.1 ▪ **Stages of passing an Act of Parliament**

health minister would introduce a Bill relevant to universal health care. The Bill is first introduced in the house of parliament in which the minister sits (excluding money and taxation Bills at the federal level, which must be introduced into the House of Representatives). Individual members of parliament can also introduce non-government Bills. These are known as private members' Bills in the House of Representatives and private senators' Bills in the Senate. Once a Bill passes through both houses, the Governor-General must grant it Royal Assent for it to become law.

The first stage of a Bill being considered by parliament is when members are given notice that at the next sitting of parliament a Bill will be introduced. Explanatory documents and a brief outline of the reasons for the Bill usually, but not always, accompany this announcement. The Bill is then placed on the agenda for the next parliamentary sitting. Unless the Bill pertains to a matter of urgency, it is not dealt with in detail at that sitting other than by way of a reading of the long title. This is known as the **first reading**. Ministers are given the documents to take away and read in preparation for the next stage. If the matter is urgent then standing orders will be suspended and the Bill will be debated and passed that day.

Under ordinary circumstances, the Bill is debated at a later date. This is referred to as the **second reading**. At that time the matter is debated and the parties in opposition may propose amendments before the Bill is passed by the house.

At the committee stage, each of the provisions of the Bill will be debated with the full house of parliament sitting as a committee. This stage of the process is a procedural mechanism and does not require the members of the parliament to operate as an investigative committee. The purpose is to consider the details of a Bill after the second reading and examine any amendments proposed by the other house of parliament if it is referred back. This process is a way of determining whether any of the provisions in the Bill fail to meet the intention of the proposed law, or if there are any unintended consequences arising from any sections of the Bill. The Bill then moves on to a **third reading** and is passed by the lower house.

The Bill is then referred to the other house – for example, if the above process took place in the House of Representatives, it is referred to the Senate – where it is examined and debated in a manner and sequence similar to that described above again. Any recommended amendments to the Bill are referred back to the other house and, if these are accepted, the Bill is presented to the Governor-General or Governor for **Royal Assent**. Once this occurs the Bill becomes an Act of Parliament. The Act may not become effective immediately because it must first be proclaimed. Sometimes the proclamation date will be mentioned in the Act but usually it will be at 'a date to be fixed'. One reason for this delay is to enable the executive government or bureaucracy to establish the necessary mechanisms for implementing the Act. Rarely will an Act take effect retrospectively. Once parliament has passed or amended laws it then becomes the responsibility of the executive government to implement the law in the spirit in which the law was intended.

Delegated Legislation

An Act passed by parliament may provide that a particular person or body – for example, a Minister of the Crown, the Governor, Governor-General or professional regulatory authority – is 'delegated power' to make rules, regulations, by-laws or ordinances ('delegated legislation') in relation to specified matters. For instance, under section 101 of the *Health Care Complaints Act 1993* (NSW), the New South Wales Parliament empowers the Governor to make regulations under the Act.

Although delegated power is derived from the parent Act and does not exist in its own right, such rules, regulations, by-laws and ordinances are binding and are to be read as one with the Act. Such delegated legislation therefore allows more detailed and precise information regarding matters such as the practical application of the Act that work together with the Act to establish the rights and obligations of those people or practices being governed.

Common Law

Australia is a 'common law' jurisdiction in which the other primary source of law is found in the decisions of judges made in court cases. Case law most often exists alongside, and/or in addition to, legislation. The relationship between statutes and judicial decisions can be complex. Statutes take precedence over the common law to the extent of any inconsistency and the legislature may decide to overrule a judicial decision by passing a law to such effect. Alternatively, a statute may be enacted that codifies a topic covered by several decisions. Pursuant to the separation of powers, the judiciary may also rule on whether the Constitution allows the government to enact a particular statute or statutory provision – that is, the judiciary may speak on whether the government is acting within its power. The judiciary may also interpret the meaning of the statutory provisions. We therefore sometimes need to look to a piece of legislation to find the rule(s) relating to a particular issue, and to case law to explain how those rules should be interpreted or applied.

If there exists no statute on an issue, a judgment on a particular issue will become the 'common law'. In common law systems, the doctrine of precedent (*stare decisis*, meaning the decision stands) operates to make judges bound to follow previous *ratio decidendi* (reason for the decision) of the court in cases with similar facts at the same level of the hierarchy or in more senior courts (refer to Fig. 1.2). This application of common law rules found in the *ratio decidendi* creates consistency within the common law. It allows for some predictability when dealing with legal matters because one is able to refer to the outcomes of similar cases that have occurred before.

All judgments, however, do not bind all courts. Nor are all judges compelled to follow all that has been set down in previous decisions. In Australia there is a hierarchy of courts within the state and territory

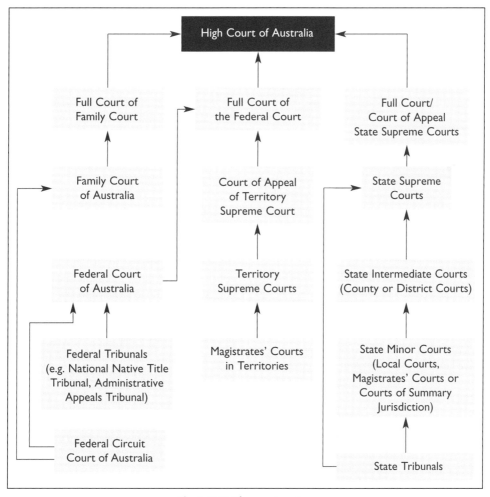

Fig. 1.2 ■ **The court system**

jurisdictions and the federal jurisdiction. Precedent can only bind if it comes from a higher court within the same hierarchy. For example, a decision in the Supreme Court of New South Wales is binding upon the District Court in New South Wales and Local Courts in New South Wales, but it is not binding on the equivalent courts in other states and territories of Australia because they are not in the same court hierarchy. Even so, a lower court in one state would be unlikely to depart from a decision taken in a higher court of another Australian state or territory where the issues are similar. Note, judgments may also contain comments that clarify a situation but do not make new law (*obiter dicta*). *Obiter dicta* from a judgment may be referred to in future cases but is not binding.

Australian courts are not bound to follow decisions made in foreign courts either, although they can influence decisions taken in Australia. This is sometimes referred to as a judgment being 'persuasive'. For example, decisions made in other common law countries such as Canada or the United Kingdom may be considered by Australian courts when making decisions.

Equitable Principles

A notable feature of the common law is that 'equitable principles' have been developed alongside the development of common law rules to address the issues of fairness and justice in those cases where common law remedies were considered inadequate. The rules of equity prevail over inconsistent common law rules. An example of an equitable maxim is, 'He who comes to equity must come with clean hands'. That is, where parties are seeking an equitable remedy, they themselves must have behaved in an honest, fair and lawful manner.

TYPES OF LAW

Law may be described as either substantive or procedural.

Substantive law is the law that regulates citizens in specific areas of their lives. Some examples of substantive law include the following:

- **Industrial (or employment) law** is where matters arising from the employer–employee relationship are identified and defined. Industrial law primarily involves agreements and awards that establish the obligations and rights of both parties in their working environment.

- **Contract law** places agreements within a formal framework that enables promises made by the parties to be enforced. Contracts of employment and contracts for the purchase and sale of goods and services are examples of contracts relevant to health practitioners.
- **Criminal law** identifies activities that the state considers unacceptable to a degree that warrants punishment. Criminal law may apply in the healthcare setting in relation to grossly unacceptable conduct or behaviour such as theft, criminal assault or murder.
- **Tort law** is concerned with civil wrongs. The word 'tort' essentially means 'twisted', and the primary purpose of tort law is to redress the wrongs suffered by a plaintiff. This is accomplished via compensation, which seeks to put the injured party in the position they would have been in had they not suffered the damage. There is rarely an element of punishment; however, one of the functions of tort law is to act as a deterrent by regulating behaviour to an acceptable standard. In the healthcare context, examples of torts are negligence, defamation and trespass.
- **Constitutional law** sets out the legal framework within which the country's political and legal systems operate.

Acts of Parliament and common law combine to produce substantive law.

Procedural law governs the way in which laws are implemented and enforced. This includes rules of the courts, rules applied to civil and criminal procedures, and rules of evidence. This aspect of law is the machinery that allows substantive law to be processed and applied. When a health practitioner brings an action for unfair dismissal against an employing healthcare facility, it is procedural law that dictates the evidence required to substantiate the claim and the appropriate legal process and remedies available.

Another significant distinction in the law is that between civil and criminal law. The common distinguishing features that differentiate civil and criminal jurisdictions include the following:

- Who can 'bring an action' (i.e. who can commence proceedings in a court or tribunal)?

In civil matters, the action involves a plaintiff – for example, a patient – bringing an action against a defendant such as a health practitioner or a hospital. In criminal matters, the action is initiated by the state in the form of the police or the public prosecutor against a defendant who has allegedly committed a crime.

■ What is the standard of proof required?

In civil law the standard of proof is *on the balance of probabilities*. That is, the judge or jury believe that one party's version of the events (based on the evidence) is more likely than the other party's version. In criminal cases the standard is *beyond reasonable doubt*. That is, to find a person guilty of a criminal offence, the judge or jury after hearing all the evidence does not have a reasonable doubt as to whether the accused has committed the criminal offence.

■ What is the purpose or intention of the two forms of action?

Essentially, civil law is about seeking a remedy for wrongs done; criminal law is about punishing wrongdoers.

GENERAL FEATURES OF THE AUSTRALIAN LEGAL SYSTEM

Adversarial and Inquisitorial Systems

One important function of the law is to resolve disputes between individuals, companies or institutions. This takes place in a court when a case is brought before a magistrate, judge or judge and jury, with the expectation that one party will be declared as having proven their case. The approach taken by the parties in common law courts is **adversarial**, each advancing their argument in an attempt to persuade the court that their claim should succeed. The role of the judge during court proceedings is to remain impartial and to ensure that the very strict procedural rules are adhered to. The judge or jury will determine the outcome of the case based only upon what the parties have presented by way of arguments and evidence.

In contrast is the **inquisitorial approach**, which is characteristic of the civil law system practised in many European countries. In that approach, the court is not confined to the evidence put before it by the police and lawyers but may seek out information

in its own right as part of the process of reaching a decision.

Within the healthcare context, cases heard before courts in Australia are adversarial. However, an exception to this is the operation of the Coroners Court. Under the respective state and territory legislation, the coroner is empowered to investigate and inquire into the death of a person for the purpose of establishing that the death has actually occurred and the identity of the deceased person, as well as the date, time and cause of the death. The parties appearing before the Coroners Court are not adversaries but rather assist the coroner, through providing evidence, to make a finding in relation to the deceased person.

Natural Justice

In a general sense the notion of natural justice ensures that the proceedings are conducted fairly, impartially and without prejudice. Natural justice is a fundamental principle that applies to all courts and tribunals. It means that the court or tribunal must give the person against whom the accusations are made a clear statement of the actual charge, adequate time to prepare an argument or submission and the right to be heard on all allegations. It is described as making two demands before a person's legal rights are adversely affected, or their 'legitimate expectations' disappointed: '(1) an opportunity to show why adverse action should not be taken …; and (2) a decision-maker whose mind is open to persuasion, or free from bias'.[7]

Presumption of Innocence

A core principle of the Australian legal system is that the law regards all accused people as being innocent until proven guilty. In criminal proceedings such a finding must be beyond a reasonable doubt. In civil proceedings the presumption operates to only allocate liability if *all* of the elements of the action are proven on the balance of probabilities. In disciplinary proceedings the complaints entity must prove that the conduct constitutes behaviour warranting professional disciplinary action.

Alternative Dispute Resolution

In all Australian jurisdictions alternative dispute resolution (ADR) is used in the civil jurisdiction as a way to assist the parties, either before or after the commencement of legal proceedings, to negotiate and resolve their dispute. ADR may assist in improving access to justice and in reducing the costs of delays. One of the most frequently used forms of ADR is mediation – a process in which the parties to a dispute are assisted by a neutral third party to identify the issues, develop options and consider alternatives, and endeavour to reach an agreement. Mediation may be undertaken voluntarily, ordered by a court or subject to an existing contractual agreement.

THE COURT HIERARCHY

The Australian court system is structured hierarchically so as to delineate the extent of authority and the jurisdictional limits of each court (see Fig. 1.2 on page 7).

Understanding Jurisdiction

The word 'jurisdiction' is relevant to the law in a number of ways. It may refer to the territory or sphere of activity over which legal authority extends; for example, federal jurisdiction applies to all of Australia, and the Supreme Court of Victoria only has jurisdiction to hear matters under Victorian law. Jurisdiction may also refer to the official power to make legal decisions and judgments. For example, the High Court of Australia has jurisdiction to hear appeals from lower court judgments.

The jurisdictional power of courts varies according to the seriousness of the offence, the amount of compensation that can be awarded, the nationality or place of residence of the parties, whether the matters are criminal or civil in nature, and even when and where the offence or event occurred. For example, a civil court has jurisdiction in relation to a claim by a person who has received healthcare services alleging negligence against a health practitioner and has the power to award a remedy in the form of monetary compensation. No other court – not a criminal court, family law court or bankruptcy court, for example – could hear this case.

Original and Appellate Jurisdiction

When a matter first appears, the court in which it is heard has what is known as 'original jurisdiction'. Before a decision may be appealed in another court, the dissatisfied party must be able to establish appropriate grounds. A decision may be the subject of an appeal, for example, when a judge has misdirected a jury or

made an error in relation to admitting or refusing to admit evidence, or when there is an issue as to the severity or leniency of the sentence. The subsequent court will be exercising its 'appellate jurisdiction'. For example, the Supreme Court may hear a matter and, if its decision is appealed, then the Full Court or Court of Appeal of the Supreme Court will hear the subsequent case using its appellate jurisdiction, where appropriate. Appellate jurisdiction is restricted to the superior courts including the District/County Court, Supreme Court, Federal Court, Family Court and High Court. In relation to the High Court, special leave (permission) must be sought before it will exercise its appellate jurisdiction.

Overview of the Courts/Tribunals

Magistrates' Courts (also known as 'Local Courts') are presided over by magistrates who are addressed during the proceedings as 'Your Worship' or 'Your Honour'. Magistrates hear cases alone because there are no juries at this level in the court structure. The jurisdiction of Magistrates' Courts is determined by the relevant legislation in each of the states and territories. These courts are the lowest courts in the court hierarchy and determine the greatest volume of cases. As a general principle, Magistrates' Courts deal with minor civil and criminal matters and with more serious criminal matters by way of committal proceedings. For example, a health practitioner may appear before a magistrate in relation to being in possession of property they have unlawfully removed from the premises of their employing hospital or health facility.

It is from this level of the hierarchy that magistrates are appointed as coroners or to preside over Children's Courts and Licensing Courts (with the exception of Victoria where the coroner and president of the Children's Court are judges of the County Court). Such courts were developed in response to the need to reduce the load from Magistrates' Courts and in recognition of the requirement for specialist knowledge.

District Courts (referred to as County Courts in Victoria) are presided over by judges who sit with or without a jury. Their jurisdiction is both original and appellate. District Courts hear and determine civil and criminal matters that are governed by the relevant legislation in each of the states and territories. As a general statement, all criminal matters other than murder, manslaughter, serious drug matters and serious sexual assault will be heard in a District Court. The judges who preside in these courts and more senior courts are referred to as 'Your Honour'.

Supreme Courts are the most senior courts in the states and territories and are presided over by a judge (referred to as 'Justice'), with or without a jury. Supreme Courts have an internal appeal mechanism referred to as the Court of Appeal or Full Court of the Supreme Court. When the court is sitting as the Full Court, there are three or more judges. While the jurisdictional limitations are determined by the relevant legislation in each of the states and territories, in civil matters they may hear claims for unlimited damages and, in the criminal jurisdiction, murder, manslaughter, serious drug matters and serious sexual assault. An appeal from a decision of a judicial member of a tribunal in relation to a professional disciplinary matter will be heard by the Court of Appeal.

The **High Court** was established under the Constitution of the Commonwealth of Australia and is comprised of the Chief Justice and six other judges (referred to as 'Justice'). The High Court is the most senior court in the Australian hierarchy. (Note: It is possible for a case to be heard by an international court or tribunal if the Commonwealth Parliament has become a signatory under an international declaration or convention.) The original jurisdiction of the High Court concerns any matters that involve interpretation of the Australian Constitution, disputes between residents of different states/territories, or disputes between states/territories and the Commonwealth government. In addition, provided leave has been obtained, appeals to the High Court can come from the Federal Court, the Family Court and the Supreme Court of any state or territory involving civil or criminal matters. The Full Bench of the High Court, comprising all seven justices, hears cases in which the principles are of great public importance, involve interpretation of the Constitution or invite departure from a previous decision of the High Court. Appeals from state and territory Family Court and Supreme Court decisions will be dealt with by the Full Court of not less than two justices. A single justice may hear and determine specified matters.

The **Federal Court of Australia** was established under the *Federal Court of Australia Act 1976* (Cth). This court was set up to further reduce the load on the High Court. Constitutional cases involving such matters as trade practices, bankruptcy and federal industrial disputes are heard. Appeals on decisions can be made to the High Court or the Full Court of the Federal Court.

The **Federal Circuit Court** (originally called the Federal Magistrates' Court) was established at the end of 1999 to deal with less complex matters that would otherwise have been heard in the Federal Court or Family Court. The jurisdiction of the Federal Circuit Court has grown since its inception and broadly includes family law and child support, administrative law, admiralty law, bankruptcy, copyright, human rights, industrial law, migration, privacy and trade practices. Approximately 90% of the court's workload is in the area of family law. The Federal Circuit Court does not hear appeals.

Tribunals can be government-sponsored or private. They can be administrative or civil. Administrative tribunals are concerned with executive actions of government. Civil tribunals are concerned with resolving private disputes. In many jurisdictions tribunals have been amalgamated, hearing both administrative and civil issues. These include the Queensland Civil and Administrative Tribunal, the Victorian Civil and Administrative Tribunal, the State Administrative Tribunal in Western Australia and the New South Wales Civil and Administrative Tribunal. Examples of other tribunals include tenancy tribunals and small claims tribunals.

Tribunals perform 'quasi-judicial' functions in that they make decisions within the ambit of their limited or specific roles. Decisions are made in a variety of ways and may involve a judge, a member or a board of specialists not qualified in law. Tribunals do not make laws that are applied by courts. While tribunals lie outside the court hierarchy, appeals from their decisions may be made into the court system if permitted under legislation. Often the role of tribunals is limited and narrowly defined.

In relation to the conduct of health practitioners, a National Board (e.g. the Medical Board of Australia, the Nursing and Midwifery Board of Australia or the Physiotherapy Board of Australia) can refer disciplinary matters to the relevant state tribunal for hearing. This happens only when the allegations involve the most serious unprofessional conduct (professional misconduct) and a National Board believes suspension or cancellation of the practitioner's registration may be warranted.

SKILLS RELEVANT TO UNDERSTANDING JUDICIAL DECISIONS AND LEGISLATION

Reading judicial decisions or legislation is not something lay people commonly do. However, it is an important skill for those wishing to find and understand the law and can assist health practitioners in understanding the law that is relevant to them in their day-to-day practice and delivery of healthcare services.

Reading Judicial Decisions (Cases)

When reading a judicial decision (case) in a law report it will have information regarding the case name, the court in which it was heard, the names of the judge(s)/justice(s) before whom the case was heard, and often further details to assist the reader. Box 1.2 provides information about what a case reference citation means.

When reading a case from a law report there may be catch words at the top of the document that highlight the important aspects of the case – for example, 'negligence', 'breach of duty' or 'failure to warn'. The report will also often include a 'headnote', which provides a summary of the case that includes facts considered by the publisher as important to that decision. The court's decision will also be noted near the top of the report, indicated by the word 'held'. This will usually contain the *ratio decidendi* (the reason for the decision). A summary of the findings of each of the judges who heard and determined the case is also provided. This may include separate reasons delivered by each of the justices or, where there is agreement (where they concur), two or more justices may hand down a joint decision. At the end of the written determination the 'orders' (the judges' final decision) handed down by the court will be reported. The full judgment, which is written by the judge(s), is then detailed.

Cases may be found in law reports, online[8] or on disk. The increasing number of cases that can now be accumulated through storage on electronic databases has resulted in unreported cases (those not formally reported in the printed volumes of the law reports) now being available. Note that the format of case reports on web-based databases differs from that of the traditional paper-based law reports. They are not allocated volume or page numbers in the report and the paragraphs are

---

BOX 1.2
HOW TO READ A CASE CITATION (AND FIND A CASE)

Example: *Harriton v Stephens* (2006) 226 CLR 52
- *Harriton v Stephens* refers to the litigants (the parties) involved in the case.
- When writing a case name the names of both litigants are italicised.
- The 'v' in the case name means 'versus'; however, in Australia the case name is read as 'Harriton and Stephens'.
- If it is the first time the case has come to court the first party named (Harriton) is the **plaintiff** and the second party (Stephens) is the **defendant**. If the case is on appeal then the first party named will be the **appellant** and the second party the **respondent**.
- (2006) 226 CLR 52 provides information on the case and the location of the full court report. The use of round brackets around the year refers only to published law reports, of which there are many in higher court jurisdictions.
- (2006) refers to the year the case was reported. When the year is in round brackets it indicates that the volume number (in the example, 226), and not the year, is the essential identifying feature of the citation.
- 226 refers to the volume number of the law report. When more than one volume is published in a particular year the volumes in that year will be numbered (e.g. 226(1), 226(2)).
- CLR is the abbreviation for the Commonwealth Law Reports series containing the report on the case of *Harriton v Stephens*.
- 52 refers to the page reference for the beginning of the case report.

Note: When the year is in square brackets it indicates that the year is the important identifying feature of the report and that the volume number is not essential, and may not even be present. An example is *X v Y* [1975] VR 1. Square brackets may also mean that the case is not found in a formal law report (i.e. it is 'unreported').

---

individually numbered for reference. Some may not have additional summary information or headnotes. As an example, the unreported case *Edwards v Kennedy*, a case involving allegations of medical negligence, is able to be located on the LexisNexis database as:

Edwards v Kennedy BC 200901404,
Supreme Court of Victoria – Common Law Division
Kaye J
5714 of 2007

26, 27 February, 12 March 2009
Citation: Edwards v Kennedy [2009] VSC 74

Statutory Interpretation

Statutes and regulations determine much of the professional activity in the delivery of health care. It is therefore important that health practitioners are both aware of, and understand, the various state, territory and Commonwealth Acts that affect their practice. There are rules governing statutory interpretation contained in various state, territory and Commonwealth interpretation Acts.[9] Such Acts enshrine common law rules of statutory interpretation, which include:

- the **literal rule**, which applies the ordinary meaning to words unless an alternative new meaning is applied (specific legal terms must be given their legal meaning)
- the **purpose rule**, which obliges one to consider the underlying purpose of the legislation when attempting to interpret it
- the **golden rule**, which addresses when any meaning applied leads to a ludicrous interpretation, allowing it to be modified to avoid inconsistency and absurdity.

Generally, when reading legislation the focus must be on the actual words used. The Act should be read as a whole to enable the context of the words to be identified. The words most often can (and should) be taken literally, but if they are unclear one may turn to considering the purpose of the Act. Explanatory notes that sometimes accompany a statute and its associated regulations will assist in determining the purpose or intention of the law and in resolving any ambiguity. Courts may interpret and clarify statutory provisions if a matter ends up before them.

Legislation may be accessed in hard copy or via the internet or other dedicated databases generated and maintained by Commonwealth, state and territory governments.[10] It is important to make sure the most recent version of the Act is being consulted.

> The format of the legislation in hard copy will differ from that available online; however, the information in Box 1.3 aims to provide a general overview to assist in reading an Act. To really understand how an Act is set out it will be useful to look at the example of the *Health Practitioner Regulation National Law Act 2009* (Qld) online or in hard copy.

Regulations

One of the last sections in an Act confers on the Governor-General or Governor the power to make regulations that may be necessary to administer the Act. Regulations provide the essential details of administration that may change more frequently than the Act can be amended by parliament. Regulations are used to set fees and charges as well as a variety of requirements necessary to enable the daily implementation of the Act. Regulations are usually drafted in the federal or a state Attorney-General's department, advised by the government department responsible for administering the Act. The regulations are tabled in parliament but do not progress through parliament in the same manner as an Act.

BOX 1.3
HOW TO READ AN ACT (LEGISLATION)

Consider the example of the *Health Practitioner Regulation National Law Act 2009* (Qld).

- An Act is referred to by its name, the year it was passed by the parliament and the jurisdiction in which it was passed. The above example is the originating legislation that provides for the national registration of health practitioners in Australia (see Chapter 4).
- The coat of arms of the particular jurisdiction usually appears at the top of the front page of an Act. The Act is also given a number that is strictly in the order in which the Acts are assented to by the Governor or Governor-General. For example, the Health Practitioner Regulation National Law Act is *Act No 45 of 2009*.
- An Act will also include a long title. For the above example, the long title is 'An Act providing for the adoption of a national law to establish a national registration and accreditation scheme for health practitioners'.
- If the date of assent is included it usually appears in brackets under the long title. This is the date on which

Continued on following page

BOX 1.3
HOW TO READ AN ACT (LEGISLATION) *(Continued)*

a Bill formally completes its passage through the parliament and meets the constitutional requirements for becoming an Act. It is not necessarily the date on which the Act comes into effect. In the above example, the date of assent is 3 November 2009.

- The Health Practitioner Regulation National Law Act, other than Part 4, commenced on 1 July 2010.
- Many Acts are divided into Parts, which are like chapters of a book and may be then further divided into Divisions and Subdivisions. For example, the Health Practitioner Regulation National Law Act is 308 pages long and contains an initial four Parts that address preliminary matters, adoption of the Health Practitioner National Law, provisions specific to the Queensland jurisdiction and amendments to the *Health Practitioner Regulation (Administrative Arrangements) National Law Act 2008* (Qld). The Schedule of the Act has 305 sections (which are also referred to as provisions) set out in 12 Parts and an additional seven Schedules. Description of the first seven Parts, by way of example, are:

- Part 1 – Preliminary comprises sections 1–10 and contains the short title, the commencement date, the object of the Act, definitions, notes and the Mutual Recognition law.
- Part 2 – sections 11–17 deal with the Ministerial Council
- Part 3 – sections 18–22 address the Australian Workforce Council
- Part 4 – sections 23–30 cover the Australian Practitioner Regulation Agency
- Part 5 – sections 31–41 deal with National Boards
- Part 6 – sections 42–51 cover accreditation
- Part 7 – sections 52–137 cover registration of health practitioners.
- Schedules to an Act contain details that supplement the provisions of the Act. For example, definitions of terms used in the Act, technical descriptions and prescribed forms may be set out in a list appended to an Act in the form of a Schedule. Sections in the Act will therefore refer to a Schedule, effectively incorporating the content of the Schedule into the law.

FURTHER READING

Carvan J. *Understanding the Australian Legal System*. 7th ed. Sydney, NSW: Law Book Co; 2014.

Creyke R, Hamer D, O'Mara P, et al. *Laying Down the Law*. 10th ed. Sydney, NSW: LexisNexis Butterworths; 2017.

Finkelstein R, Hamer D. *LexisNexis Concise Australian Legal Dictionary*. 5th ed. Sydney, NSW: LexisNexis Butterworths; 2014.

Hall K, Macken C. *Legislation and Statutory Interpretation*. 4th ed. Sydney, NSW: LexisNexis Butterworths; 2015.

Hinchy R. *The Australian Legal System: History, Institutions and Method*. 2nd ed. Sydney, NSW: Pearson Education; 2015.

Meagher D, Simpson A, Stellios J, et al. *Hanks Australian Constitutional Law*. 10th ed. Sydney, NSW: LexisNexis Butterworths; 2016.

Stellios J. *Zine's The High Court and the Constitution*. 6th ed. Annandale, NSW: The Federation Press; 2015.

ENDNOTES

1. The *Commonwealth Constitution Act 1900* (UK).
2. Parliamentary Education Office. *Governing Australia: Three Levels of Law Making*. Canberra, ACT: Australian Government; n.d. https://www.peo.gov.au/uploads/peo/docs/closer-look/CloserLook_Three_Levels.pdf. Accessed 10 March 2019.
3. United Nations General Assembly. Universal Declaration of Human Rights, Vol. 71, A/RES/3/217 A, UN GAOR, 3d Sess. Supp. No. 13, UN Doc. A/810; 1948.
4. United Nations. *International Covenant on Economic, Social and Cultural Rights*, Vol. 360, Rep No 993 UNTS 3, 6, ILM; 1966, entered into force 3 January 1976, Article 12.2.
5. United Nations General Assembly. *Convention on the Rights of the Child*, 20 November 1989, United Nations, Treaty Series, Vol. 1577, p. 3, Article 24.1.
6. United Nations General Assembly. *Convention on the Rights of Persons with Disabilities,* adopted on 13 December 2006 during the sixty-first session of the General Assembly by resolution A/RES/61/106.
7. Forbes JRS. *Justice in Tribunals*. 2nd ed. Sydney, NSW: Federation Press; 2006. p. 100.
8. Case law can be located on individual court websites in each of the individual states and territories on <www.austlii.edu.au> for all Australian jurisdictions, and in a number of legal databases.
9. *Acts Interpretation Act 1901* (Cth); *Interpretation Act 1987* (NSW); *Interpretation of Legislation Act 1984* (Vic); *Acts Interpretation Act 1915* (SA); *Interpretation Act 1984* (SA); *Legislation Act 2001* (ACT); *Acts Interpretation Act 1954* (Qld); *Acts Interpretation Act 1931* (Tas); *Interpretation Act* (NT).
10. Individual government legislation may be accessed online via the following websites (all retrieved on 1 January 2018):
    - Federal Register of Legislation: https://www.legislation.gov.au/
    - ACT Legislation Register: http://www.legislation.act.gov.au/
    - NSW Legislation: https://www.legislation.nsw.gov.au/
    - Queensland Legislation: https://www.legislation.qld.gov.au/
    - Northern Territory Legislation: https://legislation.nt.gov.au/
    - Western Australian Legislation: https://www.slp.wa.gov.au/legislation/statutes.nsf/home.html
    - South Australian Legislation: https://www.legislation.sa.gov.au/index.aspx
    - Tasmanian Legislation: https://www.legislation.tas.gov.au/.

REVIEW QUESTIONS AND ACTIVITIES

1. Identify and describe the sources of law in Australia.

2. Identify some Acts of Parliament (both Commonwealth and in your own state/territory) that regulate and control your practice as a health practitioner.
   2.1 What is the object of each Act?
   2.2 How do the provisions affect your practice?

3. Describe the significance of the doctrine of precedent to developing common law.

4. Describe the difference between an adversarial and an inquisitorial process.

5. Identify the courts in the court hierarchy in your jurisdiction. Where are tribunals located in relation to the court structures?
   5.1 If the National Board for your discipline was to initiate disciplinary proceedings, where would the proceedings be conducted?
   5.2 If a health practitioner in your jurisdiction was to be sued in negligence by a person to whom they provided healthcare services, in which court would the trial be conducted if they were seeking $500,000 in compensation?
   5.3 In what court would an inquiry to establish the cause of a patient's death be conducted?

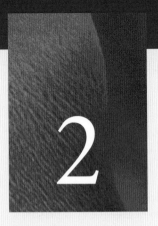

2 INTRODUCTION TO THE AUSTRALIAN HEALTH SYSTEM

LEARNING OBJECTIVES

Upon completing this chapter you should be able to:

- explain federal and state/territory government roles regarding health care in Australia
- describe the development and key characteristics of the Australian health system
- explain the Pharmaceutical Benefits Scheme, Medicare and the private health insurance rebate scheme
- describe federal, state and private sector contributions to healthcare funding
- outline the seven key rights set out in the *Australian Charter of Healthcare Rights*.

INTRODUCTION

Chapter 1 introduced the Australian legal system and the various roles and powers within it. As noted, the Australian Constitution is relevant to whether federal or state governments (or both) have the power to regulate particular issues. The Australian Constitution establishes the legal framework within which Australia's health sector operates. This chapter examines the distribution of powers between the federal and state/territory governments regarding health care. It notes that the expansion of Commonwealth powers has been highly contested, reflecting strong differences in political ideologies regarding the extent to which government should be involved with, fund and control the various aspects of health care. Within this context, the development and key characteristics of the Australian health system are examined, paying particular attention to the Pharmaceutical Benefits Scheme (PBS), Medicare and the private health insurance rebate, which together form the basis of Australia's current universal health system. Other Commonwealth, state/territory and local government responsibilities and their respective contributions to healthcare funding are noted. The chapter ends with an overview of the *Australian Charter of Healthcare Rights*.

Commonwealth Responsibility for Healthcare Services

The Commonwealth government's power and responsibility regarding health matters has expanded since the Constitution took effect in 1901. At the time of federation, the provision of healthcare services was regarded as primarily a state issue. The Commonwealth was given powers only in relation to health issues considered of national importance – for example, quarantine, invalid pensions and the repatriation of service personnel, as well as responsibility for healthcare services in the federal territories. Since then, Commonwealth powers have been expanded to create the PBS, Medicare and the private health insurance rebate to ensure that Australians have access to medicines and healthcare services in a way that meets their basic healthcare needs, and is accessible to all. This is what is meant by having a 'universal health system'.

The history and functions of the PBS, Medicare and the private health insurance rebate are further discussed below. The Commonwealth also has power and responsibility over a number of other areas that are relevant to the health system such as:

- funding supported work placements, which in turn supports having well-trained health practitioners
- ensuring safe and effective treatments and the research and development required to ensure their safety and efficacy
- funding aged care, Indigenous healthcare services and disability services
- providing accurate information about the health system to ensure it continues to work in the way it should.

A good health system reflects the capacity to respond to health emergencies. It must also be recognised that good health systems don't just treat sick people, they help to keep people healthy in the first place, preventing illness and disease.

Box 2.1 lists the Commonwealth's powers and responsibilities in this regard.

State Powers and Responsibilities Regarding the Health System

As discussed in Chapter 1, when the Australian Constitution does not explicitly grant the Commonwealth government power in relation to something, such power and responsibility falls to the states. Most regulation regarding health-related matters falls to the states. Responsibility for managing and administering public hospitals is another important example. Box 2.2 lists the main areas that state governments are responsible for in relation to health care and services.

Shared Responsibilities Between the Commonwealth and States/Territories

Some healthcare services and issues are the responsibility of both the Commonwealth and state/territory governments – that is, they have shared powers or responsibilities. Box 2.3 lists some of these areas.

Local Governments

Local governments also play an important role in the health system. They provide, for example, essential environmental health services such as sanitation, waste disposal and food safety, plus a range of community-based health and home-care services such as immunisation and

---

BOX 2.1
COMMONWEALTH RESPONSIBILITIES FOR HEALTH-RELATED SERVICES AND PROGRAMS

- After-hours general practitioner and primary care services (Medicare Locals)
- Aged care services subsidies
- Benefits for basic dental services for children and young people
- Community-controlled Aboriginal and Torres Strait Islander primary health organisations
- Health practitioner education (Commonwealth-funded university places)
- Medical research grants
- Medicare
- National coordination and leadership such as responding to pandemics and other health emergencies
- Pharmaceutical Benefits Scheme
- Regulation of private health insurers and rebates for private health insurance premiums
- Regulation of therapeutic goods and medical devices
- Subsidised hearing services
- Vaccine purchases for the national immunisation program
- Veterans' health care

BOX 2.2
STATE/TERRITORY RESPONSIBILITIES FOR HEALTH-RELATED LAW AND SERVICES

- Ambulance and emergency services
- Civil liability, criminal, guardianship and mental health law
- Food safety and handling regulation
- Funding and management of community and mental health services
- Management and administration of public hospitals
- Patient transport and subsidy schemes
- Preventive services such as breast cancer screening and immunisation programs
- Regulating on health-related matters (e.g. workplace health and safety, assisted reproduction, end-of-life decision making)
- Regulation, inspection, licensing and monitoring of health premises

BOX 2.3
**SHARED RESPONSIBILITIES
BETWEEN THE COMMONWEALTH
AND THE STATES/TERRITORIES**

- Funding of public hospital services based on an agreed national activity-based funding formula as outlined in the *National Health Reform Agreement*
- National mental health reform
- Preventive services such as free cancer screening programs including those under the National Bowel Cancer Screening Program
- Public dental clinics (state responsibility with additional Commonwealth funding provided)
- Registration and accreditation of health practitioners through the Australian Health Practitioner Regulation Agency
- Responding to national health emergencies
- Shared funding for palliative care

maternal child health programs.[1] Health practitioners may deliver such services, or help people access them, depending on what they are.

THE HISTORY OF AUSTRALIA'S UNIVERSAL HEALTH SYSTEM

As noted above, Commonwealth powers regarding health care were limited at the time of federation. This section looks at the history of how Australia's universal health system developed, and then examines in greater detail the PBS, Medicare and the private health insurance rebate. Such history is important because it illustrates tensions that have existed over the governance of health care for many years, explains the legal underpinnings of our current health system, and highlights that different political views can influence how health care is governed.

Although the regulation of many healthcare services falls to the states, ensuring access to basic healthcare services for all under a uniform, nation-wide system is favourable. However, the question over time has been how best to design such a system. The first steps towards developing a universal health system in Australia occurred in the mid-1940s when the Labor Curtin Government moved to establish a national health system. These attempts were initially thwarted by the Opposition (led by Menzies) and the medical profession protesting

against 'socialist values' and a shifting of power from doctors to the state. A High Court challenge subsequently found the Commonwealth did not have the power to establish such a system.[2] Then, in 1944, a referendum aimed at giving the government power to legislate over 14 different matters, including healthcare services, also failed.

In 1946 the Chifley Government (Chifley becoming prime minister following Curtin's death) took the issue to the people again via a referendum focused on enabling the Commonwealth to direct benefits to families and the ill. The referendum was successful, leading to the insertion of section 51(xxiiiA) into the Constitution giving the Commonwealth power regarding:

The provision of maternity allowances, widows' pensions, child endowment, unemployment, pharmaceutical, sickness and hospital benefits, medical and dental services (but not so as to authorise any form of civil conscription), benefits to students and family allowances.

The insertion of section 51(xxiiiA) complemented Commonwealth powers under section 51(xiv) to make laws concerning insurance, and section 96, to 'grant financial assistance to any state on such terms and conditions as the Parliament thinks fit', and paved the way for developing a national health system. The introduction of the PBS followed, then a variety of changing systems intended to enable access to health care ultimately resulted in the current system of Medicare and a private health insurance rebate scheme.

Access to Medicines – the Pharmaceutical Benefits Scheme

The PBS is a Commonwealth-funded scheme that allows the Australian population access to a large range of prescription drugs at a low cost through government subsidisation. It originally formed part of post–World War II general social welfare legislation, being established in 1948 to ensure all Australian residents and eligible overseas visitors had access to 'life-saving and disease preventing drugs' at an affordable price.[3] Since its introduction, the PBS has become fundamental in enabling access to medicines within Australia, evolving from supplying a limited number of drugs free of charge to the community, into a broader subsidised scheme.[4]

Under the PBS, medicines or pharmaceuticals are prescribed by doctors or authorised health practitioners who have a PBS prescriber number.[5] The medicines are then dispensed by an approved community pharmacist,[6] approved public or private hospital authority[7] or approved medical practitioner.[8] The Commonwealth subsidises around 83% of the cost of medicines and the patient funds the rest via a co-payment.[9] People who fall into concessional categories, receiving certain pensions, benefits or cards, pay less. The government subsidy occurs via cash transfers made directly to the approved dispenser of the PBS medications, who must claim on a reimbursement basis for the cost of the medications.

A safety net arrangement applies when the total amount of co-payments paid by a patient (or immediate family) in a calendar year reaches a certain threshold. In such instances, the co-payment reduces to a smaller amount, with the benefit paid to the pharmacist increasing.[10] In the case of concessional patients, the safety net threshold is lower, and when reached, no co-payment is required for the rest of the calendar year.[11]

Medicines eligible for supply under the PBS are listed in the *Schedule of Pharmaceutical Benefits*. To get on the schedule, the Pharmaceutical Benefits Advisory Committee (PBAC) assesses the conditions for which the medicines have been approved in Australia, their clinical effectiveness, their safety and their cost-effectiveness. This information is compared with other listed medicines that treat the same condition. If the PBAC recommends a drug be listed, and the Australian Government agrees, the subsidy is approved.

The PBS also provides other forms of assistance to ensure affordable access to medicines, including funding for public hospitals for certain high-cost drugs (e.g. immunosuppressants used in patients receiving organ transplantation).[12]

To ensure the integrity of the PBS, the government provides information and feedback to health practitioners and dispensers regarding 'accidental non-compliance'. The government will seek to correct behaviour when there may be innocent mistakes or errors and will enforce the law in cases of deliberate exploitation of the program. This includes, for example, using someone else's Medicare card, forging prescriptions, making PBS claims for medicines that were not supplied, falsifying authority information or deliberately prescribing outside restrictions. Professional regulatory consequences and significant criminal sanctions may apply.

Private Prescriptions

If a medicine is not listed under the PBS schedule a person will have to pay 'full price' for the medicine as a private prescription. That is, the medicine is not subsidised by the Australian Government and is considered a 'non-PBS medicine'. Note, 'full price' will be determined by both what the pharmaceutical company that produces the drug charges and what the pharmacy charges at the point of sale. Pharmacies may charge differently for non-PBS medicines, so a person who seeks a non-PBS medicine may need to shop around to find the best price. The cost of private prescriptions does not count towards the safety net threshold.

ACCESS TO HEALTH CARE – EVOLVING SCHEMES

Following the section 51(xxiiiA) amendments to the Constitution, respective Commonwealth governments continued to focus on access to healthcare services as an integral part of Australia's health system. However, systems implemented saw several major restructurings, as laws reflected significantly differing political ideologies. The changes over time include:

- 1948: The Chifley Labor Government enacted the *National Health Service Act*. The legislation was seen as an 'enabling measure' for a national health scheme, introducing a fixed schedule of fees for general practice services, with payment shared between the patient and the government. There was no compulsion on doctors or patients to join.
- 1953: The Menzies Liberal Country Party Coalition Government introduced a voluntary insurance scheme (known as the 'National Health Scheme') that provided for voluntary health insurance funds subsidised by the government, with special welfare arrangements for the needy. The scheme remained for two decades, undergoing only minor changes despite being marred by insurance companies gradually increasing their fees while also rejecting a large number of claims. Such actions left people unable to pay for both insurance and their treatment. When claims were paid, people were met

with a widening gap between the cost of treatment and what they received from their insurance company. The complexity of the system also left 15–17% of Australians uncovered by insurance and unentitled to free health care.

■ 1975: The Whitlam Labor Government introduced Medibank, a universal health insurance system.

■ 1975: The Fraser Coalition Government introduced significant changes to Medibank ranging from increases in the Medibank levy to reductions in reimbursements for services. By 1981 Medibank had been abolished and a system of voluntary private insurance subsidised by government was reinstated.

The above evolution of the health system illustrates that the governance of health care and its funding is a political issue influenced by differing ideologies. It is important to understand that such ideologies affect healthcare funding and the role of government and insurers. Thus, while the following explains further the current Medicare and insurance system, it is important to know how it evolved and to understand that it is a system that can change over time.

Medicare

In 1983, following the Hawke Labor Government coming to power, a new scheme – Medicare – was introduced via amendments to the *Health Insurance Act 1973* (Cth), the *National Health Act 1953* (Cth) and the *Health Insurance Commission Act 1973* (Cth). Medicare remains in place today, albeit having seen some changes over the years. Its broad objective is to make health care accessible, according to need, to all Australian citizens and those holding citizenship or visa status from countries with which Australia has a reciprocal healthcare agreement.

Medicare is a compulsory scheme regulated through the federal government and funded through a mix of general revenue and an income tax surcharge known as the 'Medicare levy'. The levy paid is calculated at the rate of 2% of each individual's taxable income, with an additional surcharge of 1% for high-income earners without private health insurance (this system is intended to encourage higher income earners to take out private health insurance to reduce the burden on the Medicare scheme). Low-income earners do not pay

the levy, or pay a reduced amount, depending on their income level.

Access to health care is facilitated via Medicare in two main ways:[13]

1. Benefits are provided to people for out-of-hospital medical services via the Medicare Benefits Scheme.

Such services include, but are not limited to: general practitioner and specialist services; dental care for children in some circumstances; selected diagnostic imaging and pathology services; eye checks by optometrists; and allied health services in limited circumstances.

2. Medicare guarantees free treatment of public patients in public hospitals.

Benefits paid for out-of-hospital medical services are generally 85% of the listed fee for the service in the Medicare Benefits Schedule (75% of the fee for private patients in hospital). Any 'gap' between what the healthcare service provider charges and the benefit is paid by the person who has received the service. When healthcare service providers are willing to accept the Medicare benefit as full payment for a service (i.e. without a gap payment), they bill the government directly and the person receiving the healthcare service is not charged – this is referred to as 'bulk-billing'.

'Free' treatment in public hospitals does not mean there are not any costs associated with such treatment, but rather that the Commonwealth and state governments fund public hospital care.

Private Health Insurance

The federal government also regulates private health insurance through the Health Insurance Act. This Act enables health insurance companies to offer private insurance to individuals who may choose their private provider and their level of cover. Individuals may seek cover for such services as ambulance, hospital and health care not included in the Medicare scheme (physiotherapy and dentistry, for example).

To encourage people to get hospital insurance and to keep it, there is a government initiative referred to as 'Lifetime Health Cover' (LHC). Pursuant to LHC, if a person takes out hospital cover after age 30, their base premium will be 2% more for each year they are over the age of 30 up to a maximum of 70%. Their partner will also have to pay LHC if they join after age 30. The

LHC loading ceases once a person has had private hospital cover for 10 continuous years.

LHC loading does not apply for people born on or before 1 July 1934. There are also special conditions for new migrants to Australia who are aged over the LHC deadline (1 July following their 31st birthday). New migrants to Australia do not have to pay an LHC loading if they take out hospital cover within 12 months of being registered for Medicare. After this time an LHC loading of 2% more for each year the person is aged over 30 when they take out hospital cover will apply. If an Australian citizen is overseas on their LHC loading deadline they will not pay an LHC loading if they purchase hospital cover within 12 months of the day they return to Australia (noting that they are able to return to Australia for periods of up to 90 consecutive days and are still considered to be overseas).

Note, LHC applies only to hospital cover; it does not apply to private health insurance ancillary covers (commonly referred to as 'extras').

Issues With the Current Scheme

Medicare is not without its challenges. For example, it does not cover some important services such as dental for most adults, some allied health services, and ambulance services. People are required to carry insurance or pay out of pocket for such services. This can be difficult for those who cannot afford such insurance and illustrates that the dual system of Medicare and private insurance does not serve all people. Insurance is costly and premiums continue to rise. Increasingly Australians are choosing to, or due to financial circumstances must, rely only on Medicare (44.6% of the population are privately insured for hospital cover and 53.9% for general treatment[14]).

There are also ongoing issues between the Commonwealth and states/territories regarding the shared responsibility for funding public hospitals. Complaints about long waiting lists for public hospital treatment and long waiting times for emergency services abound. This can create frustrations and may have health implications for people who can only afford public health care. As was noted above, differences in political ideologies, as well as the costs of funding the system, also mean that the structure of the health system, and its funding, may be subject to ongoing change.

The National Disability Insurance Scheme

In considering access to healthcare services in Australia it is also important to note the National Disability Insurance Scheme (NDIS). The NDIS is an insurance scheme that funds individualised support for people with permanent and significant disability aged under 65, their families and carers. To be eligible for the NDIS a person with a disability must meet certain criteria. Eligible people, known as 'participants', are given an individual plan of support tailored to suit their needs. This could include informal supports that a person receives through family or friends, mainstream services and other community services. Such support and services are not limited to healthcare services, but healthcare services and supports may be an important part of a person's individual plan.

The relevant legislation is the *National Disability Insurance Scheme Act 2013* (Cth) (NDIS Act). The NDIS Act establishes the National Disability Insurance Agency (NDIA), which has responsibility for delivering the NDIS. The functions and powers of the NDIA are set out in the NDIS Act. Subsidiary legislation is also important. That is, the NDIS rules are made under the NDIS Act and set out further laws on matters of detail in relation to the NDIS and must be read in conjunction with the NDIS Act. Notably, Australia's obligations under the United Nations *Convention on the Rights of Persons with Disabilities* are given effect via the NDIS Act in conjunction with other laws.

Aged Care

People of all ages have access to Medicare, the PBS and the private health insurance rebate described above. Aged care services provide care to people over 65 and Aboriginal and Torres Strait Islanders aged 50 years or older. The Commonwealth government has a significant role in funding and regulating formal aged care services, which include:

- **home support**, which aims to keep people living independently at home and in the community
- **home care**,[15] which relates to a range of personal care, support, clinical and other services tailored to meet the assessed needs of an individual in their home
- **residential care**,[16] which is personal care or nursing care (or both) provided to a person in a residential

facility that provides accommodation and a range of care services to people who are unable to continue to live in their own home.[17] It is not care in a person's home, in a hospital, in a psychiatric facility or for the frail, or any other care specified in the Act or its Subsidy Principles as not meeting the definition of residential care.

The *Aged Care Act 1997* (Cth) provides the legislative framework for 'home care services' and 'residential care services' and establishes who can provide care, who can receive care, the type of aged care services available and how aged care is funded. Funding is based on assessment of need, including whether such needs may be met by funded aged care services.[18] Home support is not governed by the Aged Care Act but is shaped by program guidelines and requirements specified in grant funding agreements.

Government-funded aged care operates alongside and in conjunction with other services to meet the needs of Australia's older population, including health care, disability services and specialist palliative care. As per recent changes regarding care for people with a disability, there have been changes to government policy in recent years in relation to aged care services that emphasise and encourage consumer-directed care.[19]

HEALTHCARE EXPENDITURE

Of total current health expenditure most recently measured in 2014–15, the Australian Institute of Health and Welfare reports that the Commonwealth government contributed 41%, the state/territory governments contributed 26% and non-government sources (individuals, private health insurance and other non-government sources) provided the remaining 33%.[20] The distribution of such expenditure between the various governments and the non-government sectors varies depending on the types of health goods and services being provided.

A large share of federal expenditure is directed towards medical services via Medicare and the PBS. The balance of expenditure for these services is sourced from the non-government sector either via insurance premiums or private funds. Expenditure on community healthcare services comes mostly from the state and territory governments. Expenditure on public hospital services is shared by the governments. Non-government sources account for large portions of expenditure on dental services, private hospitals, aids and appliances, medications for which no government benefit has been paid and other health practitioner services.[21]

THE CHARTER OF HEALTHCARE RIGHTS

Within the above discussed system of health care sits legal and ethical obligations and rights relevant to patients, consumers, families/carers, healthcare providers and facilities. We will consider such ethical and legal obligations throughout the rest of the book; however, it is useful here to end this chapter by noting the *Australian Charter of Healthcare Rights*, which was endorsed in July 2008 by all Australian health ministers (Commonwealth and state/territory) for use across the country. The Charter applies to all health settings anywhere in Australia including public hospitals, private hospitals, general practice and other community environments. While not law, it expresses and incorporates a number of obligations health practitioners owe patients under existing law, professional codes and employer policies.

The Charter has three guiding principles: (1) everyone has the right to be able to access health care and this right is essential for the Charter to be meaningful; (2) the Australian Government commits to international agreements about human rights that recognise everyone's right to have the highest possible standard of physical and mental health; and (3) Australia is a society made up of people with different cultures and ways of life, and the Charter acknowledges and respects these differences. Such elements reflect the ethical, legal, social and political values that have evolved since the early days of the Curtin Government.

The seven key rights within the Charter are access, safety, respect, communication, participation, privacy and comment.[22] At the time of writing this book, however, the Charter was under review, with suggested amendments to these rights for its next iteration (the second edition) to change the wording of the rights to access, safety, respect, partnership, information, privacy and give feedback.[23] The proposed changes follow public consultation that took place in 2018, with the second phase consultation on the proposed amendments closing in March 2019. The final second edition of the Charter is expected in 2020.

FURTHER READING

Australian Institute of Health and Welfare. Health Expenditure Australia 2014–15. Health and welfare expenditure series no. 57. Cat. no. HWE 67. Canberra, ACT: AIHW; 2016.

Ducket SJ, Wilcox S. *The Australian Healthcare System.* 5th ed. Melbourne, VIC: Oxford University Press; 2015.

Willis E, Reynolds L, Keleher H. *Understanding the Australian Healthcare System.* 3rd ed. Sydney, NSW: Elsevier Australia; 2016.

ENDNOTES

1. Parliament of Australia. *Health in Australia: A Quick Guide.* https://www.aph.gov.au/About_Parliament/Parliamentary_Departments/Parliamentary_Library/pubs/rp/rp1819/Quick_Guides/HealthAust. Accessed 31 August 2018.
2. *Attorney-General (Vic) (Ex rel Dale) v Commonwealth* (Pharmaceutical Benefits Case) (1945) 71 CLR 237–282.
3. Goddard MS. How the Pharmaceutical Benefits Scheme began. *Med J Aust.* 2014;201(1):23–25.
4. Biggs A. The Pharmaceutical Benefits Scheme – an overview. http://www.aph.gov.au/About_Parliament/Parliamentary_Departments/Parliamentary_Library/Publications_Archive/archive/pbs. Accessed 29 August 2017.
5. *National Health Act 1953* (Cth) s 88.
6. Ibid. s 90.
7. Ibid. s 94(1).
8. Ibid. s 92.
9. Section 89 of the National Health Act states that only an authorised pharmacist can supply PBS medicines; section 99 outlines the process of reimbursement for supply.
10. Australian Government Department of Health and Ageing. The Safety Net Scheme. http://www.pbs.gov.au/info/healthpro/explanatory-notes/section1/Section_1_5_Explanatory_Notes. Accessed 27 August 2017.
11. Financing and Analysis Branch, Department of Health and Aged Care. *The Australian Health Care System: An Outline.* Canberra, ACT: Commonwealth of Australia; 2000, pp. 13–14.
12. Ibid. p. 14.
13. Boxall A-M. Explainer: What is Medicare and how does it work? *The Conversation,* 31 January 2014.
14. APRA, Statistics: Quarterly Private Health Insurance Statistics December 2018 (released 14 February 2019)
15. *Aged Care Act 1997* (Cth) s 45-3.
16. Ibid.
17. Ibid. s 41-3.
18. Ibid. s 21.
19. Allan S, Blake M. *Australian Health Law.* Sydney, NSW: LexisNexis Butterworths; 2018.
20. Australian Institute of Health and Welfare. Health Expenditure Australia 2014–15. Health and welfare expenditure series no. 57. Cat. no. HWE 67. Canberra, ACT: AIHW; 2016.
21. Biggs A. *Health in Australia: A Quick Guide.* http://www.aph.gov.au/About_Parliament/Parliamentary_Departments/Parliamentary_Library/pubs/rp/rp1314/QG/HealthAust. Accessed 24 June 2018.
22. Australian Commission on Safety and Quality in Health Care. *Australian Charter of Healthcare Rights.* https://www.safetyandquality.gov.au/national-priorities/charter-of-healthcare-rights/. Accessed 24 June 2018.
23. Australian Commission on Quality and Safety in Health Care. *Review of the Charter of Healthcare Rights* (2nd ed). https://www.safetyandquality.gov.au/national-priorities/charter-of-healthcare-rights/review-of-the-charter-of-healthcare-rights-second-edition/. Accessed 21 March 2019.

REVIEW QUESTIONS AND ACTIVITIES

1. Describe the evolution of the health system in Australia, noting the differing political ideologies that have influenced changes and debate.

2. List five characteristics of the Australian health system.

3. Discuss the key elements of the Pharmaceutical Benefits Scheme.

4. Where do people get their health care in Australia?

5. Describe how healthcare funding and regulation is divided between the Commonwealth and the states/territories, and the constitutional basis of the divisions.

6. Identify and discuss the 'rights' patients have pursuant to the *Australian Charter of Healthcare Rights.*

3

INTRODUCTION TO ETHICS AND ETHICAL DECISION MAKING

■ ■

LEARNING OBJECTIVES

Upon completing this chapter you should be able to:

- define 'ethics'
- recognise the focus of bioethics
- describe what a code of ethics is and what it entails
- differentiate between law and ethics
- describe consequentialism, deontology, virtue ethics and a principles-based approach to ethical decision making
- outline decision-making steps that may be taken when faced with an ethical dilemma.

INTRODUCTION

Ethics and law share many similarities in that they both seek to affect or guide individual behaviour. Both also reflect, to varying degrees, the influences of religion, science and custom. Ethical principles are often evident in law makers' language and reasoning, particularly in cases where the courts or proposers of legislation have grappled with morally complex decisions such as issues related to the beginning or end of life, challenges faced throughout the life course and end-of-life decision making. Nevertheless, ethics and law are discrete disciplines, each with its own characteristics, language and aims.

The law may shape, determine or set boundaries for behaviour, but it is not always or only shaped by moral considerations. Law comprises social, cultural, economic, political and governmental influences, with the intention of providing binding determinations, including at times, sanctions or compensation. Ethics, on the other hand, refers to various ways of understanding and considering moral life,[1] it being otherwise known as 'moral philosophy'.

In settings in which healthcare services are delivered, both ethics and law play an important role and influence decision making and practice. The previous chapters having introduced readers to the law, this chapter therefore introduces readers to key concepts of ethics. It identifies differences between ethics and the law, and explores what it means to be an 'ethical' practitioner. It also lays the foundation for ethical decision making – examining a number of underpinning ethical philosophies and approaches that may be used when resolving ethical dilemmas faced by health practitioners during their day-to-day practice.

WHAT IS 'ETHICS'?

The word ethics derives from the Greek *ethikos* and the Latin *moralitas*, both meaning custom or habit. The words 'ethics' and 'morality' are commonly used interchangeably, but ethics appears to be more of a system of thinking about moral issues and can be distinguished from the personal morals an individual may have about particular matters. Simply put, ethics involves thinking not just about what we see as being right or wrong, identifying what we value and deciding upon how we should treat others or behave, it also involves systematising, defending and recommending concepts of 'right' and 'wrong' behaviour.

Ethics as a form of philosophical enquiry was influenced by ancient Greek philosophers and is seen as something that requires a 'rational' and dispassionate view in relation to human behaviour. The study of ethics has hence developed such that it is not only concerned with questions of *what* should be done but also requires individuals to critically examine the reasons and justifications for *why* they consider a particular act to be right or wrong or the reason for holding particular values.[2]

Ethical enquiries are often divided into three general subject areas: 'metaethics', 'normative ethics' and 'applied ethics'.

Metaethics investigates where ethical principles come from and what they mean. Consideration may be given to whether ethical principles are merely social inventions and whether they involve more than expressions of individual emotions. Metaethical answers to these questions focus on the issues of universal truths, the will of God, the role of reason in ethical judgments, and the meaning of ethical terms themselves.

Normative ethics takes on a more practical task, asking what people *should* do when trying to arrive at moral standards or principles that regulate right and wrong conduct, and developing theories to justify such norms. In normative ethics, questions posed, and claims made, concern how things *ought* to be, how to value them, which things are good, or what actions are right or wrong, acceptable or unacceptable. Normative claims are usually contrasted with 'constative' claims, which are factual statements that attempt to describe reality. Constative claims are capable of being factually correct or incorrect, while normative claims may be seen as a matter of opinion (even if 'rationally' or dispassionately formed) and may therefore be open to debate and different points of view. Sometimes this means knowing what to do when faced with an ethical dilemma is not always clear or agreed upon.

Finally, **applied ethics** involves examining specific controversial issues such as abortion, animal rights, assisted reproduction, euthanasia, infanticide, organ donation, medical treatment and social morality. Such issues are controversial in the sense that there are significant groups of people both for and against them. But, importantly, they also raise distinctly moral issues (the subject of applied ethics) as opposed to simply sensitive issues that are a matter of social policy. By using the conceptual underpinnings and tools of metaethics and normative ethics, applied ethics focuses on what should or should not be done in such contexts and why. Notably the 'ethical' answer to such questions is not based on individual morality but rather on various forms of reasoned decision making and is aimed at deriving universal norms and codes of conduct.

Bioethics

Ethics also has various branches or areas of focus. In the health sciences, one almost certainly will come across the term 'bioethics', which is the examination of ethics in relation to the life sciences and health care. 'Medical ethics', 'nursing ethics', 'clinical ethics' and 'psychological ethics' are all branches of bioethics.[3]

A broad view of bioethics sees it as a search for wisdom combining the fields of science and philosophy to question important issues that may affect the survival of the human species, nations and cultures.[4] A narrower view focuses on applied ethics to resolve concrete moral problems. The narrower view has tended to dominate practice, discussion and academic literature regarding bioethics in recent decades. However, broader bioethical considerations may be seen in discussions of, for example, environmental ethics or health and human rights.

Be the focus broad or narrow, bioethics, like ethics generally, is not concerned with examining personal moral values (which may be based on a person's upbringing, religion or experiences) but rather requires us to focus on formal decision-making processes regarding issues that require moral judgment. The point is to intentionally and critically evaluate the basis for such judgments in order to find reasons that support one decision over another, and that may be applied in future situations. In the professional healthcare context this is particularly important because health practitioners are accountable for their actions as *professionals*, not just personally. Patients, the general public and other professionals would not, and should not, be expected to know or be subject to each and every health practitioner's personal moral values (which may vary broadly) but rather have expectations regarding what they expect in terms of professional and ethical conduct from those who work in healthcare settings or deliver healthcare services.

CODES OF ETHICS

A 'code of ethics' may be seen as a developed set of moral rules, values or expectations devised for a particular purpose. They are often developed via a process of consultation, debate, discussion, evaluation and review over a period of time and may serve to guide behaviour, despite not having the force of the law. For example, *The ICN Code of Ethics for Nurses* was first adopted by the International Council of Nurses in 1953 and has been revised and reaffirmed at various times since, most recently in 2012.[5] From 1 March 2018 it was adopted in Australia as the applicable code of ethics for nurses.

Codes of ethics, however, should not be treated as an end in themselves. While they may guide behaviour, they are not a substitute for *behaving ethically*. In this regard codes, whether prescriptive or aspirational, may be too broad or imprecise to guide deliberations, especially when faced with the particularly complex situations such as those faced by health practitioners in day-to-day practice. Decisions made in such situations often involve fine discretionary judgments that cannot be captured via a code. They will also be influenced by other factors such as the law, which, when relevant, reigns supreme. Nevertheless, codes:

- serve as a public statement regarding the morals and values patients may expect a particular group of health practitioners to uphold
- inform those entering the profession about what is expected of them
- may 'act as catalysts for ethical conduct, both by heightening awareness of ethical priorities, and providing guidance from experienced professionals for the resolution of ethical conundra'.[6]

DISTINGUISHING BETWEEN ETHICS AND LAW

Ethics and law may overlap but they are distinct from one another. This is most apparent when considering examples in which the law may (or may not) require a given action while ethics might demand something else (or vice versa). For example, in many jurisdictions there is no legal duty to rescue. As such, one may see a drowning person but have no *legal obligation* to rescue them. A moral duty may, however, be seen to exist. Ethical decision making then comes into play; for example, a person may decide their moral duty does not involve jumping into the water (particularly if the observer cannot swim) but may involve calling for help.

Note the distinction between law and ethics is also important because ethics allows judgments about the law itself. That is, while a law may be valid and enforceable because it has been enacted by a certain government, it may not be ethically acceptable. For example, laws supporting apartheid were once valid but were contrary to the values and ethics of many. To this end, ethics allows us to question and challenge the laws that we find morally questionable or wrong. Of course, when asking questions about what the law *should* be, or why it is what it is, ethics is one (but not the only) component that may influence the answer to that question.

Table 3.1 notes some distinguishing features of law and ethics.

DECISION MAKING WHEN FACED WITH AN ETHICAL DILEMMA

When making decisions about ethical issues, there are two kinds of questions to ask. The first is, 'What is the right thing to do?' This question requires us to consider what our conduct or actions should be and leads us to think about the kinds of moral norms that we follow in our personal and professional lives. The second question is, 'Why is this the right thing to do?' This question engages with the reasons we consider an act right or wrong (or good or bad).

Although seemingly simple questions, thousands of years of scholarship concerning moral dilemmas tell us there is still no single 'right' answer that philosophers all agree on in relation to moral questions posed. However, there is a rich literature offering insights into different ways of thinking about these questions and their possible answers, and there is considerable agreement about what must be considered in developing such answers.

Here, it is worth considering four widely accepted frameworks for ethical analysis and moral reasoning and decision making. These involve looking at: (1) the *consequences* of different courses of action; (2) the *duties* or obligations of those making the decisions; (3) the *character* and virtues of the decision-maker; and (4) a *principles*-based approach.

	TABLE 3.1	
	Distinguishing Features of Law and Ethics	
Basis for Comparison	Law	Ethics
Meaning	The law refers to a systematic body of rules that governs a particular society or community, regulating the actions of its members	Moral principles and values that guide individual or group behaviour on issues of human conduct
Aims and objectives	Law is created with an intent to maintain social order and peace and to provide protection to all citizens	Ethics help people to decide what is right or wrong and how to act
Made by	Government (e.g. legislature, judiciary, authorised bodies)	Individuals, groups (e.g. professional bodies)
Influences	Culture, economics, ethics, human rights, jurisprudence, resources, social and political ideologies, values	Moral philosophy, metaethics, normative ethics, descriptive ethics, religion, morality
Expression	Expressed and published in writing in the form of statutes, regulations, ordinances and common law judgments	Often abstract; sometimes expressed in 'codes of ethics' or 'guidelines'
Violation/ enforceability	Breach of the law may result in punishment (e.g. imprisonment or a fine or both), liability to pay compensation or a court order to do or stop doing something	Generally there is no other consequence for violating ethics than personal guilt or shame, or social disapproval. If a professional does not adhere to a code of ethics, there may be a professional consequence

Consequentialism

Consequentialism is a theory that claims that an action is right or wrong depending on the outcomes (consequences) of the action. Consequentialism is very influential in medicine given the focus on patient outcomes – in general we think that we should do whatever achieves a good health outcome. This sounds fairly straightforward, but depending upon how we think about the consequences, we might get different answers to the same question. For example, a consequentialist argument in support of euthanasia might claim that it is better for a person to die when they choose rather than live a few days more in constant pain. The 'good' outcome here is the person having their preference satisfied. On the other hand, a consequentialist argument against euthanasia might claim that patients will lose trust in doctors if euthanasia is practised because patients will fear that their doctor could take the decision out of their hands and kill them. Thus the potential bad outcome here is a loss of patients' trust in doctors.

The most well known consequentialist theory is utilitarianism, which links consequences with creating the most benefit, welfare or happiness. Many people are familiar with the utilitarian saying 'the greatest good for the greatest number'. Utilitarians believe that the consequences of actions are morally important so far as they affect the welfare or happiness of the greatest number of people. However, while decisions based on a utilitarian approach may use such justifications, the approach may lead on a smaller scale to decisions that many may view as immoral. For example, not treating the severely ill or infirm in order to direct resources to those who are likely to recover well and contribute to society may serve the greatest number of people but would be morally questionable. What creates the greatest happiness for the greatest number of people isn't necessarily 'right'.

Deontology

Deontology contrasts with consequentialism in that it claims that we cannot judge the rightness or wrongness of an action solely by looking at the consequences of that action. Rather, deontologists claim that we must examine the duties and responsibilities of the person performing the action and the rights of those affected by that action. For example, in medicine doctors have a duty to avoid harm to their patients and patients have a right not to be harmed. This is an important moral consideration no matter what the circumstances. However, this may again lead to different outcomes when making ethical decisions. In relation to euthanasia, a deontologist might claim that doctors have a duty not to kill innocent people and that this duty should not be violated in any circumstances. On the other hand, many pro-euthanasia arguments claim that people have a 'right to die' at the time and place of their choosing.

Nevertheless, deontological theories take account of moral obligations, duties, motives and intentions, rather than simply the consequences of actions. In this regard we may define the broad duties of health practitioners as:

- a duty to tell the truth
- a duty to prevent harm (act with non-maleficence)
- a duty to promote good (act with beneficence)
- a duty to respect the autonomous choices of patients
- a duty to obtain informed consent
- a duty to protect patient confidentiality.

However, difficulty in applying deontological decision making to ethical issues arises when there are competing duties or rights. There is no clear process for deciding which duty or right to give preference to.

Virtue Ethics

The third approach considered here is virtue ethics. Virtue ethics focuses on the *character* and *intentions* of the person making the decision as the central tenet of decision making as well as what kind of person we are and should be. A question about the right thing to do is answered by considering what 'a good person (health practitioner) would do'. There are a number of virtues that are considered important in medicine and health care including compassion, honesty and justice. However, one can illustrate that this approach – again, like consequentialism and deontology – does not lead to one 'right' answer. In relation to the example of euthanasia, a virtue ethicist could claim that compassion for the patient is a morally good reason for providing euthanasia, while an opponent of euthanasia could argue that the virtue of prudence prohibits euthanasia.

As a decision-making tool, virtue ethics directs our attention to particular qualities and character traits that are morally relevant. This way of thinking may be familiar to health practitioners in that it is common to call on role models or mentors when faced with challenging situations or to imagine what a mentor might say or do in a particular situation. However, again, this approach is not without problems. How much useful guidance about how to act does it in fact provide, rather than simply identifying people who are considered to have acted well?

Principles-Based Approach

The final approach to be mentioned here is one found within biomedical ethics first propounded by Beauchamp and Childress.[7] They identified four core principles of biomedical ethics, which they proposed should form the basis of ethical decision making:

- **Respect for autonomy:** respecting the decision-making capacities of autonomous persons; enabling individuals to make reasoned, informed choices and emphasising self-determination
- **Beneficence:** promoting good; the health practitioner should act in a way that benefits the patient
- **Non-maleficence:** avoiding the causation of harm; the health practitioner should not harm the patient (or the harm should not be disproportionate to the benefits of treatment)
- **Justice:** patients in similar positions should be treated in a similar manner.

The principles have appeal because they are simple and reflect a certain morality that respects self-determination, seeks to do good and avoid harm, and values justice. However, while helpful to understanding issues that may arise in professional practice, and useful when drafting ethical policies, they again pose issues – particularly when applied to clinical problems in that the principles may conflict. They are very much like the deontological approach in this regard. It has also been found that while people state they value the four medical ethical principles, they do not actually seem to use them directly in the decision-making process.[8] The reasons for this may be explained by the principles being fairly abstract, which leads to an absence of true application when resolving ethical dilemmas.

DERIVING A PROCESS FOR ETHICAL DECISION MAKING

There are many other approaches to ethical reasoning and decision making. The four described above are the most widely used and, between them, are generally able to capture most of the matters that we commonly think to be morally important. In this sense it is important also to remember that each of the abovementioned approaches can make room for the other(s). Indeed, it is the more modern view that any plausible ethical decision-making process may have something to say about all of them (and others, depending on the circumstances). In recent years a number of philosophers have come to doubt that there can be only one correct theory and have said it a mistake to view the various theories as mutually exclusive claims to moral truth.[9]

Health practitioners don't routinely face ethical dilemmas in every decision they make, requiring them to stop and engage in a detailed ethical analysis. Health practitioners take for granted that they should help patients in need and that good health is valuable. The ethical ground of health care is often therefore invisible to practitioners because they are so accustomed to doing the right thing in terms of assisting patients. However, sometimes it is necessary to have to stop and ask about the right thing to do. This may occur because the treatment is unlikely to be successful or because the patient does not want to receive a potentially beneficial treatment; sometimes there are competing pressures so that helping one patient comes at a cost to others. As health practitioners become more experienced, the ethical issues often seem to loom larger. This may be because those who are experienced no longer worry about *how* to do things and are able to consider whether or not they *should* do them. Understanding what ethics is, and having an ethical framework within which to think about what one should do, and why, when faced with moral dilemmas may assist in answering such questions.

When faced with an ethical dilemma in healthcare contexts it is also useful to approach the problem by following a number of steps that will help to make clear, consistent and reasoned decisions. To this end, various models for ethical decision making are found in the literature.[10] The following sets out some basic components:[11]

1. *Identify what the ethical issue is (or issues are).* Here, one may frame the dilemma as a normative question (i.e. What *should* I do in this situation?). It will also be relevant to identify and consider any expected standards, codes and the law because there may be rules that dictate what one *must* do and such rules must be followed. However, equally there may be rules that are not clear in terms of the ethical decision to be made within their bounds, and decisions about *how* to act ethically are still pertinent.

2. *Identify personal reaction to the case.* This may involve recognising a 'gut reaction' or 'instinct' that reflects emotive reactions to the situation at hand. By identifying such reactions you may in turn reflect on the personal values, assumptions and biases that underlie them. It will also enable you to compare them with those of other professionals, who may or may not share the same views. Thinking about similarities and differences can help the critical process and lead to a choice that may be better justified than one made based on 'gut instinct'. It also enables such 'gut reactions' to be consciously set aside in order to critically analyse the situation.

3. *Gather any relevant facts regarding the situation.* It is necessary to identify all facts (and factors) that should be taken into consideration when making the decision.

4. *Identify the values at stake in the scenario.* It will here be necessary to identify values from various perspectives of any and all people (stakeholders) who may or will be affected by the decision – for example, the patient, family members, other health practitioners, management and society at large.

5. *Identify the options in the case.* Identify all possible actions and alternatives.

6. *Consider what you should do and relevant justifications for doing so (i.e. why).* Here consideration of which option should be preferred should be based on a reasoned evaluation of what is at stake. Possible actions may be considered in light of the above ethical decision-making approaches discussed, with consideration being given to the consequences of particular actions, respective duties and rights, and professional virtues. (Note: It may also involve consideration of other

approaches such as a human rights approach, a principles-based approach or an ethics-of-care approach.)

7. *Consider if the ethical problem could have been prevented.* It is important to consider whether the ethical problem could have been prevented and how. For example, consider if systemic changes can be made to prevent the problem from happening again, or whether clearer rules, guidelines, laws or otherwise are necessary to clarify what should be done in similar situations in future (and what you can do in relation to them).

We will return to such steps in Chapter 18 when we consider cases and scenarios relevant to a variety of health professions that raise ethical or legal issues.

FURTHER READING

Johnstone M. *Bioethics: A Nursing Perspective.* 5th ed. Sydney: Elsevier; 2009.

Kerridge I, Lowe M, Cameron S. *Ethics and Law for Health Professions.* Sydney, NSW: The Federation Press; 2013.

Steinbock B, London A, Arras J. *Ethical Issues in Modern Medicine: Contemporary Readings in Bio-ethics.* New York, NY: McGraw-Hill; 2013.

ENDNOTES

1. Beauchamp TL, Childress J. *Philosophical Ethics: An Introduction to Moral Philosophy.* Oxford: Oxford University Press; 1994.
2. Johnstone M. *Bioethics: A Nursing Perspective.* 5th ed. Sydney: Elsevier; 2009.
3. Kerridge I, Lowe M, Cameron S. *Ethics and Law for Health Professions.* Sydney, NSW: The Federation Press; 2013.
4. Potter V. *Bioethics: Bridge to the Future.* Englewood Cliffs: Prentice Hall; 1971, cited in Reich WT. The word bioethics: its birth and the legacies of those who shaped it. *Kennedy Inst Ethics J.* 1994;4(4):321.
5. International Council of Nurses. *The ICN Code of Ethics for Nurses.* Geneva: ICN; 2012.
6. Freckleton I. Enforcement of ethics. In: Coady M, Bloch S, eds. *Codes of Ethics and the Professions.* Melbourne, VIC: Melbourne University Press; 1996. pp. 130–165.
7. Beauchamp TL, Childress J. *Philosophical Ethics: An Introduction to Moral Philosophy.* Oxford: Oxford University Press; 1994.
8. Page K. The four principles: can they be measured and do they predict ethical decision making? *BMC Med Ethics.* 2012;13:10.
9. Steinbock B, London A, Arras J. *Ethical Issues in Modern Medicine: Contemporary Readings in Bio-ethics.* New York, NY: McGraw-Hill; 2013.
10. See, for example, Benjamin M, Curtis J. *Ethics in Nursing: Cases, Principles, and Reasoning.* 4th ed. New York, NY: Oxford University Press; 2010; Lo B. *Resolving Ethical Dilemmas: A Guide for Clinicians.* 2nd ed. Baltimore, MD: Lippincott, William & Wilkins; 2000; Purtilo R. *Ethical Dimensions in the Health Professions.* 4th ed. Philadelphia, PA: W.B. Saunders; 2005.
11. The components outlined reflect those discussed in Glover JJ. Ethical decision-making guidelines and tools. In: Harman LB, ed. *Ethical Challenges in the Management of Health Information.* 2nd ed. Sudbury, MA: Jones and Bartlett; 2006.

REVIEW QUESTIONS AND ACTIVITIES

1. What does the study of ethics address?

2. Why is it important to make a distinction between law and ethics?

3. What is bioethics?

4. Describe what a code of ethics is and what it entails.

5. Describe consequentialism, deontology and virtue ethics.

6. Research the concepts of 'respect for autonomy', 'benficence', 'non-maleficence' and 'justice', and reflect on how they may be applied in healthcare settings to guide the treatment of people seeking healthcare services.

7. Draw a matrix that outlines the decision-making steps that may be taken when faced with an ethical dilemma.

Section 2

PROFESSIONAL REGULATION AND KEY CONCEPTS RELEVANT TO HEALTHCARE DELIVERY

4 PROFESSIONAL REGULATION OF HEALTH PRACTITIONERS

Upon completing this chapter you should be able to:

- discuss the significance of the regulation of health practitioners
- describe regulatory frameworks and requirements for professions governed by the National Registration and Accreditation Scheme and those that fall outside of the scheme
- explain mandatory and voluntary reporting pursuant to the National Scheme
- identify health practitioner conduct that would provide grounds for disciplinary action
- describe the disciplinary process and possible outcomes of disciplinary hearings.

INTRODUCTION

The regulation of health practitioners is important for ensuring healthcare services are provided in a safe, professional and ethical manner. This includes, among other things, setting standards of practice for the profession, investigating complaints about members of the profession and, where appropriate, ensuring remedial action is taken and/or disciplining them. Depending on a person's area of health practice, how they are regulated may differ. This chapter will examine the regulation of health practitioners in Australia including: (1) those who fall within one of the 15 health professions currently regulated pursuant to the National Registration and Accreditation Scheme; and (2) those who are not registered or fall outside of that scheme (e.g. speech

therapists, nutritionists). It will illustrate that such regulation is a mixture of legislative provisions, guidelines, codes of practice and ethical codes that work together to create the framework for health practitioners to work within and conduct themselves in relation to their profession. Systems for complaints and modes of addressing conduct that fall short of expected standards are also discussed.

THE NATIONAL REGISTRATION AND ACCREDITATION SCHEME

Fifteen Health Professions: APRHA and the National Boards

Registration of health practitioners in Australia is underpinned by the National Registration and Accreditation Scheme ('the National Scheme'). The law governing the scheme is often referred to as the 'National Law'; however, the scheme is an agreement between all the states and territories that allowed the passage of legislation in Queensland in 2009,[1] which was then enacted in each of the other states and territories.[2] The scheme is considered national because it sets up one national registration and accreditation system, establishing a national oversight authority and the National Health Practitioner Boards ('National Boards'). However, as the scheme is state/territory-based there are some differences among jurisdictions, particularly in relation to complaints systems. Such differences are discussed further below. Table 4.1 sets out the respective state and territory laws.

TABLE 4.1	
The National Law	
Jurisdiction	Legislation
Australian Capital Territory	*Health Practitioner Regulation National Law (ACT) Act 2010*
New South Wales	*Health Practitioner Regulation (Adoption of National Law) Act 2009, Health Practitioner Regulation National Law (NSW)*
Northern Territory	*Health Practitioner Regulation (National Uniform Legislation) Act 2010*
Queensland	*Health Practitioner Regulation National Law 2009*
South Australia	*Health Practitioner Regulation National Law (South Australia) Act 2010*
Tasmania	*Health Practitioner Regulation National Law (Tasmania) Act 2010*
Victoria	*Health Practitioner Regulation National Law (Victoria) Act 2009*
Western Australia	*Health Practitioner Regulation National Law (WA) Act 2010*

Australian Health Practitioners Regulation Agency

The National Scheme established the Australian Health Practitioners Regulation Agency (AHPRA), which oversees the scheme and has protecting the public as its primary role. AHPRA has a number of functions including, but not limited to, supporting the National Boards that were also established under the scheme – for example, in developing registration standards, codes of conduct and guidelines. It manages the registration and renewal processes for health practitioners and students across Australia and publishes the national register of practitioners, making information about the registration of individual health practitioners available to the public.[3] AHPRA also provides advice to the 'Ministerial Council'[4] for the administration of the National Scheme.

AHPRA has a national office as well as offices in each state and territory[5] where the public can make a complaint about a registered health practitioner or student. It also manages investigations into the professional conduct, performance or health of registered health practitioners on behalf of the National Boards (except in New South Wales where this is undertaken by the Health Professional Councils Authority and the Health Care Complaints Commission (HCCC) and in Queensland where this may be undertaken by the Queensland Health Ombudsman). In addition, AHPRA works with the health complaints commissions in each state and territory to make sure the appropriate organisation deals with community concerns about registered health practitioners.

National Boards

In addition to establishing AHPRA, National Boards have been established for each of the professions covered by the National Scheme.[6] At the time of writing they included the:

- Aboriginal and Torres Strait Islander Health Practice Board of Australia
- Chinese Medicine Board of Australia
- Chiropractic Board of Australia
- Dental Board of Australia
- Medical Board of Australia
- Medical Radiation Practice Board of Australia
- Nursing and Midwifery Board of Australia
- Occupational Therapy Board of Australia
- Optometry Board of Australia
- Osteopathy Board of Australia
- Pharmacy Board of Australia
- Physiotherapy Board of Australia
- Podiatry Board of Australia
- Psychology Board of Australia
- Paramedicine Board of Australia.

The National Law prescribes the functions of the National Boards to include:

- registering 'suitably qualified and competent persons'
- imposing conditions on registration
- making decisions as to the requirements for registration and/or endorsement
- developing and/or approving professional standards, codes and guidelines
- approving accredited programs of study
- overseeing the management of health practitioners and students, including monitoring the conditions, undertakings and suspensions imposed on the registration of practitioners and students
- overseeing the assessment and suitability of overseas-trained applicants for registration in Australia

- overseeing the receipt, assessment and investigations of notifications made about students in the health profession or persons who are, or have been, registered health practitioners
- establishing panels to conduct hearings about health, performance and/or professional standards
- referring matters to 'responsible tribunals'
- making recommendations to the Ministerial Council about specialist recognition and approval of specialties for a profession
- giving advice, assistance and information to the Ministerial Council on issues related to registration and accreditation of health professions under the National Scheme
- in conjunction with AHPRA, keeping up-to-date national registers of health practitioners and students of the health professions and ensuring the national registers are publicly accessible
- doing 'anything else necessary or convenient for the effective and efficient operation of the National Registration and Accreditation Scheme'.[7]

The National Boards are empowered to establish state/territory-based boards (also referred to as committees) for the purpose of carrying out the functions of the National Board in 'a way that provides an effective and timely local response to health practitioners and other persons'.[8] As an example, the Nursing and Midwifery Board of Australia may establish a state board for nurses and midwives in South Australia. That body would be referred to as the South Australian Nursing and Midwifery Board of Australia.

Registration of Health Practitioners

One of the functions of the National Boards is to establish processes and standards[9] for registering health practitioners. There are several different types of registration, with eligibility and qualifications requirements set out in the National Law. Registrants must also meet any registration standards issued by the relevant board.

General Registration

Practitioners who hold general registration are required to have graduated from a board-approved, accredited program of study in the profession. They must also have completed any required period of supervised practice or internship.[10]

Specialist Registration

The Ministerial Council has approved a number of 'recognised specialties' for which 'specialist registration' may be granted under the National Law. There are **specialist titles** approved for each recognised specialty. Some practitioners may be eligible for – and may hold – both general registration and specialist registration at the same time. Others may hold specialist registration but may be limited to practising only in their specialty (e.g. people who qualified overseas and do not hold an approved undergraduate or entry-level qualification).[11]

Limited Registration

Limited registration may be granted to practitioners who do not qualify for general or specialist registration but who meet the eligibility and qualifications requirements[12] and any registration standards issued by the board. Limited registration may not be renewed more than three times, but a new application may be made.[13] There are four sub-types of limited registration:

- *postgraduate training or supervised practice* – where a practitioner holds qualifications in the profession but is required to sit an examination or assessment to qualify for general or specialist registration or to practise under supervision
- *area of need* – where an overseas-trained practitioner who does not qualify for general or specialist registration has skills and qualifications considered sufficient to work under supervision in a particular role or position in a geographic location or specific healthcare facility[14]
- *teaching or research* – where a practitioner who is not qualified for or does not intend to engage in clinical practice is qualified to fill a teaching or research position in the profession
- *public interest* – where a practitioner who does not qualify for general or specialist registration holds qualifications in the profession and is visiting from overseas for a short period to fill a locum position or to exchange practice with a local practitioner. In this case the board must be satisfied that it is in the public interest for the practitioner to practise the profession given the practitioner's qualifications and experience.[15]

Provisional Registration

Provisional registration is intended for practitioners in a profession who have completed a board-approved, accredited qualification in the profession but are required to undertake a period of supervised practice or internship to be eligible for general registration. Only three professions currently have internship requirements for general registration: medicine, pharmacy and psychology.[16]

Non-Practising Registration

Non-practising registration is available to practitioners who have previously held general or specialist registration in a profession but who do not wish to practise in the profession during the registration period. The National Boards have defined 'practising' in the profession as undertaking any role, whether remunerated or not, in which the person uses their skills and knowledge as a health practitioner in their profession and is not restricted to providing direct clinical care. Examples of using professional knowledge in a direct non-clinical relationship with clients include working in management, administration, education, research, advisory, regulatory or policy development roles, and any other roles that affect safe, effective delivery of services in the profession.[17]

Student Registration

All students (other than students of psychology, who are registered instead as a provisional psychologist) who are enrolled in an 'approved program of study'[18] for a health profession are registered under the National Scheme.

Education providers send data on the national Student Register to AHPRA and the National Boards. There is no fee attached to student registration and, unlike the registers for health practitioners, the Student Register is not publicly available.

A student's registration commences from their first year of study in an approved program of study and ceases when the student completes or otherwise ceases to be enrolled in the approved program.[19]

AHPRA and the National Boards have no role in the academic results or progression of a student. Rather, because the objective of national student registration is to promote public health and safety, the Student Register enables AHPRA and the National Boards to act on notifications of student impairment and in circumstances in which a student is convicted of an offence that may impact on the safety of the public.

Registration Standards

Included in the functions of the National Boards is the power to determine the requirements for registration and to develop and approve registration standards, codes and guidelines.[20] The National Boards have approved the following five standards as prerequisites for registering health practitioners:

- *Continuing Professional Development Registration Standard*
- *Criminal History Registration Standard*
- *English Language Skills Registration Standard*
- *Professional Indemnity Insurance Registration Standard*
- *Recency of Practice Registration Standard.*

Continuing Professional Development Registration Standard

While the National Boards have adopted this standard as a mandatory requirement for registration, the number of hours and type of professional development activities required to meet the standard differs between the professions. It is important for registered health practitioners to check with their respective boards to determine the continuing professional development expected of them.

A number of the National Boards expressly require that individual health practitioners maintain a continuing professional development portfolio for the purpose of their declaration or to produce to the National Board as part of the registration process.[21]

Criminal History Registration Standard

The terms of the *Criminal History Registration Standard* are consistent across the National Boards. A professional board will make a determination as to whether the registrant's criminal history is 'relevant to the practice of their profession' by considering the individual case against the 10 factors set out in the standard. The factors are:

1. the nature and gravity of the offence or alleged offence and its relevance to health practice
2. the period of time since the health practitioner committed, or allegedly committed, the offence

3. whether a finding of guilt or a conviction was recorded for the offence or a charge for the offence is still pending
4. the sentence imposed for the offence
5. the ages of the health practitioner and of any victim at the time the health practitioner committed, or allegedly committed, the offence
6. whether or not the conduct that constituted the offence or to which the charge relates has been decriminalised since the health practitioner committed, or allegedly committed, the offence
7. the health practitioner's behaviour since she or he committed, or allegedly committed, the offence
8. the likelihood of future threat to a patient of the health practitioner
9. any information given by the health practitioner
10. any other matter that the board considers relevant.

English Language Skills Registration Standard

All applicants for initial registration with AHPRA must be able to demonstrate proficient English language skills. This standard applies whether the professional qualified in Australia or overseas. The standards are:

- a common standard for 10 professions: Chinese medicine, chiropractic, medical radiation, occupational therapy, optometry, osteopathy, pharmacy, physiotherapy, podiatry and psychology
- a standard for Aboriginal and Torres Strait Islander health practitioners
- a standard for dental practitioners
- a standard for medical practitioners
- a standard for nursing and midwifery
- a standard for paramedicine.[22]

All the profession-specific standards share many elements with the common standard.[23] The Aboriginal and Torres Strait Islander Standard requires English language proficiency to be demonstrated through completing a Certificate IV in Aboriginal and/or Torres Strait Islander Primary Health Care Practice or a qualification the board considers to be equivalent.[24]

Professional Indemnity Insurance Arrangements Registration Standard

Consistent with the National Law, this registration standard mandates that health practitioners must be covered in the conduct of their practice by appropriate professional indemnity insurance.[25] Health practitioners are required to make a declaration as to the adequacy of their professional indemnity insurance on application for, or renewal of, their professional registration. National Boards may differ in the level of cover they require.

The Nursing and Midwifery Board Registration Standard provides an exemption from complying with the professional indemnity insurance requirement for nurses and midwives with non-practising registration and registered midwives who are practising private midwifery and are exempt under the National Law (s 284).

Students of all health professions are exempt from the professional indemnity insurance standard requirement.

Recency of Practice Registration Standard

All practising registrants are required to undertake set periods of practice in their profession to satisfy the *Recency of Practice Registration Standard* as determined by their respective professional National Board. The National Boards require, as part of the registration process, that practitioners declare that they have fulfilled the practice requirements and are thereby competent to practise in their profession. 'Practise' is not restricted to face-to-face clinical care but to applying and implementing professional knowledge and skill. The specific hours of practice required vary between the National Board standards.

Additional Standards

A number of the National Boards have developed and approved additional standards as requirements for registration. The following provides some (but not all) examples of registration standards developed and approved by specific boards:

- Aboriginal and Torres Strait Islander Health Practice Board: *Aboriginal and Torres Strait Islander Health Practice: Aboriginal and/or Torres Strait Islander Registration Standard*, Certificate IV in Aboriginal and/or Torres Strait Islander Primary Health Care (Practice) or an equivalent as determined by the board
- Dental Board of Australia: *Dental Endorsement Conscious Sedation Registration Standard, Scope*

of Practice Registration Standard, Dental Specialist Registration Standard, Dental List of Specialties Registration Standard
- Nursing and Midwifery Board of Australia: *Endorsement Nurse Practitioner Registration Standard, Registration Standard for Endorsement for Scheduled Medicines for Midwives, Registration Standard for Eligible Midwives, Nursing and Midwifery Endorsement Scheduled Medicines Registered Nurses Registration Standard*
- Optometry Board of Australia: *Optometry Endorsement for Scheduled Medicines Registration Standard*
- Psychology Board of Australia: *General Registration Standard, Provisional Registration Standard.*

Guidelines, Codes and Policies

Pursuant to section 39 of the National Law, the National Boards have jointly, and individually, developed guidelines and codes to identify the obligations and responsibilities imposed under the National Law for registered health practitioners, employers of registered health practitioners and educational providers. In addition, these guidelines and codes clarify the expectations of the National Boards as to the standards of appropriate and competent professional conduct necessary to ensure public safety and prevent the public from being at risk of harm. The development and approval of guidelines, codes and policies by the respective National Boards is, out of necessity, an ongoing and constantly evolving process. The National Boards have also jointly produced some shared codes and guidelines including guidelines regarding mandatory reporting, guidelines regarding advertising and a shared code of conduct.

Guidelines and Requirements for Mandatory Reporting

Mandatory reporting was implemented as part of the National Scheme in response to scandals in the health system that had given rise to a perception that health practitioners were often aware of colleagues' performance or conduct issues but frequently did not report concerns to an appropriate authority. The National Law therefore introduced a requirement that registered health practitioners (across all health practitioner disciplines), employers of those practitioners and education providers report certain misconduct on the part of doctors and other health practitioners to AHPRA if they have formed a reasonable belief that another health practitioner has:

- practised their profession while intoxicated by alcohol or drugs
- engaged in sexual misconduct in connection with practising their profession
- placed the public at risk of substantial harm because the practitioner has an impairment, or
- placed the public at risk of harm because the practitioner has practised in a way that constitutes a significant departure from accepted professional standards.

The justification for such provision is to ensure the safety of consumers seeking healthcare services and the public by enabling the early detection of and rapid response to concerns about a professional's conduct or performance.

The National Boards have agreed on mandatory reporting guidelines that further set out and describe the obligation for mandatory notification imposed under the National Law.[26] A mandatory notification is made to AHPRA, which subsequently forwards the notification to the relevant professional National Board. The National Law provides protection for a notifier from any civil, criminal or administrative liability where they have lodged the notification under the National Law in 'good faith'. Section 237(3) states that making a notification 'does not constitute a breach of professional etiquette or ethics or a departure from accepted standards of professional conduct', nor does it attract any liability for defamation.[27]

Contravention of the mandatory notification provision does not constitute an offence under the National Law but may amount to grounds for disciplinary action to be taken against a registered practitioner.

Exemptions arise where the practitioner making the notification:

- is employed or engaged by a professional indemnity insurer and forms the belief because of a disclosure in the course of a legal proceeding or when providing legal advice arising from the insurance policy
- forms the belief while providing advice about legal proceedings or preparing legal advice or is exercising functions as a member of a quality assurance committee, council or other similar body approved or authorised under legislation that prohibits the disclosure of the

information that someone else has already made a notification

- is a treating practitioner practising in Western Australia, or
- is a treating practitioner practising in Queensland in certain circumstances (i.e. where the practitioner providing the service reasonably believes that the notifiable conduct relates to an impairment that will not place the public at substantial risk of harm and is not professional misconduct).[28]

VOLUNTARY NOTIFICATIONS

The National Law also provides for making a voluntary notification to AHPRA by anyone (including members of the public, staff or otherwise) when a person has formed a reasonable belief that:

- a registered health practitioner's conduct, level of knowledge, skill, judgment or care is lesser than, or below, a standard reasonably expected
- the registrant is not (or may not be) a suitable person to hold a registration
- the registrant has (or may have) an impairment, or
- the registrant has (or may have) contravened the National Law or a condition of their registration or an undertaking or has (or may have) improperly obtained their registration.

Voluntary notification in relation to students may occur when the student has been charged with an offence or convicted or found guilty of an offence punishable by 12 months' imprisonment or more. A voluntary notification may also be lodged if the student has (or may have) contravened a condition or undertaking attached to their student registration.

GUIDELINES FOR ADVERTISING REGULATED HEALTH SERVICES

The National Boards have also jointly developed guidelines for advertising 'regulated health services'.[29] The guidelines apply to registered practitioners, employers of those practitioners and others who provide services through the agency of a registered practitioner. Fundamental to the guidelines are obligations imposed by the National Law that prohibit a person from advertising a regulated health service, or a business that provides a regulated health service, in a way that:

(a) is false, misleading or deceptive or is likely to be misleading or deceptive; or
(b) offers a gift, discount or other inducement to attract a person to use the service or the business, unless the advertising also states the terms and conditions of the offer; or
(c) uses testimonials or purported testimonials about the service or business; or
(d) creates an unreasonable expectation of beneficial treatment; or
(e) directly or indirectly encourages the indiscriminate or unnecessary use of regulated health services.[30]

AHPRA advises in relation to preparing or reviewing advertising that practitioners:

… should remain mindful that their audience does not have this professional background or expertise, be honest and sell services on their merits, and look at the overall impression of their advertisements, rather than whether each individual statement is correct.[31]

Breach of the National Law provisions regarding advertising may result in prosecution and a penalty of up to $5,000 per offence for an individual or $10,000 per offence for a body corporate.

Note, conduct in relation to advertising is also regulated by Commonwealth legislation including the *Competition and Consumer Act 2010* (Cth), the *Therapeutic Goods Act 1989* (Cth), the Therapeutic Goods Regulations 1990 (Cth) and relevant state/territory fair trading or consumer protection legislation.[32]

CODES OF CONDUCT

In addition to the National Law, codes of conduct form an important part of the regulation of health practitioners. A shared *Code of Conduct for Registered Health Practitioners* has been adopted by 11 of the National Boards including the National Aboriginal and Torres Strait Islander health practice, Chinese medicine, dental, chiropractic, medical radiation practice, occupational therapy, optometry, osteopathy, pharmacy, physiotherapy and podiatry boards.

The shared code of conduct aims to assist and support registered health practitioners to deliver effective healthcare services within an ethical framework and identifies standards of conduct to be applied and adhered to by registered professionals in their practice. The standards of behaviour set out in the code address the following issues:

- providing good care, including shared decision making
- working with patients or people seeking healthcare services
- working with other practitioners
- working within the health system
- minimising risk
- maintaining professional performance
- professional behaviour and ethical conduct
- ensuring practitioner health
- teaching, supervising and assessing.

The purpose of the code is to support practitioners in providing good healthcare services and to provide a framework for situations in which a registered practitioner must exercise professional judgment. In addition, the code assists the respective boards in their role of protecting the public.

The Medical Board of Australia has adopted the *Good Medical Practice: A Code of Conduct for Doctors in Australia*.[33] This code identifies and describes the principles underpinning good medical practice and provides the benchmark standards of ethical and professional conduct expected of a medical practitioner. The code is consistent with the Australian Medical Association *Code of Ethics*,[34] the *Declaration of Geneva* and the *International Code of Medical Ethics*.[35] The issues addressed by the code are broadly similar to those contained in the *Code of Conduct for Registered Health Practitioners*.

Nurses and midwives also have separate codes of conduct. From 1 March 2018, the International Council of Nurses' *The ICN Code of Ethics for Nurses* took effect for all nurses in Australia and the International Confederation of Midwives' *Code of Ethics for Midwives* for all midwives in Australia.[36] These documents replaced the *Code of Ethics for Nurses – August 2008* and the *Code of Ethics for Midwives – August 2008*.

The Psychology Board of Australia has adopted the *Australian Psychological Society Code of Ethics* for the profession.[37]

Such codes illustrate the interplay between the law and ethics and together work to determine what is expected of health practitioners when practising their professions or acting in a way that may affect their profession.

DISCIPLINARY ISSUES

The AHPRA scheme, therefore, is underpinned by the understanding that fundamental to the practice of all health practitioners is **satisfactory conduct**, which involves the due exercise of skill, judgment and care. Where a registered health practitioner practises in a manner considered below a standard acceptable to the profession, it is likely that disciplinary proceedings will be initiated.

Broadly speaking, activities that warrant initiating disciplinary action for those practising as a registered health practitioner can be categorised as 'unsatisfactory professional performance', 'unprofessional conduct' or 'professional misconduct'.

Unsatisfactory professional performance means that the knowledge, skill or judgment possessed, or care exercised, by the practitioner in the practice of the health profession in which the practitioner is registered is 'below the standard reasonably expected of a health practitioner of an equivalent level of training or experience'.[38]

Unprofessional conduct is 'conduct that is of a lesser standard than that which might reasonably be expected of the health practitioner by the public or the practitioner's professional peers. It includes:

- contravention of the National Law
- contravention of a condition to which the practitioner's registration was subject; or an undertaking given by the practitioner to the National Board that registers the practitioner
- the conviction of the practitioner for an offence under another Act, the nature of which may affect the practitioner's suitability to continue to practise the profession
- providing a person with health services of a kind that are excessive, unnecessary or otherwise not reasonably required for the person's wellbeing

- influencing, or attempting to influence, the conduct of another registered health practitioner in a way that will compromise patient care
- accepting a benefit as inducement, consideration or reward for referring another person to a health service provider or recommending another person use or consult with a health service provider
- offering or giving a person a benefit, consideration or reward in return for the person referring another person to the practitioner or recommending to another person that the person use a health service provided by the practitioner
- referring a person to, or recommending that a person use or consult, another health service provider, health service or health product if the practitioner has a pecuniary interest in giving that referral or recommendation, unless the practitioner discloses the nature of that interest to the person before or at the time of giving the referral or recommendation.[39]

Professional misconduct includes:

… unprofessional conduct by the practitioner that amounts to conduct that is substantially below the standard reasonably expected of a registered health practitioner of the equivalent level of training or experience; more than one instance of unprofessional conduct that, when considered together, amounts to conduct that is substantially below the standard reasonably expected of a registered health practitioner of an equivalent level of training or experience; and/or conduct of the practitioner, whether occurring in connection with the practice of the health practitioner's profession or not, that is inconsistent with the practitioner being a fit and proper person to hold registration in the profession.[40]

MENTAL OR PHYSICAL INCAPACITY OR IMPAIRMENT

A practitioner may also suffer from a mental or physical incapacity, or alcohol or drug addiction, that negatively affects their competency to practice. In such a situation it may be that the practitioner proceeds through the disciplinary process or is dealt with on the basis of their

health. Determinations are made on a case-by-case basis and are very much dependent on the nature of the conduct of the individual practitioner.

DISCIPLINARY PROCESS

Once a National Board receives a notification in relation to a registered health practitioner or student, the board must conduct a preliminary assessment within 60 days of receiving the notification.[41] When the nature of a notification is such that it would provide the basis for a complaint to a state or territory health complaints entity the National Board is obliged to inform the entity of the notification.[42] There is also a reciprocal obligation imposed on the state/territory-based health complaints entities to notify the relevant National Board of complaints lodged with the entity about a health practitioner.[43]

The National Board may pursue the following actions after assessing the notification:

- *Take no further action.*[44]
- *Take immediate action*[45] if the National Board reasonably believes the conduct, performance or health of the practitioner or student 'poses a serious risk to persons' and the response of immediate action is necessary to protect public health or safety. The National Board may also take immediate action in circumstances where the registration of the health practitioner was improperly obtained or the registration of the practitioner or student in another jurisdiction (not participating under the National Scheme) has been cancelled or suspended.[46]
- *Conduct an investigation* of a registered health practitioner or student if the National Board decides it is 'necessary and appropriate'.[47] After considering the resulting investigation report the National Board may decide to take no further action, take action it considers necessary or appropriate and/or refer the matter to another entity such as a health complaints commission in the relevant state/territory.
- *Require the registered health practitioner or student to undergo a health assessment* when the National Board reasonably believes the registrant has, or may have, an impairment.[48] After considering the resulting assessor's report the National Board may

decide to take no further action, take action it considers necessary or appropriate and/or refer the matter to another entity.

- *Require the registered health practitioner to undergo a performance assessment* when the National Board reasonably believes that the way the registered practitioner practises the profession is, or may be, unsatisfactory.[49] After considering the resulting assessor's report the National Board may decide to take no further action, take action it considers necessary or appropriate and/or refer the matter to another entity.
- *Take relevant action*[50] when the National Board determines the matter does not require referral to a responsible tribunal or panel. The 'relevant action' may include issuing a caution, accepting an undertaking or imposing a condition on the practitioner's or student's registration. The National Board may also refer the matter to another entity.
- *Establish a health panel*[51] when the National Board reasonably believes the registered practitioner or student has, or may have, an impairment and it is necessary and appropriate to refer the matter to a panel.
- *Establish a performance and professional standards panel*[52] if the National Board reasonably believes the way the registered health practitioner practises is, or may be, unsatisfactory or their professional conduct is, or may be, unsatisfactory and it is necessary and appropriate to refer the matter to a panel.
- *Refer the matter to a responsible tribunal*[53] in one of the participating states/territories. A board referral must take place when the board reasonably believes the registered practitioner behaved in a way that constitutes professional misconduct or has improperly obtained their registration by providing the board with documents or other information that were false or misleading. A matter involving a registered practitioner or student must also be referred to a responsible tribunal if recommended by a panel established by the board.

Decisions by Responsible Tribunals

A responsible tribunal may make a finding that the practitioner: has no case to answer; behaved in a way

that constitutes unsatisfactory professional performance, unprofessional conduct or professional misconduct; has an impairment and/or improperly obtained their registration by giving the National Board (for the particular health profession) documents or information that were false or misleading. The responsible tribunal may then do any one or more of the following under the National Law:

- issue a caution or reprimand
- impose a condition on the practitioner's registration, including a review period for that condition
- require the practitioner to pay a fine of not more than $30,000 to the particular National Board
- suspend the practitioner's registration for a specified period
- cancel the practitioner's registration.[54]

If the responsible tribunal determines that a student has an impairment the tribunal may either impose a condition on the student's registration or suspend their registration.[55]

New South Wales

In New South Wales the provisions of the National Law addressing health, performance and conduct have not been adopted. In that state, most National Boards have health practitioner councils that act in co-regulation with the HCCC regarding the handling of complaints about registered health practitioners. All complaints about health practitioners and health organisations are notified to the HCCC (including those made to a registration board or council). Mandatory notifications continue to be reported to AHPRA but are seen as complaints in New South Wales and are therefore automatically referred to the HCCC.[56]

A person is competent to practise as a health practitioner in New South Wales only if they have 'sufficient physical capacity, mental capacity, knowledge and skill to practise the profession' and have 'sufficient communication skills for the practice of the profession, including an adequate command of the English language'.[57] The National Law (NSW) provides different definitions of 'unsatisfactory professional conduct',[58] and 'professional misconduct'.[59] It is of note that additional matters may also constitute unsatisfactory professional conduct for medical practitioners[60] and pharmacists.[61] The grounds for a complaint about a registered practitioner are set out in section 144 of the National Law (NSW) and include that the practitioner:

- has, either in New South Wales or elsewhere, been convicted or made the subject of a criminal finding
- has been guilty of unsatisfactory professional conduct or professional misconduct
- is not competent to practise their profession
- has an impairment
- is otherwise not a suitable person to hold registration in the profession.

In relation to a student of a health profession, a complaint may be made if the student has been charged with an offence or been convicted of or made the subject of a criminal finding for an offence that is punishable by 12 months' imprisonment or more, whether this occurred in New South Wales or elsewhere. Complaints may also be made about an impairment, about the student contravening a condition of their registration or about an undertaking given by the student to the National Board.[62]

Complaints about registered health practitioners or students may be made to the council for the particular health profession[63] or to the HCCC.

The responses available to a council on receiving a complaint are prescribed by the National Law (NSW) and include making appropriate enquiries or referring the complaint to the tribunal (for the most serious matters), a committee (for less serious matters), the HCCC or another entity (including the National Board). Except for practitioners or students registered in the professions of medicine or nursing and midwifery, the respective council for the health profession is empowered to deal with a complaint by referring the student or practitioner for a health assessment, referring the student or practitioner to the Impaired Registrants Panel or to attend counselling.[64] A complaint about the professional performance of a practitioner may also be referred for a health assessment.[65]

On receiving a complaint about a health practitioner or student, the HCCC may decide to either:

- take no further action
- refer the complaint to the council for the health profession or the National Board
- refer the complaint for conciliation, or
- take any other action under the *Health Care Complaints Act 1993* (NSW).

When a complaint is proved against, or admitted by, the registered practitioner or student the Professional Standards Committee and the tribunal have the power to issue a caution and/or reprimand, impose conditions, order the individual to undergo medical, psychiatric treatment or counselling, complete educational courses, provide reports on the practitioner's practice, seek and take advice in relation to the management of the practitioner's practice, impose a fine, or recommend suspension or cancellation of their registration.

Queensland

In August 2013 the Queensland Government passed the *Health Ombudsman Act 2013* (Qld). This Act makes Queensland a co-regulatory jurisdiction for the purpose of dealing with complaints about regulated health practitioners practising in Queensland. The full implementation of the legislation occurred in mid-2014 with the establishment of the Office of the Health Ombudsman.

The role of AHPRA and the National Boards in relation to registering practitioners and students and accrediting programs of study and education remains unchanged under the provisions of the National Law. However, the Health Ombudsman Act amended the operation of the National Law in Queensland so the Health Ombudsman now manages all healthcare service complaints. The state thereby 'opted out' of the health, performance and conduct processes set out in Part 8 of the National Law.

The powers of AHPRA and the National Boards are restricted to dealing only with disciplinary matters referred to the agency by the Health Ombudsman. The matters to be referred can only be minor, less serious matters, with the Health Ombudsman Act expressly excluding the referral of complaints alleging 'professional misconduct' and 'serious matters'.

When AHPRA and the National Boards receive a notification (a complaint under the Health Ombudsman Act) involving professional misconduct or one based on allegations that would constitute grounds for suspension or cancellation of the practitioner's registration, the complaint must be referred to the Health Ombudsman 'as soon as practicable'. The Act is very broad in what constitutes providing a 'health service'.[66]

Consistent with the broad definition of a 'health service' are the extensive powers of the Health Ombudsman to deal with healthcare service providers who are defined under section 8 to include entities such as healthcare service organisations, individual registered health practitioners and persons who are unregistered or unregulated providers of healthcare services. The Health Ombudsman therefore, unlike AHPRA and the National Boards, has the power to deal with complaints made in relation to the conduct or practices of unregulated health practitioners and workers such as dietitians, assistants in nursing and personal care attendants.

Under Queensland's Health Ombudsman Act the reporting of 'notifiable conduct', as defined under the National Law, is to be directed to the Health Ombudsman rather than AHPRA. In addition, Part 23 of the Act removes the mandatory obligation to report 'notifiable conduct' in circumstances in which the health practitioner who is treating another health practitioner, or student of a health profession, 'forms the reasonable belief as a result of providing a health service' that the practitioner's or student's notifiable conduct '(i) relates to an impairment which will not place the public at substantial risk of harm, and (ii) is not professional misconduct'.

Disciplinary Tribunal Processes

In all Australian jurisdictions the disciplinary process is complaints-driven. The specific processing of a complaint through the National Scheme, or the New South Wales or Queensland structures is set out in the respective regulatory legislation. Under these systems the standard of proof required for findings is the civil standard; that is, the allegations must be made out on 'the balance of probabilities'. The 'clarity' of the proof required to discharge the burden must reflect the seriousness of the charge. Under the National Scheme and the New South Wales structure certain complaints about health practitioners are simultaneously referred to the relevant state complaints units or commissions, which attempt to resolve complaints. All disciplinary tribunals are bound by the requirement of recognising the right to natural justice. They are, as a general rule, not bound by the rules of practice about evidence and may inform themselves on any matter as the committee or tribunal considers appropriate.

HEALTH PRACTITIONERS NOT REGULATED BY THE NATIONAL SCHEME

While the National Scheme regulates 15 health professions, there are other health professions that are not regulated by the National Law. In such instances, they may be governed via a combination of professional self-regulation and state-based codes accompanied by healthcare complaints systems.

Self-Regulation

An example of a health profession that stipulates self-regulatory requirements is speech pathology. Speech Pathology Australia requires an accredited Australian entry-level speech pathology qualification or for the person to have successfully completed an Overseas Qualification Assessment with Speech Pathology Australia within the previous two years. Practitioners also need to meet the requirements for speech pathology practice hours and to fulfil the Professional Self-Regulation requirements to earn Certified Practising Speech Pathologist (CPSP) status. CPSP is necessary for Medicare and private health fund provider number applications.

Similarly, while professional nutritional practice is not regulated by the government and there is no legal protection over the terms 'nutritionist' or 'dietitian', the Nutrition Society of Australia, Dietitians Association of Australia (DAA) and Sports Dietitians Australia have developed credentialling systems for nutrition professionals. For example, the DAA has developed a credentialling system for the title Accredited Practising Dietitian, which is protected by law. The credential allows only qualified practitioners who have met certain requirements to use the title and requires that a tertiary-level course accredited by the DAA is completed. The title is recognised by the Australian Government, Medicare, the Department of Veterans' Affairs and most private health funds as the quality standard for nutrition and dietetic services in Australia.

Codes of Conduct

Some states have also implemented codes of conduct for 'unregistered health practitioners' and some have code-regulation regimes. For example, New South Wales' code commenced in 2008, South Australia's in 2013 and Queensland's in 2014. Acting contrary to the code can lead to complaints and disciplinary proceedings.

Work on a national code of conduct began in 2011 when the then Victorian Department of Health, on behalf of the Australian Health Ministers' Advisory Council, undertook a national public consultation on options for regulating unregistered health practitioners across the states and territories. In June 2013 health ministers agreed in principle to strengthen state and territory health complaints mechanisms via:

- a single national code of conduct for unregistered health practitioners to be made by regulation in each state and territory, and statutory powers to enforce the national code
- investigating breaches and issuing prohibition orders where a health practitioner's continued practice presents a serious risk to public health and safety
- a nationally accessible web-based register of prohibition orders
- mutual recognition of prohibition orders across all states and territories.

Following further consultation, the *National Code of Conduct* was agreed upon and is now active.

The purpose of the *National Code of Conduct* is to protect the public by setting minimum national standards of conduct and practice for all unregistered health practitioners who provide a healthcare service. As a code-regulation regime it provides:

- 'a "negative licensing" regulatory regime that does not restrict entry to practice, but allows effective action to be taken against an unregistered health care worker who fails to comply with proper standards of conduct or practice
- a set of objective and clear standards (a code of conduct) against which to assess a health care worker's conduct and practice in the event of a complaint or serious adverse event
- an independent investigator to receive and investigate complaints about breach of the National Code
- power for the independent investigator (or a tribunal) to issue prohibition orders and give public warnings about health care workers who

have failed to abide by the required standards of conduct and practice, and
- offence provisions for any person who breaches a prohibition order to be prosecuted through the appropriate court.'[67]

The National Code includes the following main clauses (further detail is set out in sub-clauses):

Clause 1: Health care workers to provide services in a safe and ethical manner
Clause 2: Health care workers to obtain consent
Clause 3: Appropriate conduct in relation to treatment advice
Clause 4: Health care workers to report concerns about treatment or care provided by other health care workers
Clause 5: Health care workers to take appropriate action in response to adverse events
Clause 6: Health care workers to adopt standard precautions for infection control
Clause 7: Health care workers diagnosed with infectious medical conditions
Clause 8: Health care workers not to make claims to cure certain serious illnesses
Clause 9: Health care workers not to misinform their clients
Clause 10: Health care workers not to practise under the influence of alcohol or drugs
Clause 11: Health care workers with certain mental or physical impairment
Clause 12: Health care workers not to financially exploit clients
Clause 13: Health care workers not to engage in sexual misconduct
Clause 14: Health care workers to comply with relevant privacy laws
Clause 15: Health care workers to keep appropriate records
Clause 16: Health care workers to be covered by appropriate insurance
Clause 17: Health care workers to display code and other information.

Who Does the National Code of Conduct Apply To?

The National Code, once enacted in a state or territory, applies to any person who provides a healthcare service and is not subject to regulation under the National Scheme. In some circumstances it also applies to health practitioners registered under the National Scheme, to the extent that they provide services that are unrelated to or outside the typical scope of practice of their registration; for example, a physiotherapist practising reiki or a general practitioner calling him/herself a 'skin cancer specialist' (which is not a protected title and not regulated as a specialty field by the Medical Board). While each state and territory's statute will identify who is subject to the National Code, health occupations likely to be captured will include (but are not limited to):

- Allied health assistants
- Art therapists
- Aromatherapists
- Assistants in nursing
- Audiologists and audiometrists
- Ayuvedic medicine practitioners
- Bioresonance practitioners
- Cardiac scientists
- Clinical perfusionists
- Complementary and alternative medicine practitioners
- Counsellors and psychotherapists
- Dental technicians
- Dental assistants
- Dietitians
- Herbalists
- Homoeopaths
- Hypnotherapists
- Lactation consultants
- Massage therapists
- Medical scientists
- Music, dance and drama therapists
- Myotherapists
- Naturopaths
- Nutritionists
- Optical dispensers
- Orthoptists
- Orthotists and prosthetists
- Pharmacy assistants
- Phlebotomists
- Reflexologists
- Reiki practitioners
- Respiratory scientists
- Shiatsu therapists
- Sleep technologists
- Social workers
- Sonographers
- Speech pathologists

Each state and territory determines the body or bodies responsible for receiving and investigating complaints about a possible breach of the *National Code of Conduct*. In most cases, this will be the state or territory's health complaints entity. For example, the *National Code of Conduct for Health Care Workers* has been adopted in Queensland and applies to health practitioners delivering a healthcare service in Queensland from 1 October 2015. The Queensland Health Ombudsman is responsible for receiving complaints. Victoria adopted the *National Code of Conduct* into its 2016 *Health Care Complaints Act 2016* (Vic), Schedule 2. Its Health Complaints Commissioner is responsible for receiving complaints under that regime.

FURTHER READING

Australian Health Practitioner Regulation Agency. Regulating Australia's health practitioners in partnership with the National Boards. https://www.ahpra.gov.au. Accessed 3 January 2018.

Forrester K. A new beginning for health complaints in Queensland: the Health Ombudsman Act 2013 (Qld). *J Law Med.* 2013;21: 271.

Grace S. CAM practitioners in the Australian health workforce: an underutilized workforce. *BMC Complement Altern Med.* 2012;12:205–29.

Hewitt J. Is whistleblowing now mandatory? The impact of mandatory reporting law on trust relationships in health care. *J Law Med.* 2013;21:82.

Kiel H. Regulating impaired doctors: a snapshot from New South Wales. *J Law Med.* 2013;21:429.

Weir M. *Law and Ethics in Complementary Medicine.* 4th ed. Sydney, NSW: Allen and Unwin; 2011.

ENDNOTES

1. *Health Practitioner Regulation National Law 2009* (Qld) ('National Law').
2. For the purposes of the discussion regarding the National Scheme and National Law, reference is here made to the provisions of Queensland law. Practitioners (and their legal representatives) should refer to the relevant law in their own state or territory.
3. Australian Health Practitioner Regulation Agency. What do we do? https://www.ahpra.gov.au/about-ahpra/what-we-do.aspx. Accessed 31 August 2018.
4. The Ministerial Council comprises the ministers of the governments of the participating jurisdictions and the Commonwealth with portfolio responsibility for health; it is also advised by the Australian Health Workforce Advisory Council, which is also established under the National Law.
5. National Law s 28.
6. Ibid. s 31.
7. Ibid. s 35(1)(q).
8. Ibid. s 36(1).
9. The registration standards developed by the National Boards must be approved by the Ministerial Council before they come into effect.
10. National Law ss 52, 53.

11. National Law ss 57, 58. See also Australia Health Practitioner Regulation Agency. Specialist Registration. https://www.ahpra.gov.au/Registration/Registration-Process/Specialist-Registration.aspx. Accessed 3 January 2018.
12. National Law ss 65–70.
13. Ibid. s 72.
14. Ibid. s 67.
15. Ibid. s 68.
16. Ibid. ss 62, 63.
17. Ibid. ss 73–76.
18. Ibid. s 5.
19. Student registration may also be required when a student, though not enrolled in an approved program of study, commences clinical training in a health profession. Students not enrolled in an approved program of study but included on the AHPRA Student Register at the commencement of clinical training will also cease to be registered at the completion of that clinical training.
20. National Law s 38.
21. For example: Aboriginal and Torres Strait Islander Health Practice Board, Chinese Medicine Board of Australia, Chiropractic Board of Australia, Dental Board of Australia, Medical Board of Australia and the Nursing and Midwifery Board of Australia.
22. Australian Health Practitioner Regulation Agency. English Language Skills. https://www.ahpra.gov.au/Registration/Registration-Standards/English-language-skills.aspx. Accessed 24 October 2018.
23. Ibid.
24. Aboriginal and Torres Strait Islander Health Practice Board of Australia. English Language Skills Registration Standard. http://www.atsihealthpracticeboard.gov.au/Registration-Standards/english-language-skills-reg-standard.aspx. Accessed 3 January 2018.
25. National Law s 129.
26. National Boards, Mandatory Reporting Guidelines. http://www.medicalboard.gov.au/Codes-Guidelines-Policies/Guidelines-for-mandatory-notifications.aspx. Accessed 3 January 2018.
27. National Law ss 237(3)(a), (b).
28. Medical Board of Australia. Guidelines for Mandatory Notifications. https://www.medicalboard.gov.au/codes-guidelines-policies/guidelines-for-mandatory-notifications.aspx. Accessed 3 January 2018.
29. Australia Health Practitioner Regulation Agency. Guidelines for Advertising Regulated Health Services. http://www.ahpra.gov.au/Publications/Advertising-resources/Legislation-guidelines/Advertising-guidelines.aspx. Accessed 3 January 2018.
30. National Law s 133.
31. Australian Health Practitioner Regulation Agency. Further Information on Advertising and the National Law. https://www.ahpra.gov.au/Publications/Advertising-resources/Further-information.aspx. Accessed 3 January 2018.
32. Fair Trading (Australian Consumer Law) Act 1992 (ACT); Fair Trading Act 1987 (NSW); Consumer Affairs and Fair Trading Act (NT); Fair Trading Act 1989 (Qld); Fair Trading Act 1987 (SA); Consumer Affairs Act 1988 (Tas); Australian Consumer Law (Tasmania) Act 2010 (Tas); Australian Consumer Law and Fair Trading Act 2012 (Vic); Fair Trading Act 2010 (WA).
33. Medical Board of Australia. Codes, Guidelines and Policies. www.medicalboard.gov.au/Codes-Guidelines-Policies.aspx. Accessed 3 January 2018.
34. Australian Medical Association. AMA Code of Ethics. https://ama.com.au/ausmed/code-ethics-revised-and-updated. Accessed 3 January 2018.
35. World Medical Association. WMA International Code of Medical Ethics. https://www.wma.net/policies-post/wma-international-code-of-medical-ethics/. Accessed 3 January 2018.
36. See: Nursing and Midwifery Board of Australia. Professional Standards. http://www.nursingmidwiferyboard.gov.au/Codes-Guidelines-Statements/Professional-standards.aspxv. Accessed 3 January 2018.
37. Australian Psychological Society. The Psychology Code of Ethics. http://www.psychology.org.au/about/ethics/. Accessed 3 January 2018.
38. National Law s 5.
39. National Law s 5.
40. National Law s 5.
41. National Law s 149(1).
42. Ibid. s 150(1).
43. Ibid. s 150(s).
44. Ibid. s 151.
45. Ibid. s 155.
46. Ibid. s 156.
47. Ibid. s 160.
48. Ibid. s 169.
49. Ibid. s 170.
50. Ibid. s 178.
51. Ibid. s 181.
52. Ibid. s 182.
53. Ibid. s 193. In Queensland the referral is to the Health Ombudsman. In other states and territories it would be to the relevant tribunal.
54. Ibid. s 196(2).
55. Ibid. s 197.
56. New South Wales Government. The National Registration Scheme for Health Practitioners: The NSW Complaints System. https://www.hccc.nsw.gov.au/Information/Information-for-health-providers/National-Registration-Scheme. Accessed 3 January 2018.
57. Health Practitioner Registration (Adoption of National Law) Act 2009 (NSW) ss 6, 6A and 6C.
58. Ibid. s 139B.
59. Ibid. s 139E.
60. Ibid. s 139C.
61. Ibid. s 139D.
62. Ibid. s 144A.
63. Councils for the individual health professions are established under the Health Practitioner Regulation National Law (NSW) s 41B.
64. National Law (NSW) s 145B.
65. Ibid. s 145E.
66. Health Ombudsman Act (Qld) s 7.
67. Council of Australian Governments (COAG). Final Report: A National Code of Conduct for Health Care Workers. https://www.coaghealthcouncil.gov.au/NationalCodeOfConductForHealthCareWorkers. Accessed 10 March 2019.

REVIEW QUESTIONS AND ACTIVITIES

1. List the health professions that are currently regulated under the National Scheme and provide three examples of health practitioners who are not regulated under the National Scheme.

2. What are the objectives of registration and regulation of health practitioners?

3. What are the mandatory reporting obligations of registered practitioners, employers of registered practitioners and education providers in relation to health practitioners and students of a health profession in your jurisdiction?

4. Explain the difference between complaints based on health concerns and those based on concerns about professional conduct and performance.

5. Describe how professional codes of ethics and codes of conduct influence standards of practice.

6. Identify the possible outcomes of disciplinary proceedings against a registered practitioner and a registered student.

5

MANAGEMENT OF HEALTH INFORMATION

LEARNING OBJECTIVES

Upon completing this chapter you should be able to:

- identify factors relevant to establishing and maintaining accurate, objective and concise records
- describe the development of a national approach to implementing digital health records
- distinguish between and explain the concepts of privacy and confidentiality in relation to health information
- identify and describe legislation and policies that support access to personal and health information.

INTRODUCTION

Documenting healthcare service provision, whether in hard copy or electronically, is fundamental to the practice of all health practitioners. The content of a person's healthcare records (variously referred to as 'health care records', 'health information'[1] and 'health records'[2]) depends not only on the particular care and treatment the person received but also on the particular institution or healthcare facility that has created and maintained the documents. In general, healthcare records include such things as a person's identifying information, health status, social, familial and health history, particular conditions and illnesses, results of examinations and tests, diagnosis of conditions, assessments of the need for treatment, treatment prescribed, information provided and the results of treatment. The record may also include the medical, nursing and research notes held by hospitals and other healthcare institutions and notes written at the preadmission or post-discharge phases of care delivery.

ESTABLISHING AND MAINTAINING HEALTHCARE RECORDS

Healthcare records serve to facilitate optimal outcomes for people who seek and receive health care provided they are accurate and up to date. They also serve as a method of communication from one health practitioner, or group of health practitioners, to another. Healthcare records may also be used for research purposes, as educational tools and as documentary evidence in legal proceedings. Health practitioners therefore have both professional and ethical responsibilities to create and maintain accurate records in relation to treatment and care provided.

In a number of jurisdictions' laws, government policies and directives mandate the requirements and standards for documentation regarding health information.[3] Key factors in maintaining clear, concise, accurate and relevant healthcare records are noted as follows.

Written entries into a person's healthcare records should be in ink. Their documentation must be 'objective, devoid of pejorative comment and worthy of independent scrutiny'.[4] This requirement is significant not only in relation to the accurate transfer of information between health practitioners but also to legal proceedings. The comments written by a health practitioner may be used as evidence regarding an allegation of negligence, malpractice or the degree of damage and disability sustained by the person they have provide healthcare services to.

Each page of a person's healthcare record must, at a minimum, identify the person by name and numerical identifier. Health practitioners must familiarise themselves with the particular policies of the employing institution about format and other inclusions. The report writer should also be clearly identified by their signature and designated position. If a student makes an entry it must be co-signed by the student's supervising clinician or the health practitioner in the clinical unit who designated the tasks to the student.

All entries must be prefaced with the complete date and time of the entry. The use of military time is most effective as a means of distinguishing whether the entry was in the 'am' or the 'pm'. Documentation of information concerning the person seeking or receiving health care should be contemporaneous with the event and recorded in chronological order. A contemporaneous recording of an event ensures greater accuracy and is more likely to be interpreted by the court as the true version.

The information must be legible and in English. There is little value in maintaining records that cannot be read or understood by others, and risks to care and safety may ensue. In legal proceedings it is imperative that documentation can be read by the court. In addition, for the purpose of the private health funds and the national health insurer the writing on the documentation must be legible for reimbursement of fees for service.[5]

The frequency of recording information in a person's healthcare file is also important. An institution or healthcare facility may have guidelines or protocols stipulating when records are to be updated or this may be left to the discretion of the particular health practitioner. As a valuable part of the total care, adequate time should be set aside to undertake the task. Even routine observations and assessments undertaken on a person must be recorded. If a person's health condition becomes unstable or deteriorates it would be necessary to carry out and document observations more frequently. When there is no entry to record observations or a change in the person's condition, the court may infer that no observations have been undertaken or that there has been an intentional omission.[6]

If a health practitioner wishes to make an addition to the records, it is acceptable to do so by clearly indicating that the addition or amendment was made. For example, the health practitioner may write the date and time and the words 'Addendum' or 'Written in retrospect' and then follow with the person's health information.

It is not acceptable to add or alter information to a healthcare record once a health practitioner becomes aware litigation has been initiated. In institutions or practices where the healthcare records are computerised there is often an 'audit trail' that will identify when the entry is made. The inclusion of forensic document experts in the pre-trial stage also increases the chances of additions and alterations to the notes regarding a person's health care being detected. A finding that a medical record has been altered will have a detrimental effect on the testimony of a health practitioner.

When an error is made in the recording of information, the policy or protocol of the health facility should be followed. The usual procedure will require that the health practitioner draws a line through the erroneous material, identifies it as having been written in error, and then dates and initials it. Errors should never be torn out, removed, erased or covered over with correction fluid. The reason for this is the possibility of inferring that the health practitioner has made an error in the treatment of the person who has received the healthcare service that they now wish to conceal.

Health practitioners should write only what they themselves have witnessed or assessed and avoid documenting information that is passed on to them by others. Each report should be an accurate record of what the person signing the entry knows to be true. If they have not directly witnessed the event, the information is hearsay evidence. If the person who received the healthcare service relates an incident that has occurred without a witness, then the records should clearly reflect that it is the person's version of the event that has been recorded. As an example, the report would state that, 'Mr Black said that he fell in the shower …' or 'Mrs Smith is complaining that her pain is becoming more severe …'.

When documenting the care or treatment of a person who is receiving a healthcare service, words such as 'appears' and 'apparently' should be avoided. As an example, the description of a person as 'appears to be drunk' does not provide objective or factual information of the person's status. It would be appropriate and preferable to write an accurate, specific and factual description of the physical condition of the person who is receiving the healthcare service such as, 'Mr X's speech was slurred and he was walking with an irregular gait'. A conclusion based on examination or next steps should also be recorded; for example, 'Mr X may have sustained a head injury and was referred for MRI'.

The records should include:

- the person's relevant health, social and familial history
- findings from any preliminary examinations
- the results of any tests performed on the person
- notes regarding discussion of possible diagnoses and a proposed management plan, including any proposed procedures or treatment options
- a record of any consent given by the person who is to receive the treatment or undergo the procedure (whether verbal or written) or, in the contrary, a record of the person's refusal to consent, undertake tests or comply with treatment
- details of any medication prescribed including the drug name, quantities, frequency of dosage, date prescribed and any repeat prescriptions
- notes regarding any further conversations or consultations (including, for example, follow-up telephone conversations, home visits, consultations in the health practitioner's office, conversations at other locations such as a hospital)
- details of any clinical opinion reached by the health practitioner.

The use of abbreviations and symbols must conform to the particular institution's policy or protocol. There is a great danger in using abbreviations that are not commonly known and understood by other health practitioners. Accurate medical terminology should be used whenever appropriate. Health practitioners must be mindful that when recording information in electronic form, the computer may have predictive text that auto-corrects technical terminology; it is important to check what has been entered.

Health practitioners must always read the healthcare records. While most hospital and healthcare facilities provide for a verbal handover (either in person or via recordings) at the change of shift, this is, by its very nature, only a summary of the events that have taken place over the preceding shift and should be treated as complementary to the written report. There is always the possibility that the professional giving the verbal handover has forgotten information or failed to recognise the significance of information that became available during the shift. As a result, information that may be critical to the person's health care and treatment will be missed.

COMPUTERISED RECORDS AND ELECTRONIC HEALTH

Hospital and healthcare facilities are increasingly adopting computerised charting and record keeping. Using information systems to create and maintain healthcare records has resulted in more accurate, easily accessed and up-to-date information on each person who seeks or is provided health care. It is proposed that the 'advantages of electronic record systems is that they allow complete, automatic and integrated entry of clinical and pathological data, rapid access to the system, users at multiple sites, and the transferring of patient information from site to site'.[7] Electronic records may also facilitate the ability of people to manage their own health care.

Technology provides obvious advantages to health practitioners in being able to efficiently access accurate, complete and up-to-date information, which may be essential to the speed with which a person is able to be treated. However, there are issues of concern when using computer technology for documenting healthcare information, including the potential threat to a person's privacy and the need to ensure that entries are checked for accuracy (and errors). Hospitals and healthcare facilities implementing electronic databases for recording and storing healthcare information need to have policies and protocols for protecting individual privacy and confidentiality regarding health information and to prevent unauthorised use. There should also be routine checking of data entry to ensure its accuracy.

National Strategy for Digital Health Records

In 2005 Commonwealth, state and territory governments committed to a national approach for recording, storing and using health information. This commitment was first implemented through establishing the National Electronic Health Transitional Authority (NEHTA), whose task it was to lead the uptake and coordination of progressing and adopting an electronic health (e-health) records system across Australia. A health identifier system was also established, in which each individual, healthcare providers and organisations that provide healthcare services are given a unique identifier aimed to ensure the right health information is associated with the right individual at the point of care.[8]

However, following a 2014 review that found little uptake of e-health, work on how to progress the government's commitment to e-health records was undertaken. On 1 July 2016 NEHTA was superseded by the Australian Digital Health Agency (ADHA).

The ADHA is currently responsible for all national digital health services and systems. Following extensive public consultation, the ADHA released *A National Digital Health Strategy* for 2018–2022, emphasising seven key strategic priority areas:

1. health information that is available whenever and wherever it is needed
2. health information that can be exchanged securely
3. high-quality data with a commonly understood meaning that can be used with confidence
4. better availability and access to prescriptions and medicines information
5. digitally-enabled models of care that improve accessibility, quality, safety and efficiency
6. a workforce confidently using digital health technologies to deliver health and care
7. a thriving digital health industry delivering world-class innovation.[9]

In 2017 the Australian Government also announced that a 'My Health Record' for every Australian would begin nationally from mid-2018. The My Health Record system is regulated via a variety of legislation, regulations and rules.[10] By law, a review of the legislation is required every three years.

The aim of the My Health Record system is to achieve a system in which healthcare providers are able to see important health information from anywhere, at any time, thus being able to better provide treatment and care to people. A My Health Record may contain information about prescribed medicines, Medicare claims history, organ donation preferences, hospital discharge, diagnostic imaging (e.g. ultrasound or x-ray results) and pathology (e.g. blood tests). An individual can also add information such as any allergies and adverse reactions and advance care planning information concerning wishes they have about their health care in the event they become too unwell to communicate.

Concerns about the My Health Record system have nevertheless been raised, in particular regarding the need for strong privacy, security and risk management to protect sensitive information. There has also been concern raised over who will be able to see such records and how they may be used. In addition, health practitioners need to understand how to use digital tools in a way that safely handles personal information, and consumers need to be educated about their privacy rights to make informed choices regarding how their health information is used.[11] There is ongoing work by the ADHA regarding how to address these issues.

Under the regime (at the time of writing), a person who has a My Health Record who decides they no longer want one can cancel it at any time. The information in the record, including any backups, will be permanently deleted from the system. A person who has cancelled their My Health Record can re-register, which will result in a new record.

PRIVACY AND CONFIDENTIALITY OF HEALTH INFORMATION

Whether information is conveyed orally, recorded electronically or written in a person's file, it is fundamental when considering the exchange or recording of health information to also consider concepts of privacy and confidentiality. Such concepts are often used interchangeably, but it should be remembered that 'confidentiality' and 'privacy' represent slightly different legal concepts.

Confidentiality

Confidentiality protects information given in confidence. It relates to the non-disclosure of *all* information that comes to a health practitioner during their relationship with a person who seeks or receives healthcare services, in whatever form. Confidentiality is important in establishing and maintaining a relationship of trust between health practitioners and people seeking healthcare services, which allows for disclosure of sensitive information that otherwise may not occur. In addition, it may be seen to respect a person's rights as an autonomous recipient of healthcare services, which includes having control over their own information and their ability to make decisions and disseminate their information at their own discretion.

The duty to maintain the confidentiality of all information obtained in the course of providing health care applies to people of any age. It is owed by the health practitioner and any staff coming into contact with the information as part of the healthcare process (e.g. administrative staff). It means that information cannot generally be released to others without the person's permission or, when incompetent, the permission of the person's substitute decision-maker (e.g. their legal guardian). In this regard, it is important to remember that health practitioners are under a strict ethical and legal duty to keep information about the people they see confidential unless the law permits disclosure. Confidentiality may be protected in equity, by the common law, via professional regulation and via statute.

Breach of Confidence

An equitable duty of confidentiality arises where three conditions are satisfied:

1. the information 'must have the necessary quality of confidence about it'
2. the information 'must have been imparted in circumstances importing an obligation of confidence'
3. 'there must be an unauthorised use of that information to the detriment of the party'.[12]

It has been accepted that information of a personal and intimate nature would satisfy the necessary quality of confidence, and that the relationship between the health practitioner and the person seeking or receiving health care constitutes a circumstance importing an obligation of confidentiality.[13] In *Breen v Williams*, Brennan CJ said, 'Equity might restrain [the doctor] from disclosing without authority any information about [the patient] and her medical condition …'.[14]

However, whether the requirement of a 'detriment' in an equitable action for breach of confidence would be satisfied if the breach did not result in an economic loss is of issue. While it has been suggested that in cases involving medical confidentiality the 'mere disclosure and its immediate consequences' is sufficient to warrant injunctive relief,[15] whether a person could recover compensation for emotional distress related to the

disclosure of health information has not been tested in an Australian court of law.[16]

Common Law Negligence

At common law if confidential information was released in a way that fell below the standard of care expected of a health practitioner, arguably a cause of action in negligence may be available. However, again, a cause of action in negligence requires that the plaintiff suffers legally compensable loss or harm. The requirement at law in this regard is that a recognised psychological injury, rather than mere sadness, embarrassment or distress resulting from the breach, or physical or economic harm, would have to occur before compensation may be awarded.

Professional Codes of Conduct and Regulation

Most often a breach of confidentiality would be dealt with under disciplinary action relevant to the registration and/or practice of a health profession. The obligation to keep information confidential is also incorporated into the codes of ethics and codes of conduct adopted by health practitioners of all disciplines. For example, the International Council of Nurses' *The ICN Code of Ethics for Nurses* provides that: 'The nurse holds in confidence personal information and uses judgement in sharing this information'.[17]

Statute

Some statutory provisions also protect confidentiality. For example, many mental health Acts protect confidentiality via what are known as 'secrecy' provisions.[18] Such provisions prevent disclosure of mental health information obtained by any reason of any function a person has, or at any time had, in the administration of the relevant mental health legislation.

Breach of confidence in this regard may again result in disciplinary proceedings under the health practitioner's regulatory statute and/or a fine where there is a contravention of a statutory duty of confidence.

The duty of confidentiality does not cease when the therapeutic relationship ends or when the client dies.

Limits of the Obligation of Confidentiality

Not all information received when providing healthcare services is confidential. For example, information that is trivial can be exempt from the duty of confidentiality.

Confidential information may also be disclosed following:

- *express or implied consent* (e.g. consent to share information may be implied when other health practitioners within the same health facility have a legitimate therapeutic interest in the care of the client)
- *pursuant to legal requirements* such as mandatory reporting regarding child abuse; certain infectious diseases; reporting cause of death; providing information pursuant to a subpoena, for example, midwives, medical practitioners and nurses are required by legislation in each jurisdiction to notify the Registrar of Births, Deaths and Marriages of any birth or death they attend; and the Coroner's Act in each state and territory imposes a legal obligation on various health practitioners to inform the coroner of any death that occurs in circumstances specified in the relevant legislation
- *on grounds of public interest* such as if there is a risk to national security and in cases of notifiable disease reporting (e.g. HIV, hepatitis C, gonorrhoea, syphilis, smallpox, typhoid, leprosy and cholera).

Privacy

At law, privacy is a separate concept to confidentiality, albeit complementary. Privacy is governed by Commonwealth and state/territory legislation, which has a much wider reach than the common law protection of confidentiality.

Commonwealth Privacy Legislation

The *Privacy Act 1988* (Cth) regulates the handling of personal information by Australian Government agencies (and the Norfolk Island Administration) as well as applying to all healthcare service providers in the private sector throughout Australia. It does not apply to state/territory public sector healthcare service providers such as public hospitals (noting the Commonwealth does not have power to regulate state/territory public agencies).

Personal information can include a wide variety of information and is not just limited to information relevant to providing healthcare services. However, pursuant to section 6 of the Privacy Act personal information includes the *collection*, *use* or *disclosure* of 'sensitive information', which includes health information.

Generally, health information should only be collected when the person about whom such information pertains has consented to its collection and when such collection is 'necessary' to provide a healthcare service. Further, only the minimum amount of information needed to provide a healthcare service should be collected.[19]

The Privacy Act includes a set of 13 Australian Privacy Principles (APPs), which guide what people handling private information must do in relation to personal information privacy, collecting personal information, dealing with personal information, maintaining the integrity of personal information and access to, or correction of, personal information. All health practitioners should be familiar with the APPs, including the *Australian Privacy Principle Guidelines* published by the Office of the Australian Information Commissioner.[20] The APPs are summarised below.

Consideration of Personal Information Privacy

APP 1: OPEN AND TRANSPARENT MANAGEMENT OF PERSONAL INFORMATION. An APP entity must have a clearly expressed and up-to-date policy about the management of personal information by the entity available for reference free of charge.

APP 2: ANONYMITY AND PSEUDONYMITY. Unless unreasonable or prohibited by law individuals must have the option of not identifying themselves, or using a pseudonym, when dealing with an APP entity.

Collection of Personal Information

APP 3: COLLECTION OF SOLICITED PERSONAL INFORMATION. An APP entity must not collect sensitive information about an individual unless the individual consents to the collection and the information is reasonably necessary for, or directly related to, one or more of the collecting agency/entity/organisation's functions or activities, and collection is authorised under an Australian law or a court/tribunal order and/or a permitted general or permitted health situation exists.

APP 4: DEALING WITH UNSOLICITED PERSONAL INFORMATION. Upon receiving personal information the entity did not solicit, the entity must within a reasonable time determine whether the information could have been collected pursuant to the APP. If not, the entity must destroy the information or ensure the information is de-identified.

APP 5: NOTIFICATION OF THE COLLECTION OF PERSONAL INFORMATION. An APP entity must at or before the time of collection or, if that is not practicable, as soon as practicable, take reasonable steps to inform the individual of the holder of the information why information is held and their entitlements.

Dealing With Personal Information

APP 6: USE OR DISCLOSURE OF PERSONAL INFORMATION. If an APP entity holds personal information about an individual that was collected for a particular purpose, the entity must not use or disclose the information for another purpose unless:

- the individual has consented to the use or disclosure
- the individual would reasonably expect the APP entity to use or disclose it for the secondary purpose and the secondary purpose is directly related to the primary purpose
- the use or disclosure is authorised by Australian law or a court/tribunal order
- a permitted general situation exists
- the APP entity is an organisation and a permitted health situation exists, or
- the APP entity reasonably believes that the use or disclosure is reasonably necessary for one or more enforcement-related activities conducted by, or on behalf of, an enforcement body.

APP 7: DIRECT MARKETING. An organisation must not use or disclose personal information for the purposes of direct marketing unless the subject has consented.

APP 8: CROSS-BORDER DISCLOSURE OF PERSONAL INFORMATION. Prior to disclosing personal information to a person in a foreign country or state, the entity must take reasonable steps to ensure the recipient does not breach the APP. (There are some exceptions listed to this within the Act.)

APP 9: ADOPTION, USE OR DISCLOSURE OF GOVERNMENT-RELATED IDENTIFIERS. APP 9 restricts the adoption, use and disclosure of government-related identifiers by organisations. It also applies to agencies in specific circumstances set out in section 7A of the Act.

Integrity of Personal Information

APP 10: QUALITY OF PERSONAL INFORMATION. An APP entity must take all reasonable steps to ensure personal information is accurate, up to date and complete.

APP 11: SECURITY OF PERSONAL INFORMATION. An APP entity must take all reasonable steps to protect information from misuse, interference and loss, as well as unauthorised access, modification or disclosure. If an entity holds information that is no longer required for the purpose it was collected, such information must be destroyed or the information de-identified.

Access to, and Correction of, Personal Information

APP 12: ACCESS TO PERSONAL INFORMATION. An APP entity must give an individual access on request to personal information related to them. There are a number of exceptions to this, which are further discussed in the section on access to information.

APP 13: CORRECTION OF PERSONAL INFORMATION. If an APP entity is satisfied personal information held is inaccurate, out of date, incomplete, irrelevant or misleading, or an individual makes a request for the entity to correct the personal information, the entity must take all reasonable steps to correct the information.

Exceptions to the Protection of Sensitive or Health Information

The protection of sensitive information or health information is not absolute. Sections 16A and 16B of the Privacy Act contain certain general and specific health situation exceptions respectively to the APPs.

Section 16A provides that the information-handling requirements regarding collecting sensitive information (APP 3), using or disclosing personal information (APPs 6 and 8) and using or disclosing a government-related identifier (APP 9) do not apply if a 'permitted general situation' exists. There are seven permitted general situations listed in section 16A:

- lessening or preventing a serious threat to the life, health or safety of any individual, or to public health or safety
- taking appropriate action in relation to suspected unlawful activity or serious misconduct
- locating a person reported as missing
- asserting a legal or equitable claim

- conducting an alternative dispute resolution process
- performing diplomatic or consular functions – this permitted general situation only applies to agencies
- conducting specified defence force activities (this permitted general situation only applies to the defence force).[21]

Therefore, for example, while APP 3 requires that a person consents to their health information being collected, section 16A would support collection without such consent if it is not reasonable or practical to obtain the individual's consent and the health practitioner reasonably believes the collection is necessary to lessen or prevent a serious threat to the life, health or safety of any individual or to the public.

Pursuant to section 16B, the information-handling requirements imposed by APP 3 and APP 6 do not apply to an organisation if a 'permitted health situation' exists. There are five 'permitted health situations' listed in section 16B regarding:

- collecting health information to provide a healthcare service[22]
- collecting health information for certain research and other purposes[23]
- using or disclosing health information for certain research and other purposes[24]
- using or disclosing genetic information to prevent a serious threat to the life, health or safety of a genetic relative[25]
- disclosing health information for a secondary purpose to a responsible person for an individual.[26]

Therefore, for example, while generally a health entity must not use or disclose private health information collected for a particular purpose for a secondary purpose, such information may be disclosed to prevent a serious threat to the life of a genetic relative.

Note, an organisation may comply with the APP requirements even though an exception applies.

Regarding *collection* of health information to provide a healthcare service, section 16B specifically provides that a permitted health situation exists if the information is necessary to provide a healthcare service to the individual and either:

- the collection is required or authorised under an Australian law, or

- the information is collected in accordance with rules established by competent health or medical bodies that deal with obligations of professional confidentiality that bind the organisation.

In addition, a permitted health situation exists if:

- it is necessary for the organisation to collect the family, social or medical history regarding a person to provide a healthcare service to them
- the health information about the third party is part of the family, social or medical history necessary for the organisation to provide the healthcare service
- the health information is collected by the organisation from the person or, if they are physically or legally incapable of giving the information, their lawful representative (such as a substitute decision-maker, next of kin or guardian).

State and Territory Health Privacy Legislation

Commonwealth privacy legislation does not govern state public agencies. Some states and territories therefore have privacy legislation that is relevant to public agencies. In some jurisdictions there is also legislation relevant to private sector health providers.

The Australian Capital Territory,[27] New South Wales[28] and Victoria[29] have specific *health* privacy legislation that governs public and private sector healthcare service providers. Private sector healthcare service providers in these jurisdictions must comply with *both* Commonwealth and state/territory privacy legislation when handling health information.[30]

The Northern Territory,[31] Tasmania[32] and Queensland[33] have privacy legislation that only applies to the public sector. In these jurisdictions private sector healthcare service providers must comply with Commonwealth legislation when handling health information.[34]

Neither South Australia nor Western Australia has specific privacy legislation; however, South Australia has administrative directions and codes that apply to public sector healthcare service providers and healthcare legislation that contains some privacy-related provisions. Private sector healthcare service providers in these jurisdictions must comply with Commonwealth legislation when handling health information. In South Australia they must also comply with relevant privacy provisions in the South Australian health legislation.[35]

COLLECTING HEALTH INFORMATION VIA A THIRD PARTY

Health practitioners must generally collect health information directly from the person about whom that information relates. However, sometimes health practitioners may collect personal and health information from a third party. This may include:

- when a person authorises collection from a third party
- when there is a reasonable belief that obtaining information from a third party is necessary to provide the service to the individual
- where it is necessary to prevent serious and imminent harm or to provide emergency care where the person is unable to respond
- to gather information about a person who is unable to understand or respond appropriately to questions or comprehend their significance and such information will aid their care
- when it is necessary for the conduct of proceedings before any court or tribunal or to comply with any applicable law.

Such information may, for example, be gathered via a relative or authorised representative. In emergency situations this might be quite common; for example, paramedics attending callouts or health staff in emergency departments might be faced with having to collect information from third parties. Healthcare service providers may also communicate health information about a person to each other – for example, when a general practitioner refers a person to a specialist or when a paramedic releases medical information to treating hospital staff so they may provide continuity of care. They may also collect information about people other than the person who is seeing them – for example, in the course of taking the family, social or medical history of a person.

In all cases, information collected from third parties about a person who requires treatment should be checked with that person as soon as practicable to ensure accurate information is held and is taken into account when considering diagnosis, treatment or advice. In addition, reasonable steps should be taken as soon as practicable to notify the person about: the organisation that collected the information; what the information will be used for; who the information is likely to be disclosed to; how the information will be stored; any law requiring the information to be collected; and their rights to access the information. These steps may include advice in person, in writing, over the phone or via documentation provided to the person about whom the information relates.

ACCESS TO HEALTH INFORMATION

While many people may believe their personal health records belong to them, at common law this has been held not to be the case. In *Breen v Williams*,[36] the High Court determined that ownership of healthcare records rested with the medical practitioner and that the patient's rights to access information contained within them was limited.[37] However, Commonwealth, state and territory legislation now provides for access to health information by the person about whom such information pertains.[38] Different legislation may apply depending on whether the information is held by a public or private sector organisation and the jurisdiction the information is in.

Commonwealth Legislation

Government Agencies

The *Freedom of Information Act 1982* (Cth) provides a legally enforceable right of access to documents held by ministers and federal government agencies, including any health-related information held by them, unless the information is exempt under the Act or subject to secrecy provisions found in other relevant Acts. From 1 November 2014 the Commonwealth Ombudsman has handled complaints about the processing of freedom of information requests.

Private Businesses

Pursuant to APP 12 in Schedule 1 of the Privacy Act, if an entity (agency, organisation, small business operator) holds personal information about a person, it must give access to that information at the person's request. There are, however, a number of exceptions to this including if the APP entity is an agency and is authorised to refuse access pursuant to a Commonwealth Act or, if the APP entity is an organisation, the entity reasonably believes providing access to that information:

- would pose a serious threat to the individual or public safety
- would have an unreasonable impact on the privacy of other individuals
- is frivolous or vexatious
- would not be accessible by discovery
- would reveal the intentions of the entity in relation to negotiations so as to prejudice those negotiations
- would be unlawful
- is unlawful because denying access is required or authorised by law or a court/tribunal order
- would prejudice the taking of appropriate action in relation to suspected unlawful activity or misconduct of a serious nature that relates to the entity's functions, or
- would prejudice an enforcement body's enforcement-related activities.

Healthcare services are able to charge a fee for accessing information, provided the fee is not excessive.

State and Territory Legislation

Access to records held in the state public sector are governed by respective state legislation. Access to private sector records is governed via state and Commonwealth legislation. It is important to note each state/territory's laws separately.

Australian Capital Territory

In the Australian Capital Territory health records are considered confidential documents and remain the property of the Government Health Directorate. Pursuant to the *Health Records (Privacy and Access) Act 1997* copies of health records will not be released to consumers or third parties without a written request and signed authorisation from the consumer. Fees apply to any such request.

Requests to access healthcare records are assessed under the Act, which contains a set of 'Privacy Principles' in Schedule 1 similar to the Commonwealth AAPs. Privacy Principle 5 requires a record keeper to provide information at the request of the person who the records are about concerning: the nature of the records or information; the main purposes for which the records are, or the information is, used; and the steps that the person should take if the person wishes to obtain access

to the records or the information. A record keeper is not required to give a person information if, under a law of the territory or a law of the Commonwealth, the record keeper is required or authorised to refuse to give that information to the person.

The Australian Capital Territory Human Rights Commission administers the legislation and handles privacy complaints regarding health information and records.

New South Wales

In New South Wales access to public and private sector healthcare records is governed under separate laws.

Access to information held by government organisations is governed by the:

- *Government Information (Information Commissioner) Act 2009*
- *Government Information (Public Access) Act 2009*
- Government Information (Public Access) Regulations 2009.

Pursuant to such legislation, all New South Wales government agencies, ministers (and their staff), local councils, state-owned corporations, courts (in their non-judicial functions) and certain public authorities (e.g. universities) are presumed to have an obligation to disclose or release information unless there is an overriding public interest against doing so.

Where information is held by private healthcare service providers, the *Health Records and Information Privacy Act 2002* (NSW) is relevant. Exemptions from having to release information apply under the Act such as if its release: might cause serious harm to life/ health; might impact on the privacy of others; relates to legal proceedings; is unlawful; or is a repeat request that has previously been reasonably denied. A fee may be applicable, but it should not be excessive. Information must be provided within 45 days of the initial request.

It is recommended that requests be put in writing. If a healthcare service provider refuses to release the information (and an exemption does not apply) a person has six months from becoming aware of the situation to make a complaint or to seek a review of the conduct. If it is a private healthcare service or organisation, complaints should be directed to the New South Wales Information and Privacy Commission. If it is a public healthcare service, the person must lodge an internal review directly to the relevant Local Health District.

Northern Territory

In the Northern Territory there is no distinct health information legislation. Rather the *Information Act* (NT) relates to information privacy generally and contains rules for applying to access or amend information held by public sector organisations, regardless of whether that information relates to health. A fee may be charged – for example, to copy documents or if the information is not just personal information – but the fee should not be excessive.

Freedom of information requests can be made directly to public sector organisations, and information will be released unless an exemption applies. An exemption may apply if, for example, releasing the information is against the public interest or if in the particular case the public interest considerations against disclosure outweigh the considerations favouring disclosure.

The Northern Territory Office of the Information Commissioner is the independent statutory body responsible for overseeing the Information Act.

Queensland

In Queensland, people have the right to access and amend personal and non-personal information held by public sector agencies pursuant to the *Right to Information Act 2009* (Qld) and by the Queensland Government pursuant to the *Information Privacy Act 2009* (Qld).

Public healthcare agencies are required to comply with Privacy Principles set out in the Information Privacy Act to:

- make people aware of what kind of personal information it holds and why (PP 5)
- tell people how they can get access to it (PP 6) (if a health agency has control of a document containing personal information it must give the person who is the subject of the information access to the document if they ask)
- tell people how they can seek to have personal information amended if they believe it is not accurate.

In addition to the legislative provisions of the abovementioned Acts, Queenslanders may request access

to their health information in accordance with the Department of Health's *Health Information: Disclosure and Access Policy*. The policy allows a person to make a request in writing to the Office of the Medical Superintendent of a public hospital or manager or director of a community health service for access to their health information. Making an application directly to a public hospital or community health service in accordance with the policy does not preclude an individual from making an application through the legislative regime.

The Queensland Office of the Information Commissioner receives complaints relevant to access to information and privacy pursuant to the Queensland Acts.

South Australia

South Australia's *Freedom of Information Act 1991* (SA) gives people the right to request access to documents held by state government agencies (including public hospitals and health units), government ministers, local councils and state universities. People may request that documents about themselves that are incomplete, incorrect, out of date or misleading are amended. People can also request a review of a decision made by a state government agency, government minister, local council or state university. Requests are made directly to the agency or body, which then has 30 days to reply.

Schedule 1 of the Freedom of Information Act also sets out certain exemptions in the case that releasing the information would (among other things): affect public safety or law enforcement; lead to unreasonable disclosure of another person's affairs; or breach parliamentary or legal privilege. Applications for an internal review of decisions can be made to any government agency from which information is requested.

The Freedom of Information Act does not apply to information held by private businesses, private doctors or health specialists, which is governed by the Commonwealth Privacy Act and APPs.

Tasmania

In Tasmania section 7 of the *Right to Information Act 2009* (Tas) provides for access to information in the possession of a public authority or a minister, provided that it is not exempt information. A fee may be charged in some circumstances but must not be excessive. The

Personal Information and Protection Act 2004 (Tas) is also relevant to access and amendment of personal information (including information that relates to health). The provisions of the Act include personal information protection principles that facilitate the correction and alteration of, and access to, personal information.

Section 3B of the Personal Information and Protection Act provides that a 'personal information custodian' may deny access to information when there are concerns about the medical or psychiatric nature of the information being 'prejudicial to the physical or mental health or wellbeing of that person' requesting their information. In such a circumstance the 'personal information custodian may direct that access to the information must not be provided to the person who made the request but must instead be provided to a medical practitioner nominated by that person'.

The Tasmanian Ombudsman is the review authority under the Right to Information Act and the Personal Information Protection Act; the Ombudsman may receive and investigate complaints in relation to those Acts.

Victoria

From 1 July 2002 section 25 and Health Privacy Principle 6 of the *Health Records Act 2001* (Vic) gave Victorians a right of access to personal health information held about them by any organisation in the Victorian private sector. If the information the person is seeking access to was collected by the organisation after 1 July 2002, then the organisation must give access in one of the following ways:

- inspecting the information
- getting a copy
- viewing the information, accompanied by an explanation by a healthcare service provider.

A fee may be charged, but legislation limits what is permitted.

Access to personal health information held by a Victorian Government department or public sector organisation (such as a public hospital) is governed by the *Freedom of Information Act 1982* (Vic). Freedom of information legislation gives people the right to request documents about personal affairs and the activities of government agencies. It also affords the right to request

that incorrect or misleading information held by an agency be amended or removed.

The Victorian Health Complaints Commissioner handles complaints about access to information, among other things.

Western Australia

The *Freedom of Information Act 1992* (WA) provides for access to, and correction of, documents held by state and local government agencies. People are encouraged to apply, in writing, directly to these agencies for information. A fee will apply. People can also apply to correct that information if it is incorrect, inaccurate, out of date or misleading.

The Freedom of Information Act is overseen by Western Australia's Office of the Information Commissioner, which deals with complaints regarding agency decisions about access applications and requests to amend personal information.

Like South Australia, the freedom of information legislation does not apply to private businesses, private doctors or health specialists who are covered by the Commonwealth Privacy Act and APPs.

GOVERNMENT POLICY

In addition to the state, territory and Commonwealth legislation, individual state health departments have developed policies and guidelines that generally recognise the right of people to access information held by the hospitals and healthcare institutions under their control.[39] Such policies emphasise the right of individuals to be self-determining consumers of healthcare services and the reciprocal right of those individuals to access the information necessary for their decision making.

Exceptions to access may (depending on specific state/territory policies) generally include situations where the application is for sensitive information – for example, where the content of the documents:

- relates to actual or suspected child abuse
- includes the deliberations of health teams dealing with suspected child abuse in relation to a particular person
- includes information in relation to testing and/ or treatment of HIV or AIDS

- includes the healthcare records of a deceased person
- includes information that is potentially prejudicial to the physical or mental health or wellbeing of a person
- includes health information that, if disclosed, may reasonably be expected to be of substantial concern to another agency
- reveals or potentially reveals a confidential source of information, or
- relates to scheduled drugs.

ACCESS PURSUANT TO THE COURT PROCESS

When healthcare records are required for litigation, the various state and Commonwealth evidence Acts and rules of court permit access to the documents. The records are obtained by subpoena or writ of non-party discovery. Where the documents have been subpoenaed, they must be produced.

STORAGE AND DISPOSAL OF HEALTHCARE RECORDS

Generally, healthcare records should be stored in a manner that: protects the confidentiality of the record; prevents damage, loss or theft of the record; and ensures that the record is reasonably accessible to allow for continuity of treatment and care. However, note that each state and territory has different requirements for retaining and storing healthcare records.

The Medical Practice Regulations 2003 (NSW) prescribe that records should be kept for at least seven years after a person's last contact with the healthcare provider or facility. In the case of a child (aged under 18 years) the records should be retained until the child reaches the age of 25 years.[40] The New South Wales Health Records and Information Privacy Act requires the practitioner to keep 'health information' for this length of time.[41]

The Victorian Health Records Act and the Australian Capital Territory Health Records (Privacy and Access) Act identify retention times similar to those in New South Wales.

The length of time healthcare records are retained in other jurisdictions may be determined by the health practitioner on a case-by-case basis.

Medical indemnity insurers state that, from a medicolegal perspective, healthcare records should be kept until such time as there is little or no risk of a claim arising from a person's treatment – this may depend on the statutory limitation period, any applicable state/ territory legislation governing the retention of healthcare records and/or whether there has been a complaint or an adverse outcome or legal proceedings have been foreshadowed. In the latter cases, it is recommended that healthcare records be kept indefinitely.[42]

Retiring or Closing a Practice

In most states and territories there are obligations imposed on health practitioners who are retiring or closing their practice. The obligations include informing the people to whom they have provided healthcare services of the impending retirement or closure including the name and address of the practitioner to whom the healthcare records will be transferred and/or providing an opportunity for people to collect their own records. The Victorian Health Services Commissioner has published guidelines for the closure or transfer of a medical practice;[43] in the Australian Capital Territory the Health Records (Privacy and Access) Act provides that on the transfer or closure of a practice the healthcare records can be transferred to the provider who takes over the practice, transferred to a record keeper for storage or to the patient or practitioner nominated by the patient. In Queensland the Australian Medical Association recommends patients be given six months' notice of an intention to close or transfer a practice.

Destroying Health Information and Records

Before destroying healthcare records, it is important to consider whether there is any reason to continue to store a person's records on the basis of their medical condition or history. For example, if the person has a genetic disorder or a chronic medical condition the records may be kept for the lifetime of the person and, in some circumstances, after their death.

The method of destroying healthcare records is determined by the healthcare facility or provider, with incineration, shredding or commercial removal and destruction being most frequently used. Whatever method is chosen it remains the legal obligation of the healthcare facility or provider to ensure confidentiality is retained until destruction is complete.

It is advisable to have a clear culling system and maintain a schedule of healthcare records that have been destroyed, noting that in Victoria and the Australian Capital Territory a *Schedule of Document Destruction* is required. This schedule contains the person's name, date of birth and date of destruction of their healthcare records. In other jurisdictions it is recommended that when health information is to be destroyed a written note is retained that includes the name of the individual to whom the information relates, the period covered by the health information and the date of deletion or destruction.

FURTHER READING

Hanna L, Gill SD, Newstead L, Hawkins M, Osborne RH. Patient perspectives on a personally controlled electronic health record used in regional Australia: 'I can be like my own doctor'. *Health Inf Manage*. 2016;46(1):42–48.

Keasberry J, Scott IA, Sullivan C, Staib A, Ashby R. Going digital: a narrative overview of the clinical and organisational impacts of eHealth technologies in hospital practice. *Aust Health Rev*. 2017;41:646–664.

Office of the Australian Information Commissioner. Privacy law. https://www.oaic.gov.au/privacy-law/. Accessed 9 March 2019.

ENDNOTES

1. *Health Records and Information Privacy Act 2002* (NSW); *Information Act 2002* (NT); *Personal Information Protection Act 2004* (Tas); *Health Records Act 2001* (Vic); *Information Privacy Act 2009* (Qld).
2. *Health Records (Privacy and Access) Act 1997* (ACT).
3. See, for example, New South Wales Department of Health. Policy Directive: Health Care Records – Documentation and Management. Document Number: PD 2012_069. 21 December 2012.
4. Dix A, Errington M, Nicholson K, Powe R. *Law for the Medical Profession in Australia*. Port Melbourne: Butterworth-Heinemann; 1996, p. 161.
5. McSherry M. Electronic health care records: perils of outsourcing and the *Privacy Act 1988* (Cth), *J Law Med*. 2004;12(1):8–13
6. *Strelec v Nelson*, unreported, 12401/90 13 December 1996.
7. Kerridge I, Lowe M, Stewart C. *Ethics and Law for the Health Professions*. 4th ed. Sydney: The Federation Press; 2013. p. 305.
8. *Healthcare Identifiers Act 2010* (Cth); Healthcare Identifiers Regulations 2010.
9. Australian Digital Health Agency. *Australia's National Digital Health Strategy: Safe, seamless and secure: evolving health and care to meet the needs of modern Australia*. Canberra ACT: Australian Government; 2018.
10. *My Health Records Act 2012* (Cth); *Healthcare Identifiers Act 2010* (Cth); My Health Records Regulation 2012; Healthcare Identifiers Regulations 2010; PCEHR (Information Commissioner Enforcement Powers) Guidelines 2013; My Health Records Rule 2016; My Health Records (Assisted Registration) Rule 2015; and My Health Records (Opt-out Trials) Rule 2016.
11. Australian Digital Health Agency, 2018.
12. *Coco v AN Clark (Engineers) Ltd* [1969] RPC 41 at 47 per Megarry J. The test was approved in Australia in *Commonwealth of Australia v John Fairfax and Sons Ltd* (1980) 147 CLR 39 at 51 per Mason J.
13. *Moorgate Tobacco Co Ltd v Philip Morris Ltd [No 2]* (1984) 156 CLR 414 at 438 per Deane J.
14. *Breen v Williams* (1996) 186 CLR 71 at 81.
15. *X v Y* [1988] 2 All ER 648 at 658 per Rose J. *The Laws of Australia*, n 45, para [5]; *Breen v Williams* (1996) 186 CLR 71.
16. *Giller v Procopets* (2008) 24 VR 1 remains the sole appellate authority for the recovery of compensation for emotional distress in a breach of confidence action. The position reached in that case has not been further tested or applied in Australia. Prior to that decision, a County Court judge in Victoria, in the 2007 case of *Doe v Australian Broadcasting Corporation*, awarded equitable compensation of $25,000 for breach of confidence, for 'hurt, distress, embarrassment, humiliation, shame and guilt' as part of a larger award for other wrongs. See http://www.alrc.gov.au/sites/default/files/pdfs/publications/final_report_123_whole_report.pdf.
17. International Council of Nurses. *ICN Code of Ethics for Nurses* (revised in 2012). Geneva: ICN; 2012.
18. For example, see *Mental Health Act 1996* (WA) s 206(1); *Mental Health Act 2007* (NSW) s 189.
19. Office of the Australian Information Commissioner. Chapter C: Permitted general situations. https://www.oaic.gov.au/agencies-and-organisations/app-guidelines/chapter-c-permitted-general-situations. Accessed 9 March 2019.
20. The guidelines are available at www.oaic.gov.au/privacy/applying-privacy-law/app-guidelines.
21. *Privacy Act 1988* (Cth) s 16A; see also: Office of the Australian Information Commissioner. Chapter C: Permitted general situations.
22. *The Privacy Act 1988* (Cth) ss 16B(1), (1A) (see also APP 3.4(c)).
23. Ibid. s 16B(2) (see also APP 3.4(c)).
24. Ibid. s 16B(3) (see also APP 6.2(d)).
25. Ibid. s 16B(4) (see also APP 6.2(d)).
26. Ibid. s 16B(5) (see also APP 6.2(d)).
27. *Health Records (Privacy and Access) Act 1997* (ACT).
28. *Health Records and Information Privacy Act 2002* (NSW).
29. *Health Records Act 2001* (Vic).
30. Office of the Australian Information Commission. Other privacy jurisdictions. https://www.oaic.gov.au/privacy-law/other-privacy-jurisdictions. Accessed 9 March 2019.
31. *Information Act 2002* (NT).
32. *Personal Information Protection Act 2004* (Tas).
33. *Information Privacy Act 2009* (Qld).
34. Office of the Australian Information Commission. Other privacy jurisdictions.
35. Ibid.
36. *Breen v Williams* (1996) 186 CLR 71.

37. In *Breen v Williams* (1996) 186 CLR 71 the High Court held that: in the absence of a formal contract between doctor and patient, there is no implied term in the contractual relationship which entitles the patient to inspect or own their healthcare records; the duty of a doctor to advise and treat a patient with reasonable care and skill does not impose a general duty to grant access to healthcare records relating to the patient; a patient has no proprietary interest in the documents comprising their healthcare records or in the information contained in those documents; and there is no common law principle in Australia of a patient's 'right to know' the content of their healthcare records.

38. *Privacy Act 1988* (Cth); *Health Records (Privacy and Access) Act 1997* (ACT); *Health Records Act 2001* (Vic); *Information Act 2002* (NT); *Personal Information Protection Act 2004* (Tas); *Health Records and Information Privacy Act 2002* (NSW); *Information Privacy Act 2009* (Qld).

39. For example, see New South Wales Department of Health, *Health Care Records – Documentation and Management* December 2012 PD 2012_069 (review date December 2017); Western Australia Department of Health, Information Access and Disclosure Policy, 2016, MP0015/16.

40. Medical Practice Regulations 2003 (NSW) reg 7.

41. *Health Records and Information Privacy Act 2002* (NSW) s 25.

42. See, for example: MDA National. Retention and Destruction of Healthcare Records. https://defenceupdate.mdanational.com.au/Articles/retention-destruction-records. Accessed 3 January 2019.

43. Victorian Health Services Commissioner. Transfer/closure of a Practice or Business of a Health Service Provider. https://hcc.vic.gov.au/sites/default/files/hra_statutory_guidelines_transfer_or_closure.pdf. Accessed 3 January 2019.

REVIEW QUESTIONS AND ACTIVITIES

1. List the factors to be considered when documenting a person's health care. Consider the significance of each of the factors.

2. Describe the procedure to follow when an error is made in a person's healthcare records.

3. Who has ownership of a person's healthcare records?

4. Identify the legislation in your state/territory that addresses information privacy.
   4.1 How may a person in your jurisdiction access their personal/health information as contained in their healthcare records?

   4.2 What other obligations are imposed on practitioners and healthcare institutions under the relevant privacy principles?

5. Discuss the legal, ethical and professional obligations of health practitioners to keep healthcare information confidential.

6. What must be considered concerning the storage and disposal of healthcare records?

6 NEGLIGENCE

LEARNING OBJECTIVES

Upon completing this chapter you should be able to:

- outline and explain key considerations regarding a cause of action in negligence
- explain vicarious liability and non-delegable duties
- discuss the law in relation to giving an apology
- discuss the open disclosure process and your role as a health practitioner
- describe alternative actions to negligence in a healthcare context.

A NOTE ON TERMINOLOGY

Note: The terms 'medical negligence' or 'medical mal-practice' are often used to refer to any healthcare-related case that involves a patient or some kind of medical mishap – be the defendant a doctor, nurse, physiotherapist or other health practitioner. Such terms serve to distinguish cases that occur in healthcare settings from those that occur in other settings (e.g. schools or sportsgrounds). In fact the legal elements needed for a cause of action in negligence (duty, breach, causation) are the same no matter what the setting, but their application to the facts takes into consideration matters relevant to the healthcare setting, standards expected of health practitioners and related evidence.

INTRODUCTION

Sometimes things go wrong when providing healthcare services. In this chapter we will examine the elements necessary to establish a civil cause of action in negligence against a health practitioner, defences to such a cause of action and compensation payable if a person is successful in their claim. This requires examining both the common law and statute. We will also consider matters related to disclosing adverse events, apologies and alternative actions to negligence.

NEGLIGENCE

Negligence is a civil action[1] in which health practitioners (and institutions) may be held liable for negligent acts or omissions that have resulted in loss or harm to a patient or client. The basis of the claim is that the conduct of the health practitioner fell below the standard of care appropriate to the particular circumstances *and*

that this conduct resulted in damage (some kind of harm or loss suffered by the plaintiff). A cause of action in negligence requires the person bringing the action to establish that:

- the treating health practitioner owed them a duty of care
- the duty was breached
- the breach caused loss or damage that was not too remote a consequence of the breach.

Courts will also consider if there are any defences to the action.

Unlike criminal proceedings, an action in negligence does not seek to punish the wrongdoer but to shift the loss from the individual who has sustained loss or harm to the individual or institution who is held to have caused the loss or harm. In doing so, compensation is awarded in order to place the injured person back in the position they would have been in had they not sustained the damage – as far as money is able to do so. Importantly, the law of negligence also has an underlying function of deterring poor behaviour (or encouraging good behaviour) via the publicity of cases and educating practitioners about what is an appropriate standard of care.

Parties

Recall that the person bringing the cause of action in a civil cause of action, in the first instance, is called a 'plaintiff'. In negligence cases relevant to health or medical contexts, the plaintiff will usually be the person who was seeking or received healthcare treatment, diagnosis or advice (or a third party) harmed as a consequence of the negligent acts or omissions of a health practitioner. Sometimes someone else may be appointed as the plaintiff's representative – for example, if the plaintiff is a child or incompetent (by way of mental illness, infirmity, senility or otherwise) – called a 'next friend' (or 'guardian *ad litem*'). The next friend or guardian *ad litem* is not a party to the court action but a representative of the plaintiff's interests.

The defendant is usually the health practitioner and/or the institution for which the practitioner works (we will discuss vicarious liability further below).

Most often the plaintiff's case will be prepared and presented by an independent lawyer. Although litigants may represent themselves, this is not common in medical negligence cases. Most often the defendant will be represented and advised by their medical/professional indemnity insurer.

Proof

To be successful in an action in negligence a plaintiff must prove every element of the action according to the civil standard of proof, which is *on the balance of probabilities*. To do this the plaintiff must adduce evidence in the form of documents, testimony from witnesses or other relevant materials sufficient to satisfy this standard. The balance of probabilities is said to require more than a 'mere mechanical comparison of probabilities independently of any belief in its realities'[2] – the court or tribunal must be persuaded as to the occurrence or existence of the fact to be proven.[3] If the plaintiff fails to prove any one of the elements to the requisite standard, the action will fail completely.

Very occasionally the fact that an accident has occurred at all may raise the inference of negligence on the part of the defendant; this is the doctrine of *res ipsa loquitur*, 'the thing speaks for itself'. This will only apply when there is no evidence or explanation as to how or why the accident occurred; the accident is such that it would not occur without negligence; and the defendant is proven to have been in control of or linked – either personally or vicariously – to the situation that caused the harm.[4] However, given there are no certainties in medical treatment, and the advances in the procedural practices of discovery and the exchange of evidence, it is more likely that the plaintiff will know, or be able to find out, what happened during his or her period of care or treatment and will need to prove negligence.[5]

ELEMENTS OF A NEGLIGENCE ACTION

Negligence has been defined by the courts as 'the omission to do something which a reasonable man, guided upon those considerations which ordinarily regulate the conduct of human affairs, would do, or doing something which a prudent and reasonable man would not do'.[6] Not every injury that occurs while a patient is under the care of a health practitioner will result from negligence, and not all acts or omissions that result in an injury will be held to be negligent.

The law governing negligence is found by reference to both the common law and civil liability statutes.[7] To succeed in a claim in negligence against a health practitioner, the plaintiff must be able to establish, on the balance of probabilities, the following elements:

- the plaintiff was owed a legally recognised **duty of care** by the defendant
- that there was a *breach* of that duty in that the defendant's conduct fell below the required standard of care
- this conduct caused the patient to suffer a **material injury/damage** that was reasonably foreseeable (not too remote).

In addition, there must not be any **defences** that the defendant may raise that would avoid liability. Note, an action will still succeed if a defence is raised that reduces rather than defeats a claim for compensation.

Duty of Care

A legally recognised duty of care between health practitioners and the people to whom they provide treatment or offer healthcare advice (i.e. their patients/clients) is generally accepted to exist in the context of that relationship.[8] The duty is one in which the practitioner must exercise reasonable care and skill in providing professional advice and treatment. It covers all the ways a practitioner is called upon to exercise their skill and judgment, extending to the examination, diagnosis and treatment of the patient and the provision of information in an appropriate case.[9]

However, if the duty of care is not evident, or the scope of the duty needs to be determined, courts have historically applied a number of tests[10] to determine whether a relationship gives rise to a duty of care and, if so, what the scope of the duty is.[11] In 'novel category' cases, the court now focuses on:

- whether it was reasonably foreseeable (i.e. was 'not unlikely') if the defendant was to do something wrong that a risk of harm may occur to the plaintiff (or a class of people to whom the plaintiff belongs)
- the relationship factors (salient features) between the plaintiff and the defendant that may give rise to a duty of care (e.g. whether the plaintiff was vulnerable and unable to protect themselves, whether they were relying on the defendant's expertise, whether the defendant had control in the situation and had knowledge of the risks)
- any broader policy implications of finding a duty of care (e.g. what the broader societal impacts of finding a duty of care would be and what the impact on the law would be).[12]

Duty to Third Parties

Although health practitioners and associated staff do not owe a duty to everyone at large, it is important to remember that a duty of care may not be restricted to the patient–practitioner relationship. For example, in the context of medical doctors, duties have been found to exist in the following circumstances:

- *To a non-patient in an emergency* – for example, a doctor was in close geographical proximity to a boy who was having an epileptic fit; there was a direct request for assistance; there was nothing impeding the doctor from helping in that he had no other patients to attend to; and the doctor knew of the harm that could arise if the boy was not treated quickly.[13]
- *To a patient's sexual partner* – in a case in which a patient had HIV, the duty of the doctor was held to be an obligation to counsel the patient to disclose their HIV status to their partner.[14]
- *To the parents of a patient who were present during a consultation* – there was a case in which a doctor advised about experimental treatment available to treat cancer in the United States. The parents took out a bank loan to fund the daughter's trip to, and treatment in, the United States. However, the treatment was also available in Australia. The court held as there existed a relationship of trust and confidence, and the parents had relied upon the doctor's advice, this gave rise to a duty of care.[15]
- *To the father of a child after a negligently performed sterilisation procedure on the mother* – the person was held liable for the costs of raising the healthy child.[16]

In another case, a receptionist in a medical practice was found to have a duty of care to make an initial assessment of a patient's condition in order to determine the urgency and schedule an appointment accordingly.[17]

Duty of Care Not Found

A duty of care has not been found to be owed by those investigating allegations of sexual abuse to parents suspected of such abuse regardless of whether the allegations are true. Courts have denied such a duty on policy grounds (the broader implications of making a decision) because it would conflict with the duty owed to the child to thoroughly investigate any allegations and to protect the child from harm. Such a duty might also create 'defensive practices', which would hamper a proper and thorough investigation of suspected child abuse.

Duty of Care Not Tested

It has not been tested in an Australian court as to whether there exists a duty of care for a health practitioner to *warn* a third party of the intended criminal activity or threats of harm of a person who the health practitioner is treating. Some practitioners may worry that warning the third party may lead to a breach of confidence, but it would be unlikely that a practitioner would be held liable for breaches of confidence for contacting the relevant authorities if there was a serious risk of harm or death to another.[18] In addition, whether or not there exists a duty of care relevant to negligence, there may be statutory obligations that require mandatory reporting in certain cases.

There is also no superior court authority that determines whether there is a duty of care owed by a health practitioner to *protect* third parties from suffering harm at the hands of a person receiving health care. However, some lower court authority exists. In the New South Wales District Court case of *Simon v Hunter and New England Area Health Service* [2012] NSWDC 19, it was found that a hospital that released a mentally ill patient into the care of a friend owed a duty to the friend because they were using him to transport the patient from New South Wales to Victoria to receive ongoing care.

In cases that concern a failure to warn about, or protect, third parties from harm by a patient, a detailed analysis of the relationship factors would be required to determine whether a duty of care was owed.

Duty to the Unborn

Health practitioners must be aware that when diagnosing, treating or advising people prior to or of fertile age that any negligence may not only affect that person but also future children conceived and born to them.[19] Courts have held that a child who suffers harm as a result of a health practitioner's negligent acts or omissions while the child is in its mother's womb, or before its conception, may, once born, claim compensation from the person whose negligence caused such harm.[20] Examples include negligently giving the incorrect blood to a woman that resulted, eight years later, in harm to a child she birthed; and a variety of cases concerning negligent prenatal advice, diagnosis or treatment. Once born alive, a child's claim in negligence for compensation would proceed as per all negligence claims, with evidence being adduced to prove liability.

Duty to Rescue

As a general proposition there is no common law obligation on an individual to render emergency aid, regardless of whether they are or are not a health practitioner.

However, in the abovementioned case of *Lowns v Wood* a doctor was found to have a duty to help a young boy having an epileptic fit in circumstances in which there existed a 'proximate relationship' – there was nothing impeding his rendering such aid, and specific provisions of the *Medical Practitioner's Act 1958* (NSW) made the failure of the medical practitioner to render assistance in an emergency unprofessional conduct. There is also a duty to rescue in the following examples:

- *The legal duty to render assistance.* For example, the Northern Territory *Criminal Code Act* provides: 'any person who, being able to provide rescue, resuscitation, medical treatment, first aid or succour of any kind to a person urgently in need of it and whose life may be endangered if it is not provided, callously fails to do so is guilty of a crime and is liable to imprisonment for seven years'.[21] Also, in each of the states and territories, when the person is the 'driver' of a motor vehicle involved in an accident, legislation may impose an obligation to stop and provide reasonable assistance.[22]
- *A person has assumed responsibility for the supervision or care of another.* In a healthcare context, this may arise in circumstances where a nurse or other health practitioner accompanies a patient on outings or appointments away from the hospital or institutional environment.
- *A person requiring assistance is in an existing and special relationship with the rescuer.* In the case of *Horsley v McLaren (The Ogopogo),*[23] Laskin J referred to the relationships of parent and child, employer and employee, doctor and patient, and passenger and carrier as giving rise to a duty to rescue.
- *An employer has, as part of the policy of the institution, a stated expectation that employees, in particular circumstances, will stop and render assistance.* For example, it is not uncommon that the respective state and territory departments of health require employees who drive departmental vehicles to stop and provide assistance should they come upon an accident while on departmental business.

(Note: There is no expectation that the health practitioner, at an accident site, could deliver the same standard of care that would be anticipated in the hospital setting.)

In Queensland the *Law Reform Act 1995* (s 16) protects medical practitioners, nurses or other people prescribed under a regulation from liability related to rendering medical care, aid or other assistance to an injured person in circumstances of an emergency and which is reasonable, given in good faith and without gross negligence or the expectation of a fee. In New South Wales the *Health Services Act 1997* protects members of staff of the New South Wales Ambulance Service and honorary ambulance officers.[24]

Civil liability statutory immunities for 'good Samaritans'[25] may also be relevant in some circumstances if, for example, a health practitioner, outside of work hours in circumstances where they are not getting paid, provides assistance, advice or care to an ill or injured person. The assistance needs only to be provided 'in good faith' (or 'honestly' in the Australian Capital Territory) and not recklessly. Except for in Victoria, the good Samaritan must not be intoxicated or impaired by alcohol or drugs.[26] In New South Wales and Tasmania, the relevant provisions require that the good Samaritan must exercise reasonable care. Good Samaritan protection does not apply in New South Wales[27] or Tasmania[28] if the person is impersonating a healthcare or emergency services worker or a police officer or is otherwise falsely representing that they have skills or expertise in connection with rendering emergency assistance. Reference to the relevant statute should be had to determine the exact scope of the protection in any particular jurisdiction.

Duty of Care: Mental Harm

Cases in which the plaintiff's injury consists of 'pure mental harm' (being a diagnosable psychiatric illness that is not consequential on some other physical injury) require special consideration in relation to duty of care. In the Australian Capital Territory, New South Wales, South Australia, Tasmania, Victoria and Western Australia legislation provides that the defendant *will not* owe a duty of care to the plaintiff unless the defendant foresaw or ought to have foreseen that *a person of normal fortitude* might suffer a mental harm if reasonable care were not taken in the circumstances of the case. Note,

the plaintiff need not be of 'normal fortitude' themselves if it is reasonably foreseeable that a person of normal fortitude would have suffered harm. In determining whether a person of normal fortitude would have suffered 'pure mental harm' in the circumstances of the case, each of the jurisdictions with legislative provisions require regard to:

- whether or not the mental harm was suffered as the result of a sudden shock
- whether the plaintiff witnessed, at the scene, a person being killed, injured or put in danger
- the nature of the relationship between the plaintiff and any person killed, injured or put in danger
- whether or not there was a pre-existing relationship between the plaintiff and the defendant.[29]

If the defendant knew or ought to have known that the plaintiff is a person of less than normal fortitude then the above factors do not affect the duty of care of the defendant to the plaintiff.

In Queensland and the Northern Territory there are no such statutory provisions and the common law applies, which does not require the 'normal fortitude' test.

Breach of the Duty of Care

Once it is established that the defendant owed a duty of care to the plaintiff it must then be proven, on the balance of probabilities, that their act or omission amounted to a breach of that duty of care. Here, one would first identify what the defendant did wrong (i.e. the alleged breach(es)). Examples of some common breaches in healthcare settings that have given rise to claims in negligence include:

- failure to warn a patient about the effects of an injury or illness
- failure to correctly provide information, advice or warnings regarding *material* risks associated with treatment
- misdiagnosis or delayed diagnosis of an injury or illness
- failure to treat an injury, illness or disability (at all or adequately)
- failure to provide a referral to a specialist
- inappropriate dosage or use of medication, or incorrect use of anaesthetic

- negligent postoperative care
- use of faulty technology, products or equipment
- errors in paediatric care (i.e. infants and children)
- failure to obtain informed consent.

A plaintiff must then establish that the wrongful act or omission satisfies the legal basis for determining a breach pursuant to the respective civil liability Acts. Generally, a person does not breach a duty to take precautions against a risk of harm unless:

- the risk was foreseeable (i.e. it is a risk of which the person knew or ought reasonably to have known)
- the risk was not insignificant
- in the circumstances, a reasonable person in the position would have taken the precautions.[30]

Considering whether the risk of harm was reasonably foreseeable, and not insignificant, are threshold tests that must be satisfied before considering what a person would have done in the circumstances. Reasonable foreseeability will be established if the defendant had actual knowledge, or constructive knowledge (ought to have known), of the risk of harm. Generally, the phrase 'not insignificant' is intended to indicate a risk that is of a higher probability than something that is reasonably foreseeable but not so high as might be indicated by a phrase such as 'a substantial' or 'significant' risk.[31]

In deciding whether a reasonable person would have taken precautions against a risk of harm, the court is then to consider (among other relevant things):

- the probability the harm would occur if the care were not taken
- the likely seriousness of the harm
- the burden of taking precautions to avoid the risk of harm
- the social utility of the activity that creates the risk of harm.

Such factors will be weighed and balanced against each other to determine whether a breach occurred – this is sometimes referred to as 'the calculus of negligence'.

When the issue involves the standard of care required of skilled professionals, as it would with health practitioners, at common law, the reasonable standard of care to be met by a professional is that of the ordinary skilled person exercising and professing to have the special skill.[32] The standard of care is that demanded by the law and is not determined by whether the conduct accorded with the practice of other professionals in the position of the defendant or of some professional body. The court will weigh relevant factors in light of the defendant being a professional.

Breach: Treatment and Diagnosis, Defence. Statutory provisions in all jurisdictions except the Australian Capital Territory and the Northern Territory then allow a defendant to adduce evidence in their defence that they acted in a way that (at the time the service was provided) was widely accepted by peer professional opinion as competent professional service.[33] The fact that there are differing peer professional opinions widely accepted by a significant number of respected practitioners in the field concerning a matter does not prevent any one or more of the opinions being relied on. The court, however, does not have to accept peer professional opinion if it is 'irrational' (in New South Wales or South Australia) or 'unreasonable' (in Victoria).

Breach: Failure to Provide Warnings or Information. At the breach stage of an inquiry in relation to failure to warn or provide information, the plaintiff must convince the court that the health practitioner did not communicate the relevant information to the patient. This will usually be adduced by considering evidence of both parties while also considering the health records.

A reasonable standard of care for a health practitioner would include providing information about procedures, treatments and risks that all people would require in the position of a person seeking or receiving health care but that also takes into account *anything that may be of particular relevance to the particular person* – something that is '*material*' to them.[34] For example, a piano player might require specific information regarding an operation on a finger that would be material to them; or a runner may require particular information regarding physiotherapy versus surgery on a sore leg. Thus, if a person makes known special needs or concerns to a health practitioner, or the practitioner is otherwise aware of such needs or concerns, the expected standard would be that they should provide information necessary to those circumstances. Another way of stating this is that a person should be warned of *material risks* related to any health care or treatment proposed.[35] Note, the duty has been found to be subject to 'therapeutic privilege', which means that a doctor would not be required to disclose information when they reasonably believe such information would prove damaging to the patient.[36]

Breach: Warnings About Obvious and Inherent Risks. The respective civil liability statutes do not generally create a proactive duty to warn of obvious risks, which are defined as risks that, in the circumstances, would have been obvious to a reasonable person in the position of that person; these include risks that are patent or a matter of common knowledge.[37] However, there is an exception to this in New South Wales, South Australia, Western Australia, Queensland and Tasmania when the defendant is a professional and the risk is a risk of death or personal injury to the plaintiff from the provision of a professional service. Health practitioners must still, therefore, provide information, advice and warnings about 'obvious risks' when there is a risk of death or personal injury in these jurisdictions.

There is also a duty to warn of inherent risks – that is, risks of something occurring that cannot be avoided by the exercise of reasonable care and skill.[38]

Breach: Assessment to Be Made With Reference to the Time of the Breach. A court's determination as to whether there has been a breach of a duty of care will require consideration of the conduct in light of the knowledge and standards of practice *at the time the incident occurred* (and not at the time of the trial).[39] If, on the evidence, it would be reasonable to assume that the competent health practitioner at the time would have known of the potential for harm from a procedure or treatment, then ignorance as to that fact will not provide a defence.

Damage

Damage is the 'gist' of an action in negligence. No matter how reckless a health practitioner may have been in the care of a person who they have treated or given advice (or failed to do so), if the person has not sustained any loss, injury or harm as a result of that conduct, there can be no claim in negligence for compensation. For example, a registered nurse, doctor or dentist may

administer the incorrect dose of a drug, breaching their standard of care. However, if the person who has received the incorrect dosage does not sustain an injury, they cannot bring a cause of action in negligence to claim compensation. Examples of the kind of loss or damage a person may suffer as a result of negligence include physical injury, psychological injury, economic loss and damage to property.

Causation

The plaintiff must establish a *causal relationship* between the negligent conduct (the breach) of the health practitioner and the damage sustained by the plaintiff, or liability will not be attributed to the defendant. In a healthcare context, causation is often the most difficult element for the plaintiff to prove. The plaintiff must be able to prove that, on the balance of probabilities, the damage has been caused by the defendant's conduct and is not the natural progression of the underlying pathology, or the result of the plaintiff's illness, disease or disorder. Questions of causation are questions of fact. Civil liability legislation addresses the issue of causation as involving two distinct inquiries: factual causation and scope of liability.[40]

Factual Causation

Factual causation requires consideration of whether the breach was a necessary condition for the occurrence of harm or loss. That is, if the breach hadn't occurred would the plaintiff have suffered loss or harm anyway? If the answer is no, then factual causation is satisfied. If some factual uncertainty exists then the court may make a value judgment regarding 'whether or not and why responsibility for the harm should be imposed on the negligent party'.[41]

Factual Causation in Failure to Give Advice, Information or Warning Cases. In determining whether a failure to provide advice, information or a warning was a necessary condition for the occurrence of harm, it is necessary to ask what the plaintiff would have done if given proper advice, information or warnings regarding risks. The matter will be determined subjectively in that it relates to what the plaintiff would have done subjectively in light of all relevant circumstances, and not to what a 'reasonable person' would have done. This is the case under statute in New South Wales,

Western Australia, Queensland, Tasmania and Victoria and at common law in the Australian Capital Territory and the Northern Territory. However, in New South Wales, Western Australia, Queensland and Tasmania, this is qualified by statute, in that the plaintiff is precluded from leading evidence that includes a statement made by the person *after* suffering the harm about what he or she would have done (i.e. retrospect is not good enough), except to the extent (if any) that the statement is against his or her best interests.[42]

Scope of Liability

The respective civil liability statutes provide that the 'scope of liability' inquiry in relation to causation encompasses considerations about whether or not, and if so why, the defendant should be found liable for the harm suffered by the plaintiff. Such an inquiry may, for example, include consideration of whether there were any new intervening acts that severed the chain of causation or whether the harm/loss suffered was too remote a consequence of the defendant's actions to attribute liability.

New Intervening Acts

The causal link between the negligent conduct and the claimed loss may sometimes be severed by an event that occurs in between that is considered the effective cause of the plaintiff's injuries. To be sufficient to sever the causal connection the intervening event must ordinarily be either human action that is properly to be regarded as voluntary or a causally independent event that is by ordinary standards so extremely unlikely as to be termed a coincidence.

When such new intervening events occur, the defendant may argue that the injury would not have occurred at all had the new intervening act not taken place or that the plaintiff's injuries would not have been as serious. In the first situation the defendant would argue that he or she should not be liable for the injuries at all; in the second, that he or she should be liable only for the initial injury but not for the injuries getting worse. However, if the event is 'in the ordinary course of things … the very kind of thing likely to happen as a result of the defendant's negligence' and the defendant's negligence created 'the very risk of injury' that has occurred,[43] it will not be deemed to break the chain of causation.

In healthcare settings the issue of 'new intervening acts' may be relevant when a health practitioner is the person who commits the initial wrong causing harm or loss and some subsequent event occurs. However, it may also be relevant when the health treatment provided to someone after they have suffered an initial injury elsewhere is alleged to have been so negligent as to be an independent cause of loss/harm suffered, or to lead to making the injury or harm worse. Usually only negligence of a gross nature would be enough to break the chain of causation, but it is possible, depending on the circumstances, that a health practitioner would be liable for the damage to the extent that he or she shared responsibility for it.[44]

Remoteness of Harm

A defendant will not be held liable in negligence if the harm suffered by the plaintiff is considered too remote a consequence. To determine remoteness, the focus is on whether *the kind of damage* suffered was *reasonably foreseeable*. This may be framed in broad terms (e.g. physical injury) and does not have to be specific (e.g. a broken leg).

However, what is referred to as the 'eggshell skull' rule provides that the precise manner in which the harm has occurred does not need to be reasonably foreseeable, nor does the extent of the damage, because the defendant must take the plaintiff as they are. Therefore, for example, provided the physical injury was foreseeable, the fact that the plaintiff has particularly brittle bones would not be considered too remote.

Defences

There are five commonly raised strategies in defending an action in negligence. Some are less frequently applicable in healthcare contexts; however, all are noted here because they are all possible.

1. Argue the Plaintiff Is Out of Time

All jurisdictions have limitation periods after which, no matter how significant and severe the injury, an action cannot be initiated. If a person is out of time, and the court will not grant an extension, a claim in negligence for personal injury will be barred. The limitation period for personal injuries in all Australian jurisdictions is three years from the date on which the cause of action accrued or the date of discovery,[45] unless there is a special situation in which a longer period may apply – such as if a person has a mental disability or is under the age of 18.[46] The court may also extend the time limit if the circumstances of the case warrant an extension.[47] Note, usually arguments that a claim is out of time will be heard in what is known as an 'interlocutory proceeding' before the main claim can proceed.

2. Deny or Rebut at Least One of the Elements of the Action

If the defendant can deny or rebut at least one of the elements of the action the whole claim will fail (noting *all* elements need to be satisfied in order to succeed in a claim). The health practitioner may therefore argue that:

- a duty of care was not owed in the circumstances (or the circumstances fell outside the scope of a recognised duty)
- the conduct and behaviour at the time of the incident was of a reasonable standard for a skilled professional
- there was no damage suffered by the plaintiff
- there is no causal link between the conduct and the damage, or
- the damage was not reasonably foreseeable.

3. Raise a Defence of Contributory Negligence

The defendant may argue that there was contributory negligence on the part of the plaintiff if the plaintiff has failed to take reasonable care of themselves and such failure contributed to the damage suffered. If proven on the balance of probabilities, then compensation payable to the plaintiff must be reduced to such extent as the court determines is 'just and equitable', having regard to the plaintiff's proportion of contribution to the damage suffered.

Note, while contributory negligence is frequently raised in personal injury claims where seatbelts or motorbike helmets have not been worn at the time of the injury, it is uncommon in a healthcare context.

4. Raise a Defence of Voluntary Assumption of Risk

The defendant may argue the plaintiff voluntarily assumed the risk of being injured by participating in the activity. A defence of 'voluntary assumption of risk' (*volenti non fit injuria*) is a complete defence meaning a defendant would not be liable at all. However, the defence is most likely not applicable to healthcare situations because patients do not enter into healthcare treatment voluntarily assuming the risk of being injured. The defence is more likely to be raised in relation to injuries that have occurred during engaging in sporting activities.

5. Join Another Defendant and Show That They Are Jointly Liable for the Damage

Finally, the defendant may join another defendant and show that the other person/institution is jointly liable for the damage. This will not negate their responsibility but will enable the court to apportion responsibility for damages between the defendants.

Damages (Compensation)

Once a plaintiff has proven their case on the balance of probabilities, and any defences have been raised, the court will decide whether compensation should be paid, and the quantum. When the defendant is found liable, compensation for the loss or harm suffered by the plaintiff may include a monetary award for such things as:

- pain and suffering (subject to caps on the amount payable)
- loss of income and superannuation
- medical treatment, rehabilitation, medication and ongoing care
- medical equipment (e.g. hoists, wheelchairs, mobility aids) and modifications to a person's home (e.g. ramps, support rails)
- domestic assistance (e.g. house cleaning services, gardening or other domestic duties the person once did but is no longer able to perform).

A plaintiff may claim for their need for services (e.g. home nursing), even if those services are provided gratuitously – for example, by a parent or spouse. All states and territories, except the Australian Capital Territory, have imposed requirements regarding the number of hours and time that such services are provided, and how the sum is calculated.

A court may also award the legal costs that have been incurred in having to bring an action to court if the matter cannot be settled outside of the court environment.

Categorisation of Damages

Damages (compensation) may be categorised in a number of ways. They may be divided into specific/special damages and general damages:

- **Specific/special damages** are the financial losses the plaintiff has incurred, such as expenditure on medications and medical expenses or lost wages as a result of the damage, from the time of the injury to the time of the trial. This portion of the damages is the amount of expenditure already incurred and can be specifically and precisely identified.
- **General damages** are estimates of expenditure in the future flowing from the injury. These will include loss of future earnings, pain and suffering, loss of enjoyment of life, loss of expectation of life, anticipated costs of medical, nursing and diagnostic services, and pharmaceutical, physiotherapy and rehabilitation costs.

They may be divided according to economic (e.g. medical expenses past and future; loss of wages) or non-economic loss (e.g. pain and suffering). Such divisions are for ease of calculation and support the requirement for courts to set out what damages have been awarded. They may also have relevance in terms of when caps to certain types of damages apply (see 'Threshold requirements and caps' below).

Quantum of Damages and Lump Sum Payments

The burden is on the plaintiff to prove the damage suffered and to provide the court with evidence regarding the quantum of compensation claimed. Besides being carefully calculated to put the plaintiff back in the position s/he was in before they were injured, damages are recovered once and forever in a lump sum award. However, because compensation is paid in a lump sum, rather than over a lifetime, the award will be reduced to account for the ability for the money to be invested and to accrue interest. A standard reduction was applied at common law to ensure a plaintiff was not over-compensated, the High Court of Australia having determined that a reasonable discount rate would be around 3% (*Todorovic v Waller*). Now, under statute, most jurisdictions apply a reduction rate of 5% or higher, which makes a significant difference to the award.

Pursuant to legislation, the court can now also approve periodic payments if parties agree to a 'structured settlement'.

Threshold Requirements and Caps

All states and territories except the Australian Capital Territory have legislation that may affect a plaintiff's final award of compensation. For example, legislation now bars recovery of compensation for non-economic loss (e.g. pain and suffering) unless the plaintiff meets some kind of threshold regarding: the severity of loss (New South Wales);[48] a requirement for the injury to be considered 'significant' (Victoria);[49] the time in which their ability to lead a 'normal life' has been affected (South Australia);[50] the amount of the award being above a prescribed minimum (Western Australia and Tasmania);[51] the percentage of impairment of the whole person (Northern Territory);[52] or the level of injury as compared with a scale (Queensland).[53] In some jurisdictions there are also caps on the amount that may be awarded for non-economic loss.

Caps on the award for loss of earning capacity also exist. Several states/territories specify in legislation a maximum amount payable based on 'average weekly earnings' (e.g. three times a person's average weekly earnings, although the specific formula for calculating this award varies).

Other Types of Damages

Aggravated Damages

Aggravated damages are awarded for substantial injuries to a plaintiff's feelings such as suffering significant humiliation.[54] They are a form of compensatory damages and so may form one of the heads of damages in this regard. They are unlikely to apply in many (if any) medical negligence cases, but such an award would always depend on the circumstances of the case. Note, while they are still allowed in Victoria, Tasmania, South Australia and the Australian Capital Territory, several other jurisdictions have abolished aggravated damages in personal injury negligence cases (as part of their widespread changes to tort law).[55]

Exemplary Damages

Exemplary damages (otherwise known as 'punitive damages') may be awarded to a plaintiff if the conduct of a defendant has been excessively outrageous, gross or wanton as to warrant a penalty and warning from the court in the form of damages. The aim is 'to teach a wrongdoer that tort does not pay' and that they may 'serve to assuage any urge for revenge felt by victims and to discourage any temptation to engage in self-help likely to endanger the peace'.[56] They are rarely awarded, and considerations that enter the assessment of exemplary damages are different from those concerning compensatory damages.[57]

While allowed in Victoria, legislation in New South Wales,[58] Queensland[59] and the Northern Territory[60] precludes the award of exemplary damages in personal injury cases where the act or omission that caused the injury or death was negligence. In Queensland, exemplary damages may be awarded if the act causing the personal injury was an unlawful intentional act that intended to cause the injury sustained, or an unlawful sexual assault or other sexual misconduct.

WRONGFUL DEATH

When the negligence of a wrongdoer causes the death of a person, a separate cause of action may be brought by the dependants of the person under wrongful death legislation for the loss they have suffered. This could include a claim for loss of financial support or caregiving from the date of death.

The person's estate can also bring a claim under 'survival of actions' legislation to recoup any financial losses the victim incurred between the date of the accident and the date of death. This might include a claim for ambulance costs or medical expenses between the date of injury and death and for funeral expenses.

APOLOGIES

Following an adverse event it had been the practice of many disciplines of health practitioners to deny any knowledge of (or involvement in) the adverse event or refuse to admit that an adverse event had occurred. This was usually due to the perception that to recognise the adverse event or involvement in an adverse outcome is an admission of liability and may be used in future legal actions.

Statutory reforms have allowed for apologies by providing that an apology made in connection with any matter alleged to have been caused by the fault of the person does not constitute an express or implied admission of fault or liability by the person in connection with that matter and is not relevant to the determination of such fault or liability. However, legislation again varies across the country. While the civil liability legislation in New South Wales and the Australian Capital Territory defines an apology in a way that includes an admission of fault, in Queensland, Tasmania, Victoria, Western Australia and the Northern Territory an admission of fault is expressly excluded. The consequences of an apology or expression of regret are listed in Table 6.1.

THE AUSTRALIAN OPEN DISCLOSURE FRAMEWORK

In addition to the abovementioned legislation, the Australian Commission on Safety and Quality in Health Care's *Australian Open Disclosure Framework* is designed to 'enable health service organisations and clinicians to communicate openly with patients when health care does not go to plan … provid[ing] a nationally consistent basis for communication following unexpected health care outcomes and harm'.[61]

Under the framework the process of 'open disclosure' is defined as 'an open discussion with the patient about an incident(s) that resulted in harm to that patient while they were receiving health care'.[62] It is incumbent on an organisation or facility to develop open disclosure policies, procedures, education and training that is most suited to their particular needs, resources, legal, regulatory and institutional context. The elements of an open disclosure include:

- an acknowledgement that the adverse event has occurred or that something did not go to plan
- an acknowledgement that the patient, their family or carers are not happy with the outcome
- an apology or expression of regret that includes words such as 'I am (we are) sorry'
- identification of the known facts and what will be undertaken in terms of ongoing care
- an indication that a review or investigation is being, or will be, conducted to determine what occurred and to prevent a re-occurrence of the adverse event
- an agreement to provide feedback as it becomes available.[63]

TABLE 6.1			
Consequences of an Apology or Expression of Regret			
Jurisdiction	Legislation	Consequence	Admissibility in Proceedings
Queensland	*Civil Liability Act 2003* s 72	Allows an individual to express regret without concern that the expression of regret will be construed or used as an admission of liability	Expression of regret is not admissible in proceedings
New South Wales	*Civil Liability Act 2002* s 69	Does not constitute express or implied admission of fault or liability Is not relevant to the determination of fault or liability	Not admissible in any civil proceedings as evidence of fault or liability
Tasmania	*Civil Liability Act 2002* s 7	Does not constitute express or implied admission of fault or liability Is not relevant to the determination of fault or liability	Not admissible in any civil proceedings as evidence of fault or liability
Western Australia	*Civil Liability Act 2002* s 5AH	Does not constitute express or implied admission of fault or liability Is not relevant to the determination of fault or liability	Not admissible in any civil proceedings as evidence of fault or liability
Victoria	*Wrongs Act 1958* s 14J(1)	In civil proceedings where death or injury is in issue or is relevant to an issue in fact or law the apology does not constitute liability for death or injury or admission of unprofessional conduct, carelessness, incompetence or unsatisfactory professional performance	Nothing in the section affects the admissibility of a statement with respect to a fact in issue or tending to establish a fact in issue
Northern Territory	*Personal Injuries (Liabilities and Damages) Act 2003* s 13		Not admissible as evidence
South Australia	*Civil Liability Act 1936* s 75	No admission of liability or fault to be inferred	
Australian Capital Territory	*Civil Law (Wrongs) Act 2002* s 14	Is not (and must not be taken as) an express or implied admission of fault or liability Not relevant to deciding fault or liability	Not admissible in any civil proceedings as evidence of fault or liability

The framework also provides that phrases such as, 'It is all my (our/his/her) fault' or 'I was (we were) negligent' should be avoided, and care must be taken not to speculate on the causes of the event or pre-empt the results of any inquiry or investigation.[64] As part of an open disclosure process, under no circumstance should a health practitioner admit liability for any harm on behalf of themselves or the organisation.[65]

Professional codes and guidelines addressing the obligations of health practitioners to disclose adverse events have also been developed by the respective National Boards under the National Law.[66] All support open and honest disclosure in communication with people who have sought or received healthcare services and recognise the professional responsibility to review what has occurred and to report appropriately.[67] However, it is of note that while the professional codes and guidelines address the requirement of full and frank disclosure, there are no provisions directed to an apology or expression of regret.

VICARIOUS LIABILITY

The doctrine of vicarious liability is a common law concept and serves to shift the financial responsibility from the individual who has been found liable for the damage to another individual or entity that has a greater financial capacity to bear the loss. The policy consideration underpinning the doctrine is the recognition that an employer will be financially more capable than an employee of meeting the cost of compensating the plaintiff. Thus, within the healthcare system, the doctrine of vicarious liability transfers the responsibility for compensating the patient's damages from the health practitioner to the employer, which will be, for example, a healthcare facility, government agency or owner of a private healthcare provider.

The doctrine applies when an employee, in the course or scope of their employment, negligently injures a patient. An employer is vicariously liable for the torts of the employees but assumes no liability for independent contractors. The two tests therefore are:

- Is the negligent individual an employee?
- Did the negligent conduct occur within the course and scope of the employment?

Whether an individual is an employee will be determined through an examination of the relationship with the employer including wide *indicia* to establish whether or not the person is an employee or an independent contractor. Elements considered by the court will include such things as whether:

- tax is taken prior to the person receiving their pay
- the person receives sick leave
- there is a superannuation contribution by the employer
- the employer provides the plant and equipment
- there is an expectation of personal service.

The liability of the employer is confined to the occurrence of the negligence in the course and scope of the person's employment. This concept is given a very broad application by the courts and includes all activities that the employee is authorised to do, even if carried out in an unauthorised manner.

It is important, therefore, for health practitioners to be clear about the activities they are and are not authorised to undertake. This will vary not only from institution to institution but also between different clinical units within the same institution. What nurses are authorised to do in an emergency department or critical care unit may well be significantly different from what they are authorised to do in a general medical or surgical ward. What an ambulance officer is authorised to do at the roadside will be different from what a nurse will be authorised to do within a hospital. Hospital protocols and policies are invaluable documents in relation to this element.

To be outside the course and scope of the employment, the health practitioner must be undertaking some activity that is so totally unrelated to the employment that they are a stranger vis-a-vis the employer.

NON-DELEGABLE DUTY OF CARE

Hospitals and healthcare facilities hold themselves out as providing a service to the consumers of healthcare services and, as such, owe a non-delegable duty of care to these consumers. This duty is based on the relationship between the institution and the person and therefore cannot be delegated to others. It is based on the notion that the person seeking or receiving treatment:

> … is usually specially dependent or vulnerable in that they have no relevant expertise and must put up with whatever the hospital subjects them to in fulfilling its undertaking. The hospital has ultimate control over what the patient is subjected to even though it does not control how the medical officers do their work.[68]

A direct action against the hospital or healthcare facility may therefore also be available for breach of a non-delegable duty.

In the healthcare context a non-delegable duty imposes on the hospital or healthcare facility the obligation to employ adequate numbers of appropriately trained and skilled staff, to ensure that the plant and equipment is operational and safe, and that patients are not exposed to any undue risk. However, statutory defences in most jurisdictions give public authorities a measure of protection from liability that results from decisions to do with allocating scarce resources.[69]

It is important to note that the scope of the non-delegable duty of care does not impose liability in relation to intentional or criminal wrongdoing. The Australian High Court in *New South Wales v Lepore*[70] held that the non-delegable duty of care did not impose liability in relation to intentional wrongdoing such as the sexual abuse of children.

ALTERNATIVE ACTIONS

Consumer Protection

Private health practitioners running a business are subject to the provisions of the *Competition and Consumer Act 2010* (Cth). Provisions against misleading and unconscionable conduct are particularly relevant including that 'practitioners must take care not to:

- mislead people in regard to fees, procedures or outcomes
- use misleading advertising relating to qualifications, area of expertise, fees, procedures or outcomes, or
- act unconscionably by acting in bad faith and deliberately taking advantage of people who are disadvantaged.

Health practitioners should also take the following steps to ensure they treat patients fairly and do not mislead them:

- use simple explanations, back up claims with facts and correct any misunderstandings fully and promptly – don't use jargon
- explain all possible alternative treatments and consequences
- explain whether a procedure is essential or elective
- when referring [people to another healthcare provider], always advise them of any actual or potential conflict of interest with the provider
- give people full contact details of other health practitioners involved in their care
- maintain full and accurate records to help clarify and resolve any issues that might arise
- if the cost of a treatment is unknown, give an estimate including all relevant information and explain the limitations of the estimate
- explain all possible additional costs, such as specialist charges and rehabilitation costs.'[71]

Complaints and Professional Regulation

A patient may also lodge a complaint against a health practitioner via the Australian Health Practitioner Regulation Agency or their state healthcare complaints commission (see Chapter 4). Such complaints, and actions in relation to professional conduct, can be made alone or in addition to pursuing common law claims for compensation.

FURTHER READING

Allan S, Blake M. *Australian Health Law*. Sydney, NSW: LexisNexis Butterworths; 2018.

Devereux J. *Australian Medical Law*. 3rd ed. Abingdon, Oxon, UK: Routledge-Cavendish; 2007.

Madden B, Cockburn T. Loss of chance in medical litigation: *Tabet v Gett* [2010] HCA 12. *J Bioeth Inq*. 2010;7(3):277–82.

Madden B, McIlwraith J. *Australian Medical Liability*. 3rd ed. Sydney, NSW: LexisNexis Butterworths; 2017.

Mahar PD, Burke JA. What is the value of professional opinion? The current medicolegal application of the 'peer professional practice defence' in Australia. *Med J Aust*. 2011;194(5):253–5.

Studdert DM, Piper D, Iedema R. Legal aspects of open disclosure II; Attitudes of health care practitioners – Findings from a national survey. *Med J Aust*. 2010;193.

Weisbrot D, Breen KJ. A no-fault compensation system for medical injury is long overdue. *Med J Aust*. 2012;197(5):296–8.

ENDNOTES

1. Negligence is an action that falls within the law of torts (meaning 'civil wrong').
2. Fleming JG. *The Law of Torts*. 9th ed. Sydney, NSW: LBC Information Services; 1998. p. 352. *Briginshaw v Briginshaw* (1938) 60 CLR 336 at 360–362.
3. Sappideen C, Vines P, editors. *Fleming's The Law of Torts*. 10th ed. Sydney, NSW: Lawbook Co; 2011. p. 357. *Briginshaw v Briginshaw* (1938) 60 CLR 336 at 361–362.
4. Sappideen C, Vines P. 2011. 362–368. See further *Cassidy v Ministry of Health* [1951] 1 All ER 574.
5. Kennedy I, Grubb A. *Medical Law: Text with Materials*. London, UK: Butterworths; 1994. p. 467.
6. *Blyth v Birmingham Water Works Co* (1856) 11 Exch 781 at 784.
7. *Civil Liability Act 2002* (NSW); *Wrongs Act 1958* (Vic); *Civil Liability Act 1936* (SA); *Civil Liability Act 2002* (WA); *Personal Injuries (Liabilities and Damages) Act 2003* (NT); *Civil Liability Act 2003* (Qld); *Civil Law (Wrongs) Act 2002* (ACT); *Civil Liability Act 2002* (Tas).
8. *Rogers v Whitaker* (1992) 175 CLR 479.
9. Per Mason CJ, Brennan, Dawson, Toohey, McHugh JJ in *Rogers v Whitaker* (1992) 109 ALR 625 at 628.
10. The 'two stage' approach, which was applied in *Anns v Merton London Borough of Merton* [1978] AC 728 and *F v R* (1983) 33 SASR 189, required determination of the first question: Was the harm to the patient reasonably foreseeable? If so, a duty of care existed unless there were grounds upon which the duty should be denied or limited. The 'proximity' test, which was applied in *Jaensch v Coffey* (1984) 155 CLR 549, required that the risk of injury was foreseeable and there was a relationship of proximity

(a closeness including physical and/or conceptual) between the defendant and the plaintiff. The 'three staged' approach required consideration of the foreseeability of damage, proximity and whether the imposition of the duty was fair, just and reasonable in the circumstances: *Caparo Industries P/C v Dickman* [1990] 2 AC 605. The 'incremental' approach applied in *Hill v Van Erp* (1997)188 CLR 159.

11. *Sullivan v Moody* (2001) 207 CLR 562.

12. Ibid. at 579–580 and *Graham Barclay Oysters Pty Ltd v Ryan* (2002) 211 CLR 540, and discussed in great detail in *Caltex Refineries (Qld) Pty Ltd v Stavar* (2009) 75 NSWLR 649 at 676 and [102]–[104] per Allsop P.

13. *Lowns v Woods* (1996) Aust Torts Reports 81-312. The decision in this case is at odds with the general common law principle that there is no duty imposed on a person who is essentially a 'stranger' to rescue another. Two of the judges referred to the proximity between the parties, which, in the particular circumstances of the case, gave rise to a duty of care. Kirby P also held that the specific provisions of the *Medical Practitioner's Act 1958* (NSW), which confirmed the failure of a medical practitioner to render assistance in an emergency amounted to unprofessional conduct, was relevant to the finding of the existence of a duty of care between the medical practitioner and the plaintiff.

14. *BT (as Administratix of the Estate of the Late AT) v Oei* [1999] NSWSC 1082. See also *PD v Dr Harvey and Dr Chen* [2003] NSWSC 487 (10 June 2003) BC200303031.

15. *McAnn v Buck* 2000 WADC 81. Note the action nevertheless failed at the breach stage of the inquiry.

16. *Cattanach v Melchior* (2003) 215 CLR 1; *McDonald v Sydney South West Area Health Service* [2005] NSWSC 924.

17. *Alexander v Heise* [2001] NSWCA 422 (27 November 2001).

18. Allan S, Blake M. *Australian Health Law*. Sydney, NSW: LexisNexis Butterworths; 2018. Skene L. *Law and Medical Practice: Rights, Duties, Claims and Defences*. 3rd ed. Sydney, NSW: LexisNexis Butterworths; 2008. [9.51]. See also: UK authority *W v Egdell* [1990] 1 All ER 835.

19. Allan S, Blake M; 2018.

20. *Watt v Rama* [1972] VR 353; *Lynch v Lynch & Anor* (1991) Aust Torts Reports 81–117, 69,091; *X & Y (By her tutor X) v Pal & Ors* (1991) Aust Torts Reports 8–098; 23 NSWLR 26.

21. *Criminal Code Act* (NT) s 155.

22. For example, see *Transport Operations (Road Use Management) Act 1995* (Qld) s 92(1).

23. *Horsley v McLaren (The Ogopogo)* [1971] 2 Lloyd's Rep 410.

24. *Health Services Act 1997* (NSW) s 67I.

25. *Civil Liability Act 2002* (NSW) ss 57–58; *Wrongs Act 1958* (Vic) s 31B; *Civil Liability Act 1936* (SA) s 74; *Civil Liability Act 2002* (WA) s 5AD; *Personal Injuries (Liabilities and Damages) Act 2003* (NT) s 8; *Civil Liability Act 2003* (Qld) ss 26–27 (note that the provision in Queensland refers to the giving of first aid or other aid or assistance given by a person while performing duties to enhance public safety); *Civil Law (Wrongs) Act 2002* (ACT) s 5; *Civil Liability Act 2002* (Tas) s 35B.

26. *Civil Liability Act 2002* (NSW) s 58(2); *Civil Liability Act 1936* (SA) s 74(4)(b); *Civil Liability Act 2002* (WA) s 5AE; *Personal Injuries (Liabilities and Damages) Act 2003* (NT) s 8(3); *Civil*

Liability Act 2002 (Tas) s 35C; *Civil Law (Wrongs) Act 2002* (ACT) s 5.

27. *Civil Liability Act 2002* (NSW) s 58(3).

28. *Civil Liability Act 2002* (Tas) s 35C(2).

29. *Civil Liability Act 2002* (NSW) s 32; *Wrongs Act 1958* (Vic) ss 72 and 74; *Civil Liability Act 1936* (SA) s 33; *Civil Liability Act 2002* (WA) s 5S, *Civil Law (Wrongs) Act 2002* (ACT) s 34; *Civil Liability Act 2002* (Tas) s 34.

30. *Civil Liability Act 2002* (NSW) s 5B(1); *Wrongs Act 1958* (Vic) s 48(1); *Civil Liability Act 1936* (SA) s 32(1); *Civil Liability Act 2002* (WA) s 5B(1); *Civil Liability Act 2003* (Qld) s 9(1); *Civil Law (Wrongs) Act 2002* (ACT) s 43(1); *Civil Liability Act 2002* (Tas) s 11(1).

31. Commonwealth of Australia, Ipp Committee. Review of the Law of Negligence: Final Report, September 2002, p. 105 and [7.15].

32. *Rogers v Whitaker* (1992) 175 CLR 479 at 483.

33. *Civil Liability Act 2002* (NSW) ss 5O(1) and 5P; *Civil Liability Act 1936* (SA) s 41(1) (in South Australia the statute is worded as 'member of the same profession' rather than 'peer'); *Civil Liability Act 2002* (WA) s 5PB(1); *Civil Liability Act 2002* (Tas) s 22(1). In Queensland and Victoria, the phrase *by a significant number of respected practitioners in the field* is added after peer professional opinion). *Civil Liability Act 2003* (Qld) s 22(1); *Wrongs Act 1958* (Vic) s 59(1).

34. *Rogers v Whitaker* (1992) 175 CLR 479.

35. Ibid.

36. Ibid. (Gaudron J dissenting on this point.)

37. *Civil Liability Act 2002* (NSW) s 5F; *Wrongs Act 1958* (Vic) s 53; *Civil Liability Act 1936* (SA) s 36; *Civil Liability Act 2002* (WA) s 5F; *Civil Liability Act 2003* (Qld) s 13; *Civil Liability Act 2002* (Tas) s 15.

38. *Civil Liability Act 2002* (NSW) s 51(3); *Wrongs Act 1958* (Vic) s 55(3); *Civil Liability Act 1936* (SA) s 36(3); *Civil Liability Act 2002* (WA) s 5P(2); *Civil Liability Act 2003* (Qld) s 16(3).

39. *Roe v Minister of Health* [1954] 2 QB 66.

40. *Civil Liability Act 2002* (NSW) s 5E; *Wrongs Act 1958* (Vic) s 52; *Civil Liability Act 1936* (SA) s 35; *Civil Liability Act 2002* (WA) s 5D; *Civil Liability Act 2003* (Qld) s 12; *Civil Liability (Wrongs) Act 2002* (ACT) s 46; *Civil Liability Act 2002* (Tas) s 14.

41. *Civil Liability Act 2002* (NSW) s 5D(2); *Wrongs Act 1958* (Vic) s 51(2); *Civil Liability Act 1936* (SA) s 34(2); *Civil Liability Act 2002* (WA) s 5D(2); *Civil Liability Act 2003* (Qld) s 11(2); *Civil Liability (Wrongs) Act 2002* (ACT) s 45(2); *Civil Liability Act 2002* (Tas) s 13(2).

42. See, for example, *Civil Liability Act 2002* (NSW) s 5D(3)(b).

43. *March v Stramare* per Mason CJ, p. 518, 519; *Mahoney v J Kruschich (Demolitions) Pty Ltd* (1985) 156 CLR 522.

44. *Mahoney v Kruschich (Demolitions) Pty Ltd* [1985] HCA 37; (1985) 156 CLR 522.

45. *Limitation of Actions Act 1958* (Vic) s 5(1A); *Limitation of Actions Act 1936* (SA) s 36; *Limitation Act 2005* (WA) s 14; *Limitations Act 1981* (NT) s 12(1)(b); *Limitation of Actions Act 1974* (Qld) s 11; *Limitation Act 1969* (NSW) ss 18A(2) and 50C; *Limitation Act 1985* (ACT) s 16B; *Limitation Act 1974* (Tas) s 5A(a).

46. Ibid. (Vic) s 27E; (SA) ss 45 and 45A; (WA) ss 30–37; (NT) s 36; (Qld) s 79; (NSW) s 52; (ACT) s 30; (Tas) s 26.

47. Ibid. (Vic) s 27K; (SA) s 48; (WA) Pt 3, Div 3; (NT) s 44; (Qld) s 31(2); (NSW) s 19; (ACT) s 36(4); (Tas) s 5A(5) and s 26.
48. *Civil Liability Act 2002* (NSW) s 16.
49. *Wrongs Act 1958* (Vic) s 28LF.
50. *Civil Liability Act 1936* (SA) s 52(2).
51. *Civil Liability Act 1936* (WA) ss 4, 9–10; *Civil Liability Act 2002* (Tas) s 27.
52. *Personal Injuries (Liabilities and Damages) Act 2003* (NT) s 27.
53. *Civil Liability Act 2003* (Qld) ss 61 and 62.
54. *Lamb v Cotogno* (1987) 164 CLR 1.
55. *Civil Liability Act 2002* (WA) s 7; *Personal Injuries (Liabilities and Damages) Act 2003* (NT) s 19; *Civil Liability Act 2003* (Qld) s 52; *Civil Liability Act 2002* (NSW) s 21.
56. *Henry v Thompson* [1989] 2 Qd R 412.
57. Brennan J in *XL Petroleum (NSW) Pty Ltd v Caltex Oil (Australia) Pty Ltd* (1985) 155 CLR 448.
58. *Civil Liability Act 2002* (NSW) s 21.
59. *Civil Liability Act 2003* (Qld) s 52.
60. *Personal Injuries (Liabilities and Damages) Act 2003* (NT) s 19.
61. Australian Commission on Safety and Quality in Health Care. *Australian Open Disclosure Framework*. Canberra, ACT: Commonwealth of Australia; 2013. p. 8.
62. Ibid. p. 4.
63. Ibid. p. 53.
64. Ibid.
65. Ibid. p. 62.
66. *Health Practitioner Regulation National Law Act 2009* (Qld) s 35.
67. See, for example, Australian Medical Association. Good Medical Practice: A Code of Conduct for Doctors in Australia. https://ama.com.au/ausmed/code-ethics-revised-and-updated. Accessed 3 January 2018.
68. Boston T. A hospital's non-delegable duty of care. *J Law Med.* 2003;10:364.
69. *Civil Liability Act 2002* (NSW) s 42; *Civil Liability Act 2003* (Qld) s 35; *Civil Liability Act 2002* (Tas) s 38; *Wrongs Act 1958* (Vic) s 83; *Civil Liability Act 2002* (WA) s 5W; *Civil Law (Wrongs) Act 2002* (ACT) s 110.
70. *New South Wales v Lepore* (2003) 212 CLR 511.
71. Australian Competition and Consumer Commission. Medical Professionals. https://www.accc.gov.au/business/industry-associations-professional-services/medical-professionals. Accessed 9 March 2019.

REVIEW QUESTIONS AND ACTIVITIES

1. Identify the elements necessary to succeed in an action in negligence.

2. What is the standard of proof required in such an action?

3. Identify the legislation in your jurisdiction that establishes the standard of care for professionals. How is the standard of care determined?

4. In relation to providing advice and information and to the disclosure of risk, what information must be given to a patient?

5. Provide examples of the types of damage (loss or harm) courts recognise for assessing compensation.

6. Discuss possible strategies a defendant may employ to defeat a claim in negligence.

7. What is meant by (a) vicarious liability and (b) a non-delegable duty of care? How do they differ?

7 INTENTIONAL TORTS

LEARNING OBJECTIVES

Upon completing this chapter you should be able to:

- discuss the civil law 'intentional torts' of 'trespass to person' and 'defamation'

- in relation to trespass to person:
  - explain when trespass to person in the form of assault, battery and false imprisonment may occur in healthcare settings and the relevant law
  - describe the importance of consent when interacting with patients
  - explain the elements necessary for legal consent
  - describe considerations for people who require supported or substitute decision making
  - describe special considerations relevant to children regarding consent
  - describe other relevant defences to trespass to person
  - discuss when adults and children may refuse treatment

- explain when defamation may occur in healthcare settings and the relevant law.

INTRODUCTION

An intentional tort describes a civil wrong that results from an *intentional act* on the part of the wrongdoer. There are many different intentional torts including those concerned with property and person. In this chapter we will consider four that are relevant to people in healthcare settings: assault, battery, false imprisonment and defamation. The first three all come under the cause of action 'trespass to person'; the fourth is a standalone action.

TRESPASS TO PERSON

Health practitioners are required, as part of their role in providing healthcare services, to come into physical contact with their patients and clients. The character of physical contact will vary depending on the patient, the severity and presentation of the illness or injury and the specific work carried out by the health practitioner. The level of physical contact required by one patient may vary greatly compared with that required by another. The type of contact that different groups of health practitioners will have with patients also varies greatly. The touching of a patient by a physiotherapist will be different from the touching required by a podiatrist, which will differ again from that of a psychologist.

In all circumstances (other than those covered by exceptions such as emergency treatment), the expectation is that a valid consent will be obtained from the patient before any touching is initiated. Underpinning this is the basic legal principle that every person's body is inviolate – each person having the right to determine what is done to them. Thus, at common law, a health practitioner may commit: an **assault**, if a patient believes he or she is going to be touched or restrained without his or her consent; a **battery** if actual touching occurs without consent or legal authority; or **false imprisonment** if the patient is unlawfully restrained without consent or other legal authority (see Fig. 7.1).

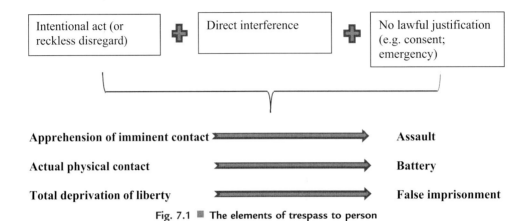

Fig. 7.1 ■ The elements of trespass to person

The emphasis on personal bodily integrity and autonomy is reinforced in the various codes of ethics and codes of conduct adopted by health practitioners. For example, the *Code of Conduct*, adopted by most of the National Boards,[1] identifies the rights of people seeking or receiving treatment (and, when relevant, their substitute decision-makers) to be autonomous and informed decision-makers about their health care and treatment. Similarly, the *Good Medical Practice: A Code of Conduct for Doctors in Australia*[2] requires that medical practitioners inform their patients and clients (and any substitute decision-maker) of 'the nature of, and need for, all aspects of their clinical management, including examination and investigations … giving them adequate opportunity to question or refuse intervention and treatment'.[3]

The following section will detail the key legal elements of the respective causes of action in trespass to person of assault, battery and false imprisonment, followed by a discussion of defences including consent, self-defence and emergency.

Assault

The intentional tort of assault involves the creation in the mind of another that imminent, unwanted physical contact may occur.[4] The threat does not need to involve any actual touching, nor does it need to be explicitly communicated. It is sufficient if the person believes, from the behaviour or conduct of the health practitioner, that they will be touched against their wishes or be subjected to some form of treatment or conduct to which they have not consented.

An example is that it is an assault to threaten to medicate a person if they do not comply with the health practitioner's request, even if they are difficult to manage. Other examples include when a person in care refuses to go to the shower or is slow to perform an activity and the health practitioner acts in a manner that leads the person to perceive some physical contact will occur to make them act or hurry up. While a health practitioner may feel pressures related to time restrictions enforced by the facility, or other patient demands, the threat to medicate to force a person to acquiesce or to make contact with a person to hurry them up constitutes an assault and is both ethically and legally unacceptable.

In considering whether an assault has occurred, consider:

- the nature of the threat (an expression of ill feeling is not an assault)
- the content of the threat (it is a threat of battery i.e. that bodily contact will occur)
- the means of making the threat (by words or conduct)
- whether the threat is conditional (e.g. 'If you do *x*, then I will do *y*') or unconditional.[5]

An allegation of assault is substantiated when the plaintiff knows of the threat, had a reasonable belief that the defendant intended to carry out the threat (and had the actual or apparent ability to do so) and can establish that the defendant's conduct caused him or her to experience an apprehension of physical contact. The focus is on the plaintiff's mindset and not whether the defendant was going to carry out the threat. It is enough if the person knew and expected that contact was about to take place, provided the apprehension was reasonable (i.e. a reasonable person in the plaintiff's position would have apprehended contact). Note, it is not necessary to prove that the person alleging assault was put *in fear*.

Battery

Battery, the actual physical contact with the person of another, does not require the plaintiff to prove that such contact was harmful or offensive,[6] nor is there a requirement for the plaintiff to have suffered harm. That is, unlike negligence, where the damage is the 'gist' of the action, there is no requirement that the plaintiff sustain any injury because of the unlawful touching. It is the actual touching of the person without their consent that is unlawful and forms the basis of the action. However, it is unlikely that the plaintiff would receive anything more than nominal damages where no injury has been sustained.

In cases of battery in a healthcare setting the touching of the patient must be intentional (or occur with reckless disregard). The requirement of intention distinguishes the deliberate action from the accidental physical contact that occurs as a part of everyday life and that would not constitute an action in battery. It is not a defence for the health practitioner to claim that they touched the patient to bestow some benefit, nor for a health practitioner to form the opinion that they know what is in the best interests of the patient and to proceed to undertake treatment or procedures without obtaining prior consent.

While the touching must be intentional, the person does not need to be aware at the time that they were touched. A person may be asleep, comatosed or anaesthetised when the unlawful touching occurs; for example, there would be grounds for an action in trespass to person if a health practitioner or student, without the person's prior consent and for no therapeutic reason, undertook a physical examination of a person while they were anaesthetised.

All health practitioners involved in implementing a therapeutic intervention without consent are equally liable. Thus, the doctor who extends an operative procedure beyond that consented to by the person being operated on and the nurse who participates in the extended operative procedure may be equally liable.

There are common law and legislative provisions that deem consent in cases where a person is unconscious or requires treatment as an emergency measure.

False Imprisonment

All adults of sound mind have the right not to be unlawfully detained against their will. Where a patient alleges that a health practitioner has interfered with their freedom of movement, the action is referred to as false imprisonment. False imprisonment is defined as the unlawful, intentional and complete application of restraint upon a person that restricts their freedom to move from one place to another or causes them to be confined to a place against their will.[7] No physical contact is required, it being sufficient if the patient fears some harm should they refuse to remain.

The restriction on the freedom of movement must be total. That is, there must be no means by which the patient can exit. Note, the presence of an exit that is not known to the patient, or not reasonable for the patient to attempt to use, still amounts to a restraint on movement for which the patient will have a cause of action. In healthcare settings, restraint may involve physical, mechanical or environmental restraint. When exercised without lawful authority or consent, any such restraint may amount to false imprisonment. Thus, in addition to the abovementioned examples, false imprisonment may include: preventing a person from leaving their bed or ward area or the hospital; acts such as applying wheelchair brakes to prevent a person from moving from one place to another; placing a person in physical restraints (such as strapping them to a chair or a bed or placing them in a restraining jacket); and using therapeutic devices such as intravenous fluid therapy, and the attendant machinery that goes with it, for no purpose other than to restrict the person's freedom of movement. Actions to restrict the freedom of movement of people may also include: administering drugs prescribed deliberately to control and restrict their freedom, such as sedatives prescribed outside recommended therapeutic guidelines and administered to restrict the person's freedom of movement; and placing a person in seclusion in a room or area they cannot leave.

There is no need for the person to know, at the time, that they have been detained. For example, in the New

South Wales Supreme Court case of *Hart v Herron*[8] a person who had undergone deep sleep therapy at the Chelmsford Hospital was held to have been falsely imprisoned during the time he had undergone the treatment, for which he had not given his consent. The court held that he had been falsely imprisoned even though he had no recollection of his time in the hospital, or that he had been detained.

Most hospitals and healthcare facilities have policies, procedures and guidelines on the use of physical, chemical, mechanical or environmental restraint on patients. These generally include express requirements for health practitioners regarding ordering the restraint, documenting the restraint and reviewing how the person is managed during the period of the restraint. The person's next of kin must also be notified about the use of physical or chemical restraint, and the restraint decision must be reviewed frequently and at predetermined intervals including a full assessment of the person restrained.

Clearly, such restraint must adhere to any relevant laws. For example, legislation that allows people to be legally detained includes crimes legislation permitting police powers of arrest and restraint, mental health legislation where a person can be made an 'involuntary patient', the *Biosecurity Act 2015* (Cth) and, in some instances, public health legislation. Any lawful restraint also must be proportional to what is needed (cannot be excessive), and there must be no reasonable alternative.

Defences to Trespass to Person

The most common defence to a cause of action related to trespass to person is consent. It is therefore important to understand what constitutes a legally valid consent and special considerations in relation to the giving of consent. Other defences may include statutory authority, self-defence, defence of other persons or property, and emergency (or 'necessity').

Defence: Consent

As a general principle, obtaining the consent of a person before commencing a procedure or treatment is respectful; however, it is also a legal requirement and is a defence to the abovementioned torts. The law seeks to protect the right of people seeking or receiving health care via legislation and the common law to choose what is done

to their bodies.[9] The legal requirement for a valid consent by a person prior to any interference applies regardless of whether they would benefit from the treatment or be harmed by refusing the procedure. A person therefore has the right to choose what treatment they will undergo and to refuse treatment they don't wish to have.

For consent to be valid in a healthcare setting, the person must:

- have the legal capacity to make a decision about the treatment
- be informed of and understand the broad nature or character of the treatment and its effects
- give consent that relates specifically to the proposed treatment or intervention
- have made the decision voluntarily and without pressure, coercion, misrepresentation, duress or fraud.

Capacity. Every adult of sound mind is presumed to have 'capacity' or to be legally 'competent' to provide a valid consent or to refuse to consent to treatment, unless there is evidence otherwise.[10] The legal capacity to consent is defined at common law and in various ways by statutes relevant to specific situations (e.g. mental health, guardianship and blood alcohol legislation; legislation regarding protecting children at risk). Generally, capacity is defined as:

> … *the ability to understand the specific situation, relevant facts or basic information regarding the decision and choices that may be made; evaluate reasonable implications or consequences regarding the decision and choices; use reasoned processes to weigh the risks and benefits; and communicate relatively consistent or stable decisions and/or choices.*[11]

Note, decision-making capacity may vary, depending on the simplicity or complexity of the decision to be made. Incapacity is also not tied to the 'status' of a person, such as having a disability or diagnosis. Rather, the focus is on whether the person has the cognitive abilities to make the treatment decision required. This may occur along a continuum, in that a person may be able to make some treatment decisions but not others. For example, they may be able to make simple decisions but need support when making more complex decisions. The law also makes provision for a substitute decision-maker when a patient, due to age, mental or intellectual incapacity, may not have the capacity to provide a valid consent.

The absence of capacity does not invalidate the need for consent; the health practitioner will need to seek consent via interacting with the person and their substitute decision-maker. (See also discussion below regarding substitute decision-makers.)

Provision of Information. When providing information to a person seeking or receiving health care it is incumbent on the health practitioner to ensure that, before obtaining consent, the patient understands the nature and effect of the information that has been given.[12] In circumstances where the person is not fluent in English, where there are communication needs or where an explanation involves highly technical language, the health practitioner must take steps to help the person to understand the information presented. For example, the health practitioner may call on a translator or use diagrams to assist. The health practitioner should also check the understanding of the patient – for example, by asking the person to explain in their own words what they have understood.

Consent Relates to Specific Treatment or Procedures. Consent for one treatment or procedure does not extend to carrying out a different treatment or procedure.[13] When obtaining consent from a person, health practitioners must discuss the specifics of the proposed treatment or procedure. Should the health practitioner consider that it is necessary to undertake a different procedure, they must again obtain valid consent. That it was convenient to carry out the procedure at the same time will not suffice.

Consent Must Be Voluntary. While it is common for a person to discuss treatment options with family, friends and health practitioners as a legitimate part of their decision-making process, consent to treatment must be given voluntarily and freely. This means that consent cannot and should not be coerced, induced by fraud/ deceit, brought about by constraint on a person's freedom of will or be the result of a power relationship between the person who is 'consenting' (the patient)

and the health practitioner. Also, consent should not be obtained in cases where drugs may be impairing a person's faculty of reason. Such factors, when present, mean that a decision no longer truly represents the person's will, and any consent given in such circumstances will not be valid.

The case of *Dean v Phung*[14] illustrates the above principles. Mr Dean, who had suffered chipped frontal teeth due to a workplace accident, was subjected to extensive unnecessary dental treatment. The court held that the dentist, Dr Phung, was motivated by financial gain in carrying out the treatment and that Mr Dean's consent pertained only to necessary treatment, not to the additional unnecessary work. As a result, the treatment constituted a trespass to person in the form of battery.

Special Considerations: Supported or Substitute Decisions. The threshold test of capacity, which is the determinative factor as to whether a substitute decision-maker is required, is whether the adult is able to understand the nature and effect of their decision, make that decision voluntarily and of their own free will, and communicate the decision to another.[15] When a person lacks the requisite capacity to decide in part or in whole for themselves, guardianship legislation outlines criteria for appointing a substitute decision-maker, the hierarchy of possible decision-makers and the scope of their powers. In all Australian states and territories, such legislation provides that a decision-maker can make health decisions for the person as long as the person is unable to make decisions for themselves and the substitute decision-maker is either:

- chosen by the person (e.g. an enduring guardian)
- assigned under legislation (e.g. a spouse, close friend or relative)
- legally appointed (e.g. by a court).[16]

(See further discussion in Chapter 12.)

Refusal to Consent. Adults of sound mind have the legal capacity not only to consent to the treatment recommended by a health practitioner but also to withhold their consent. A person has the legal right, even after giving a valid consent, to withdraw it and refuse to continue to undergo a procedure. Provided a person is competent, they have the right to refuse all treatment regardless of whether the refusal will result in permanent physical injury or death. See further discussion in Chapter 12.

Consent to Research. Any research that requires contact with its subjects will necessitate the researcher to obtain the consent of the participants before beginning the study or project. Where research is conducted without a legally valid consent, it gives rise to the possibility of a subject suing in negligence or civil assault. While the courts have not considered the precise depth and extent of the information necessary to obtain a valid consent for research purposes, it is accepted that the extent of the information is greater than that required in the treatment situation.[17]

Within the healthcare context it is also important that health practitioners clearly identify to patients the distinction between the role of health practitioner and that of researcher. That is, where health practitioners are seeking participants in research projects from their patient and client load, they must identify, before obtaining a consent, that participation or non-participation will not alter the therapeutic relationship that already exists.

Ethics again also plays an integral role. The National Health and Medical Research Council publishes the *National Statement on Ethical Conduct in Human Research*, which should be referred to by all researchers in Australia. In addition, in conjunction with the Australian Research Council and with Universities Australia, the National Health and Medical Research Council publishes the *Australian Code for the Responsible Conduct of Research*, which guides university and other public sector organisations in responsible research practices and promotes research integrity.

Forms of Consent. Consent may be **implied**, for example, rolling up a sleeve to expose an arm ready to receive vaccination, or **express** – given verbally or in writing.

IMPLIED CONSENT. A patient's consent to routine care interventions such as wound dressings and the administration of medications is often implied through the patient's behaviour. However, in all but the most obvious of situations there are difficulties in relying on non-verbal communication as a method of obtaining a consent.

Situations where it would be unwise for a health practitioner to rely solely on the behaviour of a person as indicative of consent include:

- at the initial presentation in an emergency department
- when a person is a new admission to a clinical unit
- when a person is anxious, in pain or distressed
- when a person is from a different cultural or ethnic background from the health practitioner.

In circumstances where a person has not undergone a procedure or treatment previously, it is good practice to seek a very clear direction from them that they are indeed communicating their consent. Health practitioners in clinical practice must ensure their own understanding of what a person has consented to is consistent with the understanding of that person.

The mere fact that a person presents to a hospital or healthcare facility does not in itself provide a valid consent for health practitioners to initiate diagnostic procedures or treatments. For example, in the above-mentioned case of *Hart v Herron* the plaintiff attended the admission unit of a psychiatric hospital in an agitated state to seek information from his medical practitioner about a procedure he was to undergo. He was offered medication to 'calm him down' and later was administered narcosis (deep sleep) treatment and electroconvulsive therapy without his consent. He sued both the hospital and the psychiatrist in negligence, assault, battery and false imprisonment. The hospital argued that the plaintiff, through his presentation to the admission unit, had consented to the treatment; however, the court rejected this argument.

VERBAL CONSENT. A more frequent and meaningful form of consent occurs when agreement to treatment is stated by a person. In a clinical situation, health practitioners obtain a person's consent by explaining what is about to occur and allowing the person to consider the information before verbally agreeing or refusing. Ideally, this should occur in most healthcare communications. In relation to more invasive procedures, verbal consent generally takes place in the physician's or surgeon's rooms or an outpatients department before admission. The medical practitioner will discuss the procedure, and the person has the option to refuse or to agree to the specified treatment. Where the procedure is invasive, this type of exchange is commonly followed by completing a written consent form.

WRITTEN CONSENT. In line with legislative require-ments[18] or as part of a health department or hospital policy, a consent to invasive procedures may have to be obtained in writing and witnessed. Where this is the case, it is the responsibility of the health practitioner carrying out the procedure to ensure that a *valid* consent is obtained. The written consent is most important when non-routine treatments or procedures that have risks and complications attached to them are to be carried out. The benefit of having the consent in writing lies in the fact that it provides documentary evidence of the consent.

An important function of a consent form is that it provides documentary evidence of consent for a treat-ment to proceed, or refusal of such treatment. However, mechanically recording consent in writing, or obtaining a signature on a consent form, does not in itself con-stitute a valid consent. If the process is defective, the consent will be held to be invalid or non-existent. Therefore, even when patients have signed the consent form, they are not precluded from initiating an action in trespass to person or negligence if they were insuf-ficiently informed, did not understand the content or did not have the risks explained.

Consent forms also do not usually indicate the process by which a person has been sufficiently informed. Evidence of this should be available from some other source – for example, in the progress notes of the person's medical or nursing history.

Blanket consents and 'catch all' clauses within consent forms are of limited legal value and their use should be avoided.[19]

Note again that a person can withdraw consent at any time.

Special Considerations: Consent to Healthcare Treatment in Relation to Children

PARENTAL DECISION-MAKING AUTHORITY. As a general principle, a parent (or appointed guardian) has the main decision-making authority in relation to medical and dental treatment for their child. People who are caring for children on a casual basis, such as babysit-ters, friends, relatives and schoolteachers, have no such authority unless expressly provided by a parent or legal guardian.

Parental decision making in relation to the health care of their child must be in the child's *best interests*. If it is not considered to be so (e.g. by the health practitioners treating the child), the matter may be referred to a court of law. Parents are also not able to consent to treatment made illegal by statute (e.g. genital mutilation) or to certain procedures or treatments that are considered 'special' and need court approval (e.g. sterilisation of a person with a disability).

THE ROLE OF THE COURTS. In Australia the Family Court has special welfare provisions, and the Supreme Court in each state and territory has '*parens patriae*' jurisdiction that enables the respective courts to make decisions about medical treatment/procedures for minors. The power of the courts is superior to that of parents and may be exercised to ensure decisions about treatment are in the 'best interests' of a child or young person. It may also override the decision of a 'Gillick competent' child (see further below).

When a procedure that is considered by a court to be a **special medical procedure** is proposed the decision may only be made by a court. These include procedures that are invasive, irreversible or 'non-therapeutic', meaning it is not for the purpose of curing a malfunction or disease. Special medical procedures also include procedures in which there is a significant risk of making the wrong decision, either about a child's present or future capacity to consent or about what are the best interests of a child who cannot consent and where the consequences of a wrong decision are particularly grave.

In New South Wales the law also requires that some treatments have the consent of the Guardianship Tri-bunal. For children aged under 16 years, the tribunal must approve:

- treatment that is intended or is reasonably likely to result in permanent infertility (not being consequent on some other life-saving treatment)
- any treatment for the purposes of contraception or menstrual regulation declared to be a 'special medical treatment'
- vasectomy or tubal occlusion
- treatment that involves the administration of a drug of addiction over a period of more than 10 days in any 30-day period
- any experimental procedures that do not conform with the National Health and Medical Research

Council's statement on research (discussed under 'Consent to research' on page 84).

CHILDREN AND CAPACITY TO CONSENT TO HEALTHCARE DECISIONS. When a person reaches the age of 18 years, they are considered at law to have legal capacity.[20] Prior to this age, there may be *both* common law and legislative indicators regarding when a child will be deemed capable or legally competent to give a valid consent.

The common law is silent on a specific age at which a minor is competent to give a valid consent. However, if a child is 'Gillick competent' (referring to the United Kingdom case in which the issue was comprehensively addressed)[21] they can decide for themselves whether they consent to or refuse treatment in many circumstances. Gillick competence means a child has sufficient understanding and intelligence to enable them to understand fully what is proposed.

Two states also have legislation that specifically addresses some aspects of healthcare treatment decision making by minors. In South Australia the *Consent to Medical Treatment and Palliative Care Act 1995* (SA) stipulates that people aged 16 years or older can make decisions about their own medical treatment except in the case of making an advance care plan/directive or appointing an agent to consent to treatment. In New South Wales the *Minors (Property and Contract) Act 1970* (NSW) provides that consent of a child aged 14 years or older has effect in relation to a claim by him or her for assault or battery in respect of anything done during that treatment as if, at the time when the consent is given, he or she were aged 21 years or older. The same applies if a parent of a child aged under 16 years consents to the treatment. Note, the legislation, while implying a child aged 14 may make such a decision, does not set the age for doing so, and a child's capacity would still need to be assessed. In the Australian Capital Territory, New South Wales and Tasmania, legislation differentiates between a 'child' and a 'young person'. In the Australian Capital Territory the *Children and Young People Act 2008* (ACT) defines a 'child' as being under the age of 12 years and a 'young person' as being aged 12–18 years.[22] In New South Wales the *Children and Young Persons (Care and Protection) Act 1998* (NSW) defines a child (for purposes other than employment) as a person under the age of 16 years and a young person as being 16–18 years.[23] In Tasmania the *Children,*

Young Persons and their Families Act 1997 (Tas) defines a young person as either 16 or 17 years of age.[24] This may be relevant to, but is not decisive in, determining whether Gillick competence exists, which requires determining the individual child's capacity and is not based on his or her age.

Note, a child's capacity to consent does not mean that the parent loses their authority. If there is disagreement between the parent and a Gillick-competent child as to the treatment that the child is, or is not, going to undertake, while a competent child's preferences will generally prevail, the courts may exercise a general supervisory role to act to protect the best interests of the child, particularly in the face of refusal of life-saving treatment.[25]

Defence: Emergency

When a person requires emergency treatment, and is so incapacitated as to be incapable of giving a valid consent, a health practitioner may initiate treatment that they honestly believe is reasonable and necessary in the circumstances under the common law 'doctrine of emergency'. This is also sometimes referred to as the 'doctrine of necessity', though it has been suggested that the 'necessity principle is separate from that of emergency and is wider in application'.[26] The doctrine effectively provides the health practitioner with a defence to an action in assault and battery for the treatment given at the time.

To satisfy the common law doctrine of emergency, the treatment must be necessary 'to save life' or to 'prevent serious injury to health'.[27] The circumstances must indicate that the treatment is not merely convenient, and the medical practitioner must take only 'such steps as good medical practice demands'.[28]

Note, it is important to distinguish the legal position in an emergency where a person is unconscious or not capable of consenting due to the severity of the injuries, from the situation where an adult person of sound mind refuses emergency treatment. Where the latter is the case, it is a battery to initiate or continue treatment once the person has refused to consent.

Defence: Statutory Authority

Statutory authority may provide a defence to the tort of battery when legislation provides for treatment without consent. For example, in addition to the above common law provision, in some jurisdictions, legislation applicable to emergency situations also permits the treatment of patients by medical practitioners without their consent.[29] While in a number of states and territories the authorisation applies only to doctors, in other jurisdictions it also covers a more diverse group of health practitioners.[30]

The lawful authority to treat children in an emergency is very similar to that which applies to adults. If the parent of the child, or the legally responsible adult, is not contactable and the treatment is necessary to save the child's life, or prevent serious harm, then the health practitioner may proceed with the medical intervention without consent.[31] There are also provisions that serve to override the refusal to consent by a parent when the treatment is life-saving (e.g. in relation to blood transfusions). In most cases the legislation applies to treatment that is 'necessary to save the child's life' or required as 'a matter of urgency', or specifically applies to the transfusion of blood. Such legislation is listed in Table 7.1.

Defence: Self-Defence or Defence of Another Person

The final defences to trespass to person to be noted here are self-defence or defence of another person. A person who is attacked, or threatened with an attack, may use reasonable force to defend themselves. In each case the force used must be proportional to the threat; it must not be excessive. A person may also use reasonable force to defend a third party where he/she reasonably believes that the party is being attacked or being threatened.[32]

Damages

Damages for trespass to person range from a nominal amount to recognise the violation of a person's rights, to the full range of damages including aggravated and exemplary damages. A plaintiff can claim any economic or pecuniary loss that results from injury or harm suffered as well as non-economic losses. Non-economic losses include pain and suffering, disgrace and humiliation. **Aggravated damages** are awarded when the behaviour of the defendant has occurred in particularly humiliating and malicious circumstances. **Exemplary damages** are awarded to punish and/or to make an example of the defendant to others and, again, are only awarded in the most egregious of circumstances.

In cases of false imprisonment, the compensatory damages will be assessed by reference, among other things, to the duration of the deprivation of liberty in addition to any injury to the plaintiff, be that physical or psychological injury that results in economic loss or non-economic loss related to any mental suffering, disgrace or humiliation suffered because of the false imprisonment.

DEFAMATION

The second intentional tort to be examined in this chapter is 'defamation'. It is relevant in healthcare settings both in relation to what is said or otherwise published about patients to other people and to what is published about health practitioners – for example, by way of online reviews of services or in discussions about a practitioner's quality of care.

Defamation is the publication of false information that tends to lower the person (the subject of the communication) in the estimation of their peers. It may lead to a civil action that seeks to protect the reputation of the natural or legal person. A company, government department or hospital may, for example, sue in relation to its trading reputation or to protect its reputation in terms of its goods and services. For a defamation action to be successful the plaintiff must prove that the communication:

TABLE 7.1	
Legislation Authorising Medical Intervention for Children and Young People	
Jurisdiction	**Legislation**
Australian Capital Territory	*Transplantation and Anatomy Act 1978* s 23
New South Wales	*Guardianship Act 1987* s 37 *Children and Young Persons (Care and Protection) Act 1998* s 174
Northern Territory	*Emergency Medical Operations Act 1973* ss 2, 3
Queensland	*Transplantation and Anatomy Act 1979* s 20
South Australia	*Consent to Treatment and Palliative Care Act 1995* s 13
Tasmania	*Human Tissue Act 1985* s 21
Victoria	*Human Tissue Act 1982* s 24
Western Australia	*Human Tissue and Transplantation Act 1982* s 21

- identifies (or is about) the plaintiff
- has been published to at least one other person
- is defamatory.

A cause of action must be made within a year of the defamatory publication.

Note, defamation law is very complex, requiring a difficult balance between freedom of speech and protection of reputation. It is governed via 'Uniform Defamation Laws' enacted across the states and territories that took effect on 1 January 2006. Such laws mean that defamation law in each state and territory is substantially the same, although there are some differences. For example, in New South Wales, the Northern Territory, Queensland, South Australia, Tasmania, Victoria and Western Australia, the separate torts of libel (which relates to written communications) and slander (which relates to oral communications) have been abolished and replaced with the single tort of defamation.[33] In the Australian Capital Territory, the separate torts remain in existence; however, there is no longer any practical distinction between them.

Categories of Defamatory Statements

There are three categories of defamatory statements:

- statements that lower the reputation of the person in the perception of the community
- statements that are likely to injure the plaintiff's reputation in their profession or trade
- statements that are likely to result in the plaintiff being shunned, avoided or ridiculed.

Elements of a Defamation Action

The following are the elements of a defamation action.

1. There Must Be a Statement of Fact or Opinion

The form of the communication may be permanent or non-permanent. The relevant factor is that the assertion was made, either expressly or by implication, that the person defamed deserves to be held in low esteem.

2. The Statement Must Be Published

The statement must have been communicated to a third party. The concept of 'publication' means that the statement must have been made to more than the person to whom the statement refers but does not require that

it be made to the entire community. The third party to whom the statement is communicated must be capable of understanding the defamatory nature of the content. This issue is raised in relation to the publication of a statement in a context where the recipient either has no understanding of the content (as an example, due to language differences) or the person is unknown to them. Where a person republishes the defamatory material, that person becomes a new publisher for the purposes of any legal action.

It is important to note that liability for defamation can arise as a result of a mistake or error. The publisher does not have to have intentionally defamed the person named in the published information.

3. The Statement Must Refer to the Person Alleging the Defamation (i.e. the Person Must Be Identified)

The content of the statement must refer to the person claiming to have been defamed. This is most straightforward when the plaintiff is named. However, it is not necessary for the person to be named specifically nor that there be an intention to defame. Even the use of a false name may amount to defamation if the plaintiff can be identified by other means.

In *Hutton v Jones*[34] an article of fiction was published in the newspaper referring to a person named Artemus Jones, a church warden in Peckham, who conducted an inappropriate liaison with a woman who was not his wife. There was in fact an actual person whose name was Artemus Jones who was a barrister and did not live in Peckham; however, several people still thought that the content of the article referred to him. The question for the court was whether the newspaper article was reasonably referrable to the plaintiff and was therefore defamatory. The court held that the real Artemus Jones was entitled to recover damages because people reasonably believed that the article referred to him.

It is not possible to claim defamation in relation to a group or class of people. However, a statement that refers to or identifies a particular member or members of a group may be defamatory.

4. The Statement Must Harm the Person's Reputation

The test is whether the statement of the defendant in its ordinary and natural sense defamed the plaintiff by lowering or harming the plaintiff's reputation, holding the plaintiff up to ridicule or leading others to shun and avoid the plaintiff. This is determined by using the standard viewpoint of the reasonable person in the community. This standard may vary from one community to another.

In an action for defamation before a judge and jury, the judge will determine whether the statement is capable of being defamatory and the jury will determine whether, in the circumstances, it was defamatory.

Defences to an Action in Defamation

Consent

If the defendant is able to establish that the plaintiff in fact consented to the publication of the defamatory statement, this will operate as a complete defence to the action.

Justification/Truth

The Uniform Defamation Laws provide that a complete defence to defamation will exist if the defendant can prove the material published was substantially true.

Honest Opinion (Defence of Fair Comment at Common Law)

Pursuant to the Uniform Defamation Laws the defence of honest opinion requires the defendant to prove that: (1) the communication was an expression of opinion rather than a statement of fact; (2) the opinion related to a matter of public interest; (3) the opinion was based on 'proper material' (material that is substantially true; contained in public documents; or published on an occasion that attracted the protection of absolute or qualified privilege); and (4) the facts upon which the opinion is based are stated unless they are widely known (so that the readers/viewers/listeners can form their own views on the facts).

The opinion can be extreme, provided it is honestly held.

The defence of honest opinion is similar (although not exactly the same) to the common law defence of fair comment.

Absolute Privilege

Absolute privilege applies only to statements made by members of parliament in the course of parliamentary proceedings or statements made in legal proceedings. It provides a complete defence to defamation.

Qualified Privilege

Qualified privilege can be raised as a defence if the defendant reasonably believed:

- the statement was true
- the person had the legal, moral or social duty to make it
- the recipient has a corresponding interest in receiving it.

Complaints by patients to a complaints authority, a regulatory body (a medical council or board), employer or the owner of a medical practice about the actions of a doctor would, for example, fall within this defence. For this defence to apply, the matter must have been published to the recipient in the course of giving the recipient information on the subject and the conduct of the defendant in publishing the matter must have been reasonable in the circumstances. The defence of qualified privilege does not apply if the defamation is proven to have been motivated by malice.

Triviality

A defence of triviality may be raised if the defendant can prove that the plaintiff was unlikely to sustain any harm to their reputation as a result of publishing the statement. However, courts don't commonly recognise the defence of triviality, and it is uncertain when such a defence applies.

APOLOGIES

If a plaintiff fails to accept a reasonable offer to 'make amends', this can cause their action to fail or can result in a successful plaintiff not being granted an order in which the defendant pays the costs of the court case (a 'costs order'). This is intended to encourage plaintiffs to accept an apology and/or to settle for damages and for legal costs to be paid rather than pursuing legal action. An offer to make amends must include an offer to publish or join in publishing a reasonable correction regarding the defamatory statement; this correction must also be brought to the attention of third parties. Courts will consider the prominence of the correction, how much time has passed, the seriousness of the defamatory accusations, what steps the publisher has taken to correct the matter with third parties and any compensation offered. If an offer to make amends is accepted the plaintiff cannot later pursue a court action.

DAMAGES AND COSTS

A person claiming defamation can seek compensation for non-economic loss (such as pain and suffering) and for economic loss suffered because of the defamatory statement. Damages for non-economic loss are generally capped at $250,000, although the maximum damages amount can be changed by executive order.

Exemplary or punitive damages that aim to make an example of or punish the defendant cannot be awarded. Aggravated damages may be awarded, however, if the court is satisfied that additional compensation is warranted due to the plaintiff having suffered exceptional harm as a consequence of the defamatory publication.

An apology or publication of a correction of the defamatory matter will be relevant to the mitigation of damages.

An award of costs will usually be made in favour of the successful party in any defamation action, subject to the court considering how the parties to the proceedings conducted their case.

FURTHER READING

Butson L, Shircore M, Butson B. A right to refuse: legal aspects of dealing with intoxicated patients who refuse treatment. *J Law Med.* 2013;20:542.

Callaghan S, Ryan CJ. Refusing medical treatment after attempted suicide: rethinking capacity and coercive treatment in light of the Kerrie Wooltorton case. *J Law Med.* 2011;18:811.

Chan J, Le Bel J, Webber L. The dollars and sense of restraint and seclusion. *J Law Med.* 2012;20:73.

George P. *Defamation Law in Australia.* Sydney, NSW: LexisNexis Butterworths; 2006.

McSherry B. Legal capacity under the Convention on the Rights of Persons with Disabilities. *J Law Med.* 2012;20:22.

Sullivan D. A new ball game: the United Nations Convention on the Rights of Persons with Disabilities and assumptions in care of people with dementia. *J Law Med.* 2012;20:28.

ENDNOTES

1. For example, see Aboriginal and Torres Strait Islander Health Practice Board of Australia, *Code of Conduct*; 2014. https://www.atsihealthpracticeboard.gov.au/Codes-Guidelines-Code-of-conduct.aspx. Accessed 27 March 2019.
2. Medical Board of Australia. *Good Medical Practice: A Code of Conduct for Doctors.* Melbourne, VIC: Medical Board of Australia;

2014. http://www.medicalboard.gov.au/Codes-Guidelines-Policies/Code-of-conduct.aspx. Accessed 22 June 2018.
3. Ibid. p. 3.3.
4. *Collins v Wilcock* [1984] 1 WLR 1172.
5. Allan S Health Law Central: Trespass to Person. http://www.healthlawcentral.com/decisions/trespass-person/. Accessed 22 June 2018.
6. *Hart v Herron* (1984) Aust Torts Reports 80–201.
7. *Symes v Mahon* [1922] SASR 447; *The Balmain New Ferry Co Ltd v Robertson* (1906) 4 CLR 379.
8. *Hart v Herron* (1984) Aust Torts Reports 80–201.
9. *Department of Health and Community Services (NT) v JWB (Marion's case)* (1992) 175 CLR 218.
10. See comments in *Marion's case* at 233 and in *Rogers v Whitaker* at 193. See also the more recent decisions of *Hunter and New England Area Health Service v A* (2009) 74 NSWLR 88; [2009] NSWSC 761 and *Brightwater Care Group (Inc) v Rossiter* (2009) 40 WAR 84; [2009] WASC 229, which have expressly acknowledged this point in the context of dealing with the refusal of life-sustaining treatment.
11. Allan S, Blake M. *Australian Health Law.* Sydney, NSW: LexisNexis Butterworths; 2018. [6.31]–[6.32].
12. See, for example, the case of *Ljubic v Armellin* [2009] ACTSC.
13. *Candutti v ACT Health and Community Care* [2003] ACTSC 95.
14. *Dean v Phung* [2012] NSW CA 223.
15. For examples of legislative definitions in this regard see *Guardianship Act 1987* (NSW) s 33(2); *Guardianship and Administration Act 2000* (Qld) Sch 4; *Powers of Attorney Act 1998* (Qld) Schedule 3; *Guardianship and Administration Act 1995* (Tas) s 36(2); *Guardianship and Administration Act 1986* (Vic) s 36(2).
16. South Australia has legislation specific to consent to medical treatment, which provides for medical powers of attorney: *Consent to Medical Treatment and Palliative Care Act 1995* (SA).
17. *Chatterton v Gerson* [1981] 1 All ER 257.
18. For example, see *Transplant and Anatomy Act 1978* (ACT) ss 8, 9; *Human Tissue Act 1983* (NSW) ss 23(3)(b), 21X; *Transplantation and Anatomy Act* (NT) s 8; *Transplantation and Anatomy Act 1979* (Qld) ss 10, 11; *Transplantation and Anatomy Act 1983* (SA) ss 9, 10; *Human Tissue Act 1985* (Tas) ss 7, 8; *Human Tissue Act 1982* (Vic) ss 7, 8; *Human Tissue and Transplantation Act 1982* (WA) ss 8, 9.
19. *Holland v Hardcastle* unreported, 16 December 1997, District Court of Western Australia, No. 970403.
20. *Law Reform Act 1995* (Qld); *Minors (Property and Contract) Act 1970* (NSW); *Age of Majority (Reduction) Act 1971* (SA); *Age of Majority Act 1973* (Tas); *Age of Majority Act 1977* (Vic); *Age of Majority Act 1972* (WA); *Age of Majority Act 1974* (ACT); *Age of Majority Act 1974* (NT).
21. *Gillick v West Norfolk and Wisbech Area Health Authority* [1986] AC 112.
22. *Children and Young People Act 2008* (ACT) ss 11, 12.
23. *Children and Young Persons (Care and Protection) Act 1998* (NSW) s 3.
24. *Children, Young Persons and Their Families Act 1997* (Tas) s 3.
25. *Secretary, Department of Health and Community Services v JWB and SMB (Marion's case)* (1992) 175 CLR 218. Note, the preceding

cases determined by the Family Law Court had not given a clear principle on the issue. In *Re a Teenager* (1989) FLC 92-006 and *Re S* (1990) FLC 92-124 the court held the parents of the respective children could give a valid consent. However, in *Re Jane* (1989) FLC 92-007 and *Re Elizabeth* (1989) FLC 92-023 the sterilisation of the child required a court order.

26. Skene L. *Law and Medical Practice: Rights, Duties, Claims and Defences.* Sydney, NSW: Butterworths; 1998. p. 83.

27. Wallace M. *Health Care and the Law.* 3rd ed. Sydney, NSW: Law Book Co; 2001. p. 79.

28. *T v T* [1988] FamD 2 WLR 189.

29. *Guardianship and Management of Property Act 1991* (ACT) s 32N; *Guardianship Act 1987* (NSW) s 37(1); *Emergency Medical Operations Act 1973* (NT) s 3(1); *Guardianship Act 2000* (Qld) ss 63, 64; *Consent to Medical Treatment and Palliative Care Act 1995* (SA) s 13(1); *Guardianship and Administration Act 1995* (Tas) ss 40, 41; *Guardianship and Administration Act 1986* (Vic) s 42A; *Guardianship and Administration Act 1990* (WA) s 110 ZI.

30. For example, see the *Guardianship and Administration Act 2000* (Qld) s 63.

31. *Transplantation and Anatomy Act 1978* (ACT); *Children and Young Persons (Care and Protection) Act 1998* (NSW); *Guardianship Act 1987* (NSW); *Transplantation and Anatomy Act 1989* (NT); *Emergency Medical Operations Act 1973* (NT); *Transplantation and Anatomy Act 1979* (Qld); *Consent to Medical Treatment and Palliative Care Act 1995* (SA); *Human Tissue Act 1985* (Tas); *Human Tissue Act 1982* (Vic); *Human Tissue and Transplantation Act 1982* (WA).

32. *Fontin v Katapodis* [1962] HCA 63.

33. *Defamation Act 2005* (NSW) ss 6–7; *Defamation Act 2006* (NT) ss 6–7; *Defamation Act 2005* (Qld) ss 6–7; *Defamation Act 2005* (SA) ss 6–7; *Defamation Act 2005* (Tas) ss 6–7; *Defamation Act 2005* (Vic) ss 6–7; *Defamation Act 2005* (WA) ss 6–7.

34. *Hutton v Jones* [1910] AC 20.

REVIEW QUESTIONS AND ACTIVITIES

1. Describe the legal elements necessary to establish a cause of action in trespass to person for (a) assault, (b) battery and (c) false imprisonment, and the possible defences that may be raised in answer to a claim.

2. Discuss ethical and legal principles relevant to consent to health care.

3. What considerations need to be had in relation to consent when the person who may receive treatment is a child?

4. Explain what must be proven to satisfy a cause of action in defamation and any defences that may be raised.

5. Provide examples of actions that may be considered defamatory within a healthcare setting. Would a clinical supervisor providing a negative report about their student's performance to their university be considered defamatory?

8 CRIMINAL LAW AND ISSUES RELATED TO HEALTH CARE

LEARNING OBJECTIVES

Upon completing this chapter you should be able to:

■ discuss the features that distinguish the criminal law from civil law

■ describe the elements of a crime

■ outline the features of homicide and discuss the circumstances in which healthcare delivery may be associated with homicide

■ discuss the law of assisted death and the meaning of the term euthanasia

■ identify areas of the law designed to protect the fetus.

INTRODUCTION

This chapter provides a basic introduction to the criminal law and the criminal law issues of importance to health practitioners, as opposed to the civil causes of action in negligence and the intentional torts of trespass to person and defamation covered in the preceding chapters. Notably, in criminal law, the State brings the action, while in civil cases an individual plaintiff brings the action. In addition, while civil law remedies often focus on compensation (or an order to stop engaging in a particular behaviour), the aim of criminal law is punishment, retribution, deterrence and rehabilitation. If a person is convicted of a crime, the result will be a penalty such as a prison sentence, fine, court order for probation or bond. The standard of proof in criminal cases is 'beyond reasonable doubt'.

While in everyday clinical practice health practitioners tend not to consider the criminal law, it is nevertheless relevant to matters that sometimes occur in healthcare settings. For example, it is important to understand the law of homicide in relation to euthanasia and the legal justification for administering large, potentially deadly quantities of morphine to a patient. Health practitioners should also be able to distinguish between conduct that lawfully assists patients and conduct that is illegal.

WHAT IS A CRIME?

When attempting to describe a crime, it is common to refer to activities that are considered 'wrong'. Hence, criminal acts are usually identified as activities that justify punishment. However, there are activities that are morally reprehensible but are not criminal. For example, watching a person drown would generally be considered morally wrong but would not amount to a crime in most jurisdictions of Australia.[1]

What is considered 'criminal' differs across time and from one society to another. Moreover, the type of activity incorporated into the criminal law is vast and ranges from serious harms such as murder to less serious harms such as traffic offences. Professor Glanville Williams provides a succinct definition of a crime: 'A crime (or offence) is a legal wrong that can be followed by criminal proceedings which may result in punishment'.[2]

The fact that the State enforces the criminal law reinforces the idea that crimes are public wrongs. This is in contrast with civil wrongs, which are generally considered to be private matters occurring between individuals or individual entities such as corporations.

A public wrong is an act that has a detrimental effect on the public and extends beyond private rights. Thus, criminal law determines the duties individuals owe to the entire community.

For many people, the fact that the activity is classified as a criminal offence may be sufficient to prevent their participation. However, the addition of punishment to criminal activity is considered an effective deterrent. Sanctions also provide respect for the law and allow criminal activity to be openly condemned. Criminal punishments are divided into two broad categories:

- custodial sentences, which include imprisonment or detention (e.g. in a psychiatric institution in the case of the criminally insane)
- non-custodial sentences, which include monetary penalties, supervised releases (such as probation), suspended sentences and community service orders or non-supervised releases such as good behaviour bonds.

SOURCES OF CRIMINAL LAW

The criminal law has developed over many centuries of English law and is firmly entrenched in the common law. During the 12th century, rules relating to serious offences were called felonies. During the 14th century, less serious offences evolved and were referred to as misdemeanours. Where there is legislation, many of the common law principles have been incorporated into the provisions.

Of the eight Australian jurisdictions, four have codified the criminal law. This is a process in which definitions of criminal activity and existing common law are written into legislation called a 'code'. The jurisdictions that have opted for codes are Queensland, the Northern Territory, Tasmania and Western Australia.[3] In the remaining jurisdictions (the Australian Capital Territory, New South Wales, South Australia and Victoria) the common law continues to exist together with legislation. When researching the law in these jurisdictions, it may be necessary to examine the criminal legislation and the common law. For example, in Victoria and South Australia the criminal legislation refers to the crime of murder; however, as the definition of murder is not stated, one must seek the definition in the common law.[4] This may be contrasted with New South Wales, which has included a statutory definition of murder in its *Crimes Act 1900*.[5]

FEATURES OF THE CRIMINAL LAW

Several features distinguish the criminal law from other areas of law, particularly the civil law. The features are grouped together and briefly introduced below:

- *Terminology related to the parties in a criminal offence.* The parties to a criminal action are known as the accused (the person who allegedly committed the crime), the prosecution (the police or the public prosecutor) and the offence (the defined criminal activity).
- *Initiation of the action.* The prosecution is responsible for initiating the action. The prosecution comprises the police force and the Department of Public Prosecutions. The burden rests with them to show, using the evidence collected, that the accused committed the crime. This is called the 'burden of proof'. Every aspect of the specific crime must be proven. For example, the offence of theft includes the removal of an object belonging to another, with the intention of permanently depriving the owner of it. Each component of the crime must be addressed by the prosecution (see 'Elements of a crime' below).
- *The standard of proof.* The prosecution must establish that the elements of the crime have been proven 'beyond reasonable doubt'. This is an onerous task for the prosecution. For example, there may be insufficient evidence or the evidence may be too reliant upon conjecture and suggestions regarding the surrounding circumstances. In civil cases the plaintiff must prove the case on the 'balance of probabilities' – that is, it was more probable than not that the actions of the defendant amounted to negligence. This is a much lower standard to prove compared with the criminal standard of 'beyond reasonable doubt'.
- *The presumption of innocence.* A fundamental principle in common law countries is that innocence is to be assumed unless guilt is proven by the prosecution or admitted by the accused.
- *Liability.* In civil law cases vicarious liability (see Chapter 6) ensures the employer is also responsible

and may be at fault, together with the person who created the damage, but the criminal law operates on an individual basis. Thus, in the criminal law, vicarious liability does not apply and the liability for the offence remains with the accused.

- *Ignorance of the law.* It is not acceptable for a person to argue that they were not aware of the law. As mentioned earlier, the criminal law is concerned with protecting society from public wrongs. To argue that one was not aware that the act was criminal will not prevent the possibility of guilt. Provided the prosecution can show that the accused intended to do the activity that they later discovered amounted to a crime, this will suffice.
- *Tried only once.* When a verdict has been reached by a court in a criminal matter, the accused cannot be tried again. This principle applies when the accused pleads guilty and sentence is passed or when the accused pleads not guilty and the court either acquits or finds the accused guilty of the crime. There must be a conclusion to the charge. This common law principle recognises that a person should not be punished more than once for the same offence.
- *A charge for an offence cannot be retrospective.* The specific crime must be established at law before a person can be charged with the offence. The accused cannot be charged and the crime then established at a later point in time.
- *Indictable and summary offences.* Most jurisdictions classify crimes, making a distinction between minor and major crimes. An offence that is listed as a summary offence is considered a minor breach of the law and covers violations including some traffic law breaches such as not wearing a seatbelt. Other public behaviour considered a summary offence includes shoplifting and less serious assault. Indictable offences are serious breaches of the criminal law and include serious assault, sexual offences and homicide. For many health practitioners a charge within the indictable offence class of crime can automatically affect professional registration and the consideration of a regulatory board for professional misconduct (see Chapter 4).

ELEMENTS OF A CRIME

The traditional approach to describing criminal liability is to address the two components that make up a crime. For a crime to be committed the accused must first have completed the activity or conduct that makes up the offence and, second, must have the intention referred to as the 'guilty' state of mind. The conduct is called the *actus reus* and the mental element of intention is known as the *mens rea*. Note, however, there are some crimes where only the *actus reus* needs to be proven (see 'Strict liability' below).

Actus Reus

Actus reus refers to the activity or conduct that constitutes the offence. It is often referred to as the physical act constituting the crime. A number of components are associated with the *actus reus*:

- *Voluntary.* It must be established that the act or conduct was voluntary or willingly carried out; that is, the conduct must be done with a conscious mind, and of the accused's own volition. If the act was done due to an involuntary muscle spasm or in a concussed or intoxicated state, it may be possible to argue it was involuntary.
- *Omission.* Failure to act may in some situations give rise to an *actus reus*. Liability in these cases will be dependent on the wording of the legislation – for example, the wilful neglect of a person by another who is responsible for their care. At common law, an omission may be relevant when the accused's omission includes a failure to act when a recognised duty exists or the accused has created a dangerous situation. In these situations an accused will be liable for an omission to act if they are under a legally recognised duty to do so. The duty to act may be implied and hence it is important to determine the existence of a recognised duty. In this situation the omission will be the relevant *actus reus*. The accused is meant to act as a reasonable person would in the circumstances, but not to endanger their own life.
- *Causation.* The causative component of the *actus reus* can be fulfilled only when a causal link between the conduct and the specific outcome can be established. For example, in homicide the conduct must be the cause of the death. If other

factors have contributed to the death then the question is whether the conduct of the accused amounts to a 'substantial' cause of the death. For example, V becomes involved in a fight and is hit on the head with an iron bar by A. V collapses and is taken to the hospital. He then falls from the transporting trolley and again hits his head. He later dies from a subarachnoid haemorrhage. For the causation factor to be satisfied to find A liable, it must be shown that the original blow to the head by A, not the fall from the trolley, was a contributory and substantial cause of V's death.

Mens Rea

Once the *actus reus* is determined the prosecution will need to establish the *mens rea* (the mental element). The mental element may include a variety of states such as intent, recklessness or negligence. Usually the mental element or 'guilty mind' is a subjective test; that is, the prosecution must establish that the accused deliberately performed the unlawful act. The guilty mind can include the accused's intention to undertake the unlawful conduct or that the accused's state of mind was 'reckless' as to the outcome of their conduct. A 'reckless' mental state refers to a high degree of reprehensible behaviour, which should be punished as if the conduct had been done with intent or knowledge.

CRIMINAL NEGLIGENCE

Where negligence occurs, and befits a particular crime, the prosecution does not have to establish the accused's state of mind. The *mens rea* is no longer a subjective test but becomes an objective one. Hence, it is sufficient to ask what would have been in the 'ordinary reasonable person's mind' at the time, rather than what was in the accused's mind. The conduct of the accused will then be compared with what is reasonable in the circumstances. If it can be shown that the conduct was a gross departure from that which would be considered reasonable, then a charge of criminal negligence may result.

STRICT LIABILITY

Offences known as strict liability offences occur when there is no requirement to establish the *mens rea*, it being sufficient to prove only the *actus reus*. Strict liability offences are commonly observed in motor traffic regulations where, for example, to drive without a seatbelt is an offence. The driver's *mens rea* does not have to be proven, merely that the driver's conduct or actions satisfied the *actus reus* of the offence. Within the healthcare context, occupational health and safety legislation contains examples of strict liability offences.

PARTIES TO OFFENCES: ACCOMPLICES

The person who has committed the offence is referred to as the principal, while the term 'accomplice' is a broad description that applies to people who take part in some way in the commission of the crime. The activity of the accomplice may include encouragement and facilitation to plan the offence, or assistance at the time the crime is committed or after the crime has occurred. A health practitioner may be charged as an accomplice if they assist in the removal of life support in circumstances where the principal is later charged with the murder of the patient.

To Aid, Abet, Counsel or Procure a Crime

The general rule is that accomplices who have some input before or during the commission of the criminal offence become parties to it and are, like the principal, subject to the maximum penalties. Someone who assists after the crime has been committed usually attracts a lesser penalty. To 'aid and abet' describes any conduct that contributes in some way to the commission of the offence – conduct that assists or incites the principal. This often includes the accomplice's presence at the scene of the offence. To 'counsel or procure' is to encourage and assist the bringing about of the offence. This often includes behaviour prior to the commission of the crime. The New South Wales Court of Criminal Appeal held that presence at the actual scene could be broadly interpreted in the following way:

> The concept of being 'present' is somewhat elastic; an accessory may be actually present (in the sense of being within sight and sound of the crime) or constructively present (in the sense of being sufficiently near as to be able to readily go to the assistance of the principal offender, should the occasion arise).[6]

In addition, for a health practitioner to supply materials or information for use in a crime could also render that professional an accomplice.

Omission to Act

To be an accomplice usually requires some type of positive activity; one is not usually considered to be an accomplice for a failure to prevent the offence from occurring. However, where a duty is owed to protect the victim from harm (either at common law or by legislation) and a person fails to do so, this may amount to assistance of the crime. In *R v Russell*,[7] a father stood and watched his wife drown their two children and then drown herself. The husband was held to be liable as an accessory for three counts of manslaughter. He could also have been found guilty of manslaughter by criminal negligence in that he failed to assist his wife and children when he had a common law responsibility to do so. By analogy, a health practitioner who fails to provide resuscitation when there is a duty to act may similarly be accused.

Intent to Assist

The accomplice's action must include in some way the intention of assisting or helping the principal to commit the crime. The intention to assist may be inferred by proof that the accomplice knew their activity would support the principal. If the accomplice's actions are reckless or negligent, this does not usually result in the person being charged as an accomplice, particularly if the accomplice is unaware of the circumstances that surround the principal's activities. Hence, the accomplice must knowingly aid the principal.

CRIMINAL LAW DEFENCES

An accused may raise several defences. They exist either at common law or are included in the relevant legislation.

Provocation

The defence of provocation is a partial defence in that it reduces what would normally be considered murder to the offence of manslaughter. It is therefore relevant to sentencing. The defence assumes that what would normally constitute the crime of murder is less blameworthy because the accused is 'transported by passion and was not master of himself or herself'.[8] The accused must argue, based on the evidence, that they were acting under provocation that would have had the same effect on a reasonable person standing in the accused's position. It is a controversial defence that, over time, has been amended or repealed in many states and territories because it was unintendedly used by men who had murdered other men in relation to non-violent sexual advances or murdered their partners due to possessiveness or sexual jealousy.

The defence of provocation has been abolished in Tasmania, Victoria and Western Australia. The Australian Capital Territory and the Northern Territory have amended the law to exclude non-violent sexual advance as a sufficient basis to raise the defence. New South Wales laws were amended in 2014 to refer to 'extreme provocation' and to require the accused to have been responding to conduct of the deceased that was an indictable offence;[9] non-violent sexual advance to the accused does not constitute extreme provocation.[10] In New South Wales the provocation does not need to have occurred immediately before death to allow the defence for victims of long-term abuse. In 2011 section 304(1) of Queensland's *Criminal Code*, which provided for the partial defence of provocation, was amended to reduce the scope of the defence.

Health practitioners would be expected to accommodate a broad range of patient behaviour. For example, when a patient is mentally impaired, the health practitioner would not be able to argue they assaulted a person seeking health care due to provocation.

Self-Defence

This is a defence that operates in the case of assault and murder. One person may be acting to fend off an attack from another person. The important issue is that the accused's response must be 'proportionate' to the attack or threatened attack. In other words, the accused must use no more force than is reasonable in the situation. This is measured by considering the entire circumstances surrounding the activity of self-defence, not merely making a judgment in hindsight. A health practitioner who punches an elderly, frail patient because the patient was shaking his fists is responding inappropriately and disproportionately and the defence would not be available.

Insanity

One significant purpose of the criminal law is to provide retribution. It has been recognised that if an accused is unable to understand the reason for the punishment then the role of retribution is redundant. If an accused claims insanity, the 'M'Naghten rule' (named after a case in England in which the defendant was M'Naghten) provides the basis for the defence.[11] To argue insanity successfully, the accused must demonstrate that they are suffering from a disease of the mind that gave rise to a defect of reason and that as a result they did not know the nature of the act or did not know that it was wrong. It has been argued that the test does not cover various forms of mental disorders including that of a psychopath (due, for example, to their not being delusional).[12] Furthermore, while a successful defence would result in a finding of not guilty, the accused may be indefinitely incarcerated in a psychiatric institution 'at the Governor's pleasure'. With the abolition of the death penalty this defence is less commonly argued; instead, other defences that affect the mind such as automatism or diminished responsibility may be argued.

Automatism

Automatism is where the state of mind of the accused is impaired for some reason – for example, due to the ingestion of alcohol or drugs. In such circumstances there is no link between the mind and the actions of the body. The defence relies on the argument that the accused did not act voluntarily. This is similar to an insanity plea in that the accused's state of mind is such that they were not aware of the nature or quality of the act or were unable to judge that it was wrong. Voluntariness in the defence of insanity is not the relevant issue. If automatism is successfully argued, it will result in a verdict of not guilty and a complete acquittal.

Diminished Responsibility

The common law defence of diminished responsibility is available in some jurisdictions.[13] It is available where the accused is charged with murder and has the effect, if successful, of reducing the offence to manslaughter. This defence was developed when the sentence for murder was a mandatory death sentence. Where it could be shown that the accused's state of mind was impaired to

an extent that it did not amount to insanity, a finding of diminished responsibility potentially resulted in a conviction and sentence. However, this would not be a death sentence. The justification for the defence was the need to recognise that the abnormal state of mind should be associated with a reduction in guilt or blameworthiness.

In *R v Byrne*,[14] an abnormality of the mind was considered to be 'a state of mind so different from that of ordinary human beings the reasonable man would term it abnormal'. This includes the inability to judge what is right or wrong or to form a rational judgment. It may include a mental illness; however, a person does not have to be mentally ill to argue the defence. Other examples include post-traumatic stress disorder, depression and neurosis.

HOMICIDE

Homicide refers to the killing of a person and includes murder, manslaughter and infanticide. There is considerable overlap between potential homicide and the withdrawal of medical treatment. It is useful to briefly consider the crimes of murder and manslaughter to enable the reader to identify healthcare activities that may amount to homicide. Ideally, health practitioners should have a clear grasp of the law in relation to both refusal of treatment (discussed in Chapter 12) and the law of homicide.

Murder

Murder is regarded as the most serious crime and usually attracts a longer penalty of imprisonment than any other. The earliest accepted common law definition of murder was stated by Sir Edward Coke in 1797. A modified version reads:

> *Murder is when a man of sound memory, and of the age of discretion, unlawfully kills … any reasonable creature in being, under the King's peace, with malice aforethought, either express or implied by law, so as the party wounded, or hurt … dies within a year and a day after the same.*[15]

The elements of this crime include the necessary *actus reus* (the act of killing) and the *mens rea* (the malice aforethought).

The additional features include the following.

- *Sound memory and age.* This requires the accused to have legal capacity in the sense that they are of sound mind and are of an age to understand the crime. The common law has held that a child under seven years of age is not capable of committing a crime. In several jurisdictions this has been raised to 10 years of age. The common law also requires that, until the child attains 14 years, the prosecution must show the accused knew that the act was wrong.
- *Unlawfully kills.* Before a person can be found guilty of homicide, there must be no lawful justification for the killing. While this would seem obvious, in nearly all situations killing will amount to homicide provided the other requirements are made out. The killing must be done without lawful justification. From a healthcare perspective, this could include actively assisting a patient to die, despite the intention to remove suffering.
- *The victim must be a reasonable creature 'in being'.* A fetus becomes a human being when it is born alive and is separate from its mother, although the umbilical cord may not have been cut. It is not murder if a fetus dies in utero because it is not recognised as a human being. If a child is born alive but later dies due to injuries inflicted in the antenatal period, then murder or manslaughter may be found. The crime of infanticide, in which special circumstances exist, also amounts to homicide.

In relation to death it is well recognised that patients can be artificially kept alive by life-support systems. The definition of death enables health practitioners to disconnect life-support machines once it is established that death (the irreversible cessation of circulation or brain function) has occurred. Thus, for the purposes of homicide, the health practitioner is not killing a 'human being'.

Manslaughter

The requirements necessary for a charge of murder are identical for a charge of manslaughter, with the exception of the mental element. It is the *mens rea* that distinguishes murder from the lesser crime of manslaughter.

Manslaughter is divided into two types:

- **Voluntary manslaughter** occurs when the accused intended to kill or cause serious harm but liability is reduced because of a relevant defence that provides some justification for the action. It does not matter that the accused did not foresee the possibility of death. The intention to create the serious harm is sufficient. For example, self-defence and provocation are defences that reduce an offence of murder to manslaughter.
- **Involuntary manslaughter** occurs when the accused was killed as a result of an unlawful or dangerous act, or is reckless or grossly negligent. The unlawful and dangerous act does not have to amount to a specific crime. For example, the unlawful administration of drugs, whereby a drug is administered without an appropriate order and death results, may be considered sufficient to establish involuntary manslaughter. The act must also be considered dangerous. What amounts to dangerous is not the subjective belief of the accused but rather an objective test of what a sober and reasonable person would consider to be dangerous. Diminished responsibility may also amount to involuntary manslaughter if the accused is suffering from a substantial mental impairment.

Negligent manslaughter occurs when the accused owes a duty to the victim and the accused's conduct significantly departs from the reasonable standard of care. In recklessness the accused is aware that their behaviour is justifiably risky but decides to continue with that activity anyway. To establish manslaughter by criminal negligence, the prosecution must show that the act was carried out by the accused voluntarily and consciously; there does not need to exist the intention of killing, but the actions must have fallen significantly short of the requisite standard of care a reasonable person would have exercised and involved a high degree of risk of death.

EUTHANASIA

The word 'euthanasia' is not a legally recognised word for the purposes of criminal law; there is no crime of euthanasia. The word loosely means 'good death', and while the definition of euthanasia can be broadly interpreted, the word has been used differently in varying contexts, which has led to confusion because some actions are legal and other actions or activities sit within the criminal law. For example, 'euthanasia' has been used to describe the death of a person who wishes to be helped to die or when a person is disconnected from a life-support machine. It has also been used in situations where patients refuse treatment and subsequently die.

Terms Used to Describe Euthanasia

For many people, 'euthanasia' pertains to the actual assistance given to patients to help them to die. However, for others, it is common parlance to refer to 'voluntary', 'involuntary', 'active' and 'passive' euthanasia.

Voluntary euthanasia usually refers to mentally competent patients who can make their own decisions regarding treatment and its refusal. In this situation a competent patient can refuse active treatment. However, unless legislative provision exists a person cannot request to be assisted to die; this would be considered 'assisted suicide' (see discussion below).

Non-voluntary euthanasia relates to situations where patients do not have legal capacity and life is terminated. It may be that the incompetent person, who now is unable to make a decision, previously indicated that treatment not be continued in certain circumstances (see Chapter 12).

Active euthanasia applies in situations where a patient wishes to die and requires active assistance, sometimes referred to as physician-assisted suicide. Conversely, **passive euthanasia** suggests treatment is omitted or withdrawn from the patient to allow death to occur.

Involuntary euthanasia is the decision to end a patient's life without or against their consent.

While these descriptions provide some idea of the various settings in which euthanasia may be considered, they are not particularly precise or exhaustive. For example, the difference between active and passive actions can be difficult to differentiate. Is switching off a life-support machine an active step or merely the passive withdrawal of futile treatment?

Distinguishing Euthanasia and Homicide

The varied uses of the word 'euthanasia' in the context of the criminal law and current healthcare practices often create confusion. There is also an absence of clear Australian judicial authority regarding acceptable practice. It is the intent to kill or cause serious bodily harm to another that forms the *mens rea* of murder. Neither the motive nor the reason behind the intention are supposed to be relevant. However, this reasoning has been distinguished from cases where the principle of 'double effect' has been argued. That is, it is not murder when the doctor's intention is to relieve pain, despite the fact that the pain-relieving drugs may hasten death.

Assisted Dying

The ability of competent patients to be assisted to end their life is legal in some parts of the world. Belgium, Luxembourg, Netherlands, Switzerland and the American states of Montana, Oregon, Vermont and Washington all permit assisted suicide or voluntary euthanasia. Organisations such as Dignitas (Switzerland), Dying with Dignity (UK) and Exit International (Australia) provide assistance for mentally competent people who wish to die. These organisations provide services to people who wish to control their time of death and be assisted to do so. For example, to utilise the services of Dignatas the necessary prerequisites must be met: the person must be of sound mind and must have either a terminal illness or unendurable incapacitating disability, or be in unbearable or uncontrollable pain. In addition, there must be a personal signed request stating the reasons for wanting to use the services of Dignitas, a detailed current medical report, together with two or three older reports and biographical information. Once the request is assessed there are further consultations required with the Swiss doctors.

Australia

Traditionally suicide, where a person intentionally takes their life, formed part of the criminal law. Where a person survived a suicide attempt, they were guilty of the crime of 'attempt'. Suicide is no longer a criminal offence, and legislation in several jurisdictions provides justification for a person who uses reasonable force to prevent a suicide.[16] Where two or more people agree and intend to take their lives at the same time, this is referred to as a 'suicide pact', and in three jurisdictions, while the conduct is an offence, a survivor cannot be charged with murder.[17] However, for health practitioners it is highly relevant that it is an offence in all Australian jurisdictions except Victoria to assist a person to commit suicide.[18]

Assisted suicide is any act that intentionally helps another person kill themselves – for example, by providing them with the means to do so (most commonly through prescribing a lethal medication). The last act is that of the patient. The term 'assisted dying' is more commonly used in recent dialogue, most usually in situations where the person being assisted is terminally ill.[19] The legislative provisions in relation to assisting in a suicide must be considered in light of the refusal of treatment requirements, discussed in Chapter 12.

Australia's first assisted dying legislation was the *Rights of the Terminally Ill Act 1995* (NT). It existed as law for less than a year before the federal government enacted legislation to overturn it, using its power under section 122 of the Constitution. The Northern Territory Act allowed doctors to assist their patients to die, provided certain requirements were fulfilled. A list of requirements had to be satisfied before the patient could be assisted by a doctor. For example, the patient had to be assessed by three doctors (one of whom had to be a psychiatrist), the patient had to be an adult, the illness had to be considered terminal and be causing severe pain, and specific aspects of consent, including a certificate and witnesses, were necessary requirements. There was also a timeframe, whereby the doctor could not assist before 48 hours from the time the patient had signed the certificate of request. The legislation provided that a doctor's actions in providing assistance could not be counted as homicide. During the relatively short period the law was in operation three people were assisted to die.

In Victoria, following the *Final Report of the Victorian Inquiry into End of Life Choices* in June 2016, the Andrews Government enacted the *Voluntary Assisted Dying Act 2017* (Vic). The law allows 'assisted dying' from June 2019, which involves the person seeking assistance being able to access a 'voluntary assisted dying substance' through a medical treatment process. The person seeking assistance is required to execute the 'death-causing' act. The person seeking to access voluntary assisted dying must have full decision-making capacity.[20] Section 6 of the Act provides for the circumstances under which a person can access voluntary assisted dying. These include that the person has:

- made a first and final request
- executed a written declaration to that effect
- been assessed as 'eligible for access' by two medical practitioners.

The eligibility criteria are set out in Part 2 of the Act and require that the person:

- be ordinarily resident in Victoria
- be over 18 years of age
- has been diagnosed with a disease, illness or medical condition that is incurable, advanced, progressive and will cause death
- is expected to die from that condition within a period not exceeding six months
- is suffering from the condition that cannot be relieved in a manner considered tolerable by the person.[21]

The six-month period may be extended to 12 months in the case of people who have been diagnosed with a neurodegenerative disease such as motor neurone disease.[22] The Act does not allow people to access the voluntary assisted dying scheme through the execution of an advance care directive; this is implicit in the requirement that the person must have current capacity when making the request.

Note that Victoria is the only jurisdiction in Australia with such legislation, and in other states and territories assisted dying may amount to an offence. For example, in the Queensland Supreme Court case of *R v Nielson*[23] a man travelled overseas to obtain a drug (Nembutal) to give to a friend to enable the friend to suicide. The friend took the medication and died soon afterwards. The court imposed a six-month custodial sentence. The court highlighted that the deceased was mistaken as to his actual illness (he was not terminally ill) and the accused had obtained a financial gain because the deceased had changed his will in favour of the accused.

Principle of 'Double Effect'

As mentioned above, the courts have recognised that where patients are terminally ill and require pain relief, the giving of large doses of analgesia, which will hasten death, does not necessarily amount to homicide. The basis for this was explained in *Bland's* case by Lord Goff of Chieveley:

[It is] the established rule that a doctor may, when caring for a patient who is dying of cancer, lawfully administer pain killing drugs despite the fact that he knows that an incidental effect of that application will be to abbreviate the patient's life. Such a decision may be properly made as part of the care of the living patient, in his best interests; and on this basis, the treatment will be lawful. Moreover, where the doctor's treatment of his patient is lawful, the patient's death will be regarded in law as exclusively caused by the injury or disease to which his condition is attributable.[24]

The treatment must be appropriate in the circumstances and not excessive. At times, the doses and combinations of drugs may well appear to be excessive; however, with the advent of palliative care programs, the drug regimens administered to relieve pain and suffering are unique to each individual. It would be the responsibility of the prosecution to show that the drug regimen was not reasonable or not in the patient's best interests. As for other types of care that may hasten death, the law has difficulty in establishing clear boundaries.

In Queensland, the *Criminal Code* through the insertion of section 282A, confirms that a person is not criminally responsible for providing palliative care to another person where the incidental effect of providing such care hastens the patient's death. The provisions of the section require the treatment and care to be given in good faith with 'reasonable' care and skill either by a doctor or on the written order of a doctor. The provision of palliative care is only 'reasonable' if it is in the context of good medical practice, which is defined as practice that recognises the ethical standards and practices of the medical profession in Australia.

CHILD DESTRUCTION AND FETICIDE

The criminal offence of child destruction exists in all Australian jurisdictions except New South Wales and Victoria. The offence involves the deliberate destruction of a fetus during the mid- to latter part of the pregnancy when the fetus is assumed to be advanced in gestational age. The offence is meant to ensure that the person responsible for destroying a mature fetus does not escape liability for homicide. It was created

to cover the situation in which the child is neither a fetus (whose destruction is an abortion) nor a legal person (whose destruction is murder).[25]

In the Northern Territory an offence exists for killing an unborn child, or for preventing a birth, where a person is about to birth a child.[26] The Australian Capital Territory, Western Australia and Queensland criminal codes also make it an offence to 'stop the child being born alive'[27] or, in Tasmania, 'to cause the death of a child which has not become a human being in such a manner that he would have been guilty of murder'.[28]

In these jurisdictions the focus of killing seems to be at the time the child is delivered. For example, in Queensland, section 313 of the Criminal Code (Qld) provides for a maximum penalty of life imprisonment for: (1) any person who prevents a child from being born alive when a female is about to be delivered of a child – if they commit an act or omission of such a nature that if the child had been born alive and then died, the person would be deemed to have unlawfully killed the child (noting the provision does not apply to cases of lawful termination of pregnancy); and (2) any person who unlawfully assaults a pregnant female and destroys the life of, or does grievous bodily harm to, or transmits a serious disease to, the child before its birth. (Note, the provisions do not apply in cases of lawful termination of pregnancy.)

In South Australia the separate offence of 'child destruction' is committed when a person 'destroys the life of a child capable of being born alive, by any wilful act, or unlawfully causing such child to die'.[29] There is recognition that the offence is not substantiated if a doctor acts in good faith for the purpose of preserving the life of the mother.

The legislation emphasises the deliberate intention of the person undertaking the act of 'destruction'. There is also some concern regarding the meaning of 'a child capable of being born alive'. The presumption is that the gestational age of a fetus capable of being born alive is 28 weeks or more. However, as medical knowledge of premature neonates is expanded, fetuses of less than 28 weeks' gestation will be capable of being born alive.

There has been no judicial interpretation of the above provisions in Australia, perhaps reflecting the lack of prosecution under these provisions.[30] The cause of action is most often mooted in relation to drug or drink drivers who cause car accidents resulting in the death of a child in utero, or a violent assault on a pregnant woman that causes the same. Some have argued the offence 'creates serious legal uncertainty as to what constitutes a lawful medical abortion; in essence, the maintenance of the offence may serve to make the lawful unlawful'.[31] However, there have been no prosecutions in relation to lawful medical abortion for child destruction.

Infanticide

Infanticide is an offence that relates to the killing of the newborn child by its mother. In any other situation the offence would be murder; however, it is considered that, in the specific situation of such a death, special circumstances may apply due to distress related to pregnancy, birth or puerperium. Specific statutory offences exist in New South Wales, Tasmania and Victoria.[32] If a child is born alive and then dies because of injuries that were inflicted by the mother, the special charge of infanticide is made.

Many jurisdictions have a similar offence known as 'concealment of birth'.[33] The features of the offence include the secret disposal of the body of a child and/ or the deliberate concealment of the birth. In any event, it would be possible to raise either offence against a mother who has killed her child, provided the woman has recently (the presumption is within 12 months) delivered her child and the child was capable of a separate existence from its mother (see also the section on child destruction on page 101).

ADDITIONAL CRIMINAL OFFENCES

Assault

For the purposes of the criminal law, while the difference between assault and battery exists, the legislation and the case law tend to no longer make the distinction. The criminal offence of assault generally includes both the threatened and the actual application of force to a person without their consent, whereas in the civil law, assault and battery remain separate actions. Refer to Chapter 7.

For the purpose of the criminal law, the offence must include *actus reus* and *mens rea*. *Actus reas* is the creation of apprehension in the mind of the victim of imminent physical violence and/or the actual application of force or touching of the victim. *Mens rea* includes the subjective test that the accused either intended to create fear in the mind of the victim or was reckless about whether fear and apprehension were created. If the apprehension is recklessly created, then it must be shown that the accused foresaw that it was 'possible' the victim would be fearful.

Within the healthcare setting this may occur when a health practitioner shouts at a patient in an abusive manner or threatens the patient under their care in order to obtain compliant behaviour. The touching, grabbing or striking of a patient with malice amounts to a criminal assault.

Not all situations will give rise to a successful claim of assault, as in the case where behaviour is recognised as being within the limits expected in ordinary social contact. For example, section 182(3) of the Tasmanian *Criminal Code* excludes from the crime of assault any act that is 'reasonably necessary for the common intercourse of life … and which is not disproportionate to the occasion'. This equates with the common law position.

One significant difference in the application of the criminal law relates to the seriousness of the assault. When the assault goes beyond the threat or application of force and involves actual harm, the criminal law has developed a number of categories of assault according to the degree of harm that may result – these include common assault, assault causing bodily harm, grievous bodily harm and wounding. **Common assault** would include the creation of apprehension or actual touching without the individual's consent. **Bodily harm** describes harm that is designed to interfere with the health of the victim and must be 'more than merely transient or trifling'.[34] **Grievous bodily harm** includes injuries of a very serious nature that are not fatal. Each offence has an *actus reus* and *mens rea* that must be satisfied, and the elements of each offence vary. There are also distinctions between the descriptive terms used to describe criminal assault in the legislation of each state and territory.

Rape

The law in this area is complex and has been in the process of reform for some decades. The original common law definition of rape and the application of the law were particularly narrow. First, only a woman could be raped; this excluded rape as a crime in relation to men. Second, rape within marriage was not recognised as a crime and the *actus reus* of the offence was limited to penetration of the penis into the vagina. Modern expectations have broadened the offence to include the possibility of males or females as victims, together with somewhat broader definitions in most jurisdictions to include 'female genitalia' and other orifices such as the mouth and anus. Some jurisdictions have included the offence of rape together with other offences of a sexual nature and collectively called them 'sexual offences'.

What is of particular note is the requirement of consent, which remains an intrinsic part of the *mens rea*, *actus reus* and surrounding circumstances for rape and sexual assault. The act must occur without the consent of the complainant, and the consent to participate in the sexual activity may be withdrawn at any time. Courts will attach significance to the complainant's conduct to ascertain whether consent was given. Much of the law reform has aimed at modifying presumptions that inactivity or passivity equate to consent.

While the codified states do not require proof of *mens rea* for rape, the defence of 'honest and reasonable mistake' is available to the accused. Mobilio's case (see below) highlighted the need to reform the law in relation to consent to treatment and the provision of care where the professional's intention was questionable.

FRAUDULENT CONSENT AND THE PROVISION OF HEALTH CARE – MOBILIO'S CASE

Mobilio was a radiographer who was convicted of three counts of rape in 1991 after he conducted internal ultrasounds on women fraudulently. It was argued that the women had apparently consented in that they did not refuse the internal examination. The prosecution argued their consents were not 'real' because each woman consented for diagnostic purposes and Mobilio had introduced the transducer solely for his own gratification. The referring doctors in each of the cases had requested that their patients undergo external ultrasound examinations. It was not considered necessary, nor was it requested, that an internal ultrasound be conducted for the purpose of confirming a diagnosis.

The Court of Criminal Appeal overturned the conviction.[35] The court took a very narrow approach as to what constituted consent in this particular situation. The women consented to introducing the transducer into their vaginas, and this was considered by the court to amount to consent. The fact the accused may have undertaken the act with

a different intention to that of the women's understanding was considered irrelevant.

Subsequently, the Victorian law was amended to provide clarification and to avoid a repeat of the Mobilio situation. The legislation provides that where a woman's consent is induced by fraud as to the medical nature of that activity, the consent is invalid.

Current Categories of Rape

The common law, together with statutory modification in many jurisdictions, includes circumstances where a person does not freely agree to an act. These include where:

- the person submits through force, fear or unlawful detention
- a person is unconscious or incapable of understanding the sexual nature of the act, or
- a person is mistaken about the sexual nature of the act or mistaken about the medical or hygienic purpose of the act.[36]

For health practitioners, clear, detailed and accurate communication to ensure consent is obtained and justification of the activity on diagnostic and medical grounds will be relevant considerations of whether there has been a sexual assault.

Female Genital Mutilation

Several Australian jurisdictions have introduced the offence of female genital mutilation into the criminal law.[37] In Victoria, for example, the enactment of the *Crimes (Female Genital Mutilation) Act 1996* criminalises unacceptable circumcision practices on female children. The legislation expressly prohibits a number of practices including: the removal or cutting of the clitoral hood or any part of the genital area (excise); stitching up of the genital area (infibulate) of a girl or female baby; or cutting the clitoris or damaging the female genital area in any other way.

While the legislation is specific to Victoria, it provides that when the baby or child lives in Victoria, it is illegal to have female genital mutilation performed on her in another country or another part of Australia. Penalties are directed to the person who performs the procedure or arranges for someone else to perform the procedure. Female genital mutilation constitutes child abuse in

Victoria, and many health practitioners would be mandated to report the injuries (see Chapter 16).

FURTHER READING

King M. Non-adversarial justice and the coroner's court: a proposed therapeutic, restorative, problem solving model. *J Law Med.* 2008;16:442–57.

Lu Oam D, McKenna J. Recent coronial comments on the physical restraint of mental health patients. *Aust Health Law Bull.* 2013;21(5):353–5.

Marino G. NSW coronial inquest into the death of Michael Sutherland – the pitfalls of a lack of empathy. *Aust Health Law Bull.* 2011;19(9):138–41.

Oam A, Harris C. When time is of the essence – inquest into the death of Veronica Campbell. *Aust Health Law Bull.* 2011;19(4):58–61.

ENDNOTES

1. Failing to help a person in danger is a crime in the Northern Territory. Clause 155 of the *Criminal Code Act* imposes a general duty to rescue, stating that any person who is able to provide rescue, resuscitation, medical treatment, first aid or succour of any kind to a person who is urgently in need of it and whose life may be endangered but 'callously fails to act' is committing an offence. The maximum penalty is seven years' imprisonment.

2. Williams G. *Textbook of Criminal Law.* 2nd ed. London, UK: Stevens and Sons; 1983, p. 27.

3. *Criminal Code Act 1983* (NT); *Criminal Code 1899* (Qld); *Criminal Code Act 1924* (Tas); *Criminal Code of Western Australia 1913* (WA).

4. *Criminal Law Consolidation Act 1935* (SA) s 11; *Crimes Act 1958* (Vic) s 3.

5. *Crimes Act 1900* (NSW) s 18.

6. *R v McCarthy and Ryan* (1993) 71 A Crim R 395 at 409.

7. *R v Russell* (1933) VLR 59.

8. Waller L, Williams C. *Criminal Law: Text and Cases.* 8th ed. Sydney, NSW: Butterworths; 1997, p. 472.

9. *Crimes Act 1900* (NSW) s 23(2)(b).

10. Ibid. s 23(3)(a).

11. M'Naghten, who suffered from delusions of persecution (and likely had schizophrenia), had hatched a plan to shoot a Mr Peel, but the plan failed when he mistakenly shot Edward Drummond, Peel's secretary, who later died from the bullet wound. M'Naghten was charged with murder, which carried the death penalty. His defence was that he was suffering from a mental illness. He escaped the murder charge and was committed to a 'lunatic asylum' where he died at age 52 from diabetes. The M'Naghten case is one of the most influential in relation to criminal insanity and has been discussed and applied in courts all over the world.

12. Barnes SD. Psychopaths and Insanity: Law, Ethics, Cognitive Neuroscience and Criminal Responsibility. PhD thesis. Manchester, UK: University of Manchester; 2014.

13. *Crimes Act 1900* (ACT) s 14; *Crimes Act 1900* (NSW) s 23A; *Criminal Code 1899* (Qld) s 304A.

14. *R v Byrne* (1960) 2 QB 396.

15. Coke E. *Coke's Institutes of the Laws of England.* vol. 7. London, UK: E & R Brooke; 1794.

16. For example, the *Crimes Act 1958* (Vic) s 463(B).

17. Note in New South Wales that section 31B of the *Crimes Act 1990* provides the survivor is not to be charged with murder or manslaughter; however, may be charged under section 31C (aiding). See also Victoria (*Crimes Act 1958* s 6B(1), (1A)) and South Australia (*Criminal Law Consolidation Act 1935* s 13A(3)).

18. *Crimes Act 1900* (NSW) s 31C; *Criminal Code 1899* (Qld) s 311; *Criminal Law Consolidation Act 1935* (SA) s 13A(5); *Criminal Code* (Tas) s 163; *Crimes Act 1958* (Vic) s 6B(2); *Criminal Code 1913* (WA) s 288; *Crimes Act 1900* (ACT) s 17; *Criminal Code 1983* (NT) s 168.

19. See, for example, Lewis P. *Assisted Dying and Legal Change.* Oxford, UK: Oxford University Press; 2007.

20. *Voluntary Assisted Dying Act 2017* (Vic) s 4.

21. Ibid. s 9.

22. Ibid. s 9(4).

23. *R v Nielson* [2012] QSC 29.

24. *Airedale National Health Service Trust v Bland* (1993) 1 All ER 821.

25. McIlwraith J, Madden B. *Healthcare and the Law.* Pyrmont, NSW: Thomson Reuters; 2010, p. 537.

26. *Criminal Code Act 1983* (NT) s 170.

27. *Crimes Act 1900* (ACT) s 42; *Criminal Code Act 1995* (Qld) s 100; *Criminal Code 1913* (WA) s 290.

28. *Criminal Code Act 1924* (Tas) s 290.

29. *Criminal Law Consolidation Act 1935* (SA) s 82.

30. Allan S, Blake M; 2018.

31. Rankin MJ. The offence of child destruction: issues for medical abortion. *Syd Law Rev.* 2013;35(1):1–26.

32. *Crimes Act 1900* (NSW) s 22A; *Criminal Code Act 1924* (Tas) s 165A; *Crimes Act 1958* (Vic) s 6.

33. For example, *Criminal Law Consolidation Act 1935* (SA) s 83; *Criminal Code Act 1924* (Tas) s 166; *Crimes Act 1900* (NSW) s 85; *Crimes Act 1900* (ACT) s 45.

34. *R v Donovan* (1934) KB 498.

35. *R v Mobilio* (1991) 1 VR 339.

36. Bronitt S. The direction of rape law in Australia: toward a positive consent standard. *Crim Law J.* 1992;18:249–253. Reproduced with permission of Thomson Reuters (Professional) Australia Limited, legal.thomsonreuters.com.au.

37. *Crimes Act 1900* (ACT) ss 92V–Z; *Crimes (Female Genital Mutilation) Amendment Act 1994* (NSW); *Criminal Code Act 1983* (NT) ss 186A–D; *Criminal Law Consolidation Act 1935* (SA) s 33; *Children's Protection Act 1993* (SA) ss 26A–B, 27; *Crimes (Female Genital Mutilation) Act 1996* (Vic).

REVIEW QUESTIONS AND ACTIVITIES

1. Outline four distinguishing features of the criminal law.

2. Describe the terms *mens rea* and *actus reus*.

3. What is the difference between euthanasia and homicide?

4. Discuss the differences between murder and manslaughter. Identify clinical practice examples that could lead to a charge of either crime.

5. Discuss the criminal, civil and professional ramifications for sexual misconduct or rape of a person by a health practitioner.

6. What crimes exist to protect an unborn or newly born child?

7. Discuss laws relevant to genital mutilation.

Section 3   MATTERS OF LIFE AND DEATH

9 REGISTRATION OF BIRTHS AND DEATHS AND THE CORONERS COURT

LEARNING OBJECTIVES

Upon completing this chapter you should be able to:

- identify why the registration of births is important and the purposes it serves
- identify the agency responsible for recording births and deaths in your jurisdiction
- outline the requirements for registering births and deaths across Australia
- identify the functions of the coroner
- describe the distinguishing features of the Coroners Court.

INTRODUCTION

The previous chapters have introduced key areas of ethics and law relevant to the regulation and practice of health care in Australia. This chapter examines the law regarding notification and registration of births and deaths in the respective states and territories. It also identifies the role and function of the coroner in relation to health care. The Coroners Court ('Coroner's Court' in some jurisdictions) is the court most commonly visited by health practitioners who appear as witnesses. It requires particular attention because it is a specialised court that functions quite differently from other courts in the Australian hierarchy.

NOTIFICATION AND REGISTRATION OF BIRTHS AND DEATHS

The notification and registration of births plays an integral role in supporting a child to gain access to

schools, health care, legal protection and legal standing.[1] It may also serve as a tool to prevent child exploitation, enabling authorities to be aware of children in existence. The notification and registration of births and deaths also provides an avenue to collect vital statistics about the health and longevity of people – serving an important public health function by providing a basis for planning, implementing and monitoring health policies and programs.[2]

Each state and territory of Australia has laws that establish a register of births, deaths and marriages.[3] The Registrar of Births, Deaths and Marriages is the central authority in each jurisdiction that keeps records of all births, deaths, marriages and adoptions. Health practitioners working in particular practice environments have a responsibility to report appropriate information regarding these events.

Births

Birth notification and registration is the process by which a child's birth is recorded on a civil register held and maintained by the Registrar of Births, Deaths and Marriages. It includes entry onto the register of the date and place a child's birth occurred, the names of the parents and the name and sex of the child. Registration of births and stillbirths[4] in all states and territories is compulsory.

The 'person responsible' for notification of the birth is the chief executive officer of the hospital.[5] Where the birth occurred outside a hospital the responsibility lies with the doctor or midwife who attended the birth. Notification must be in the prescribed form.[6] The parents of the child would subsequently 'register' the birth by also filling in a birth registration form and supplying it to the relevant state/territory births, deaths and marriages register within a designated timeframe.

There is a specified time limit within which a birth is required to be notified by the 'person responsible' to the Registrar of Births, Deaths and Marriages and then subsequently registered by the parents (although provision is made for late registrations). Table 9.1 sets out the laws and timeframes for birth notification in each jurisdiction relevant to when a child is born in a hospital.

Doctors must also certify stillbirths. A **stillbirth** is defined as a child who is of at least 20 weeks' gestation (22 weeks in the Australian Capital Territory) or weight of at least 400 grams (500 grams in the Australian Capital

Territory) and who has not breathed (New South Wales, the Northern Territory, South Australia, Victoria) and/or has had no heartbeat (New South Wales, the Northern Territory, Queensland, South Australia, Tasmania, Victoria) after delivery. The registration is to be completed in the same manner as if the child had been born alive, except in Tasmania where the registration is completed as a perinatal death (see further below) and Queensland[7] where it is recorded as a death.

In Victoria sections 43 and 44 of the *Child Wellbeing and Safety Act 2005* also require notification of the birth within 48 hours to the municipal district in which the mother of the child usually resides (or where the birth takes place if unknown). Notification is intended to ensure that the local maternal and child health centre is aware of the birth and can monitor and assist with the child's health needs after birth.

Perinatal Data Collection

The registration and notification of births and perinatal data can facilitate:

- research into the incidence and causes of maternal deaths, stillbirths and the deaths of children
- research into the incidence and causes of obstetric and paediatric morbidity
- a perinatal data collection to collect, study and research information on births
- research into perinatal health, birth defects and disability
- planning of neonatal care
- research into the epidemiology of birth defects and disability.

It also makes available information to health service providers about obstetrics and paediatrics, enabling them to develop strategies to improve obstetric and paediatric care.

The National Perinatal Data Collection is a national population-based cross-sectional collection of data on pregnancy and childbirth. The data is based on births reported to the perinatal data collection in each state and territory in Australia. Midwives and other birth attendants complete notification forms for each birth using information obtained from mothers and from hospital or other records. A standard de-identified extract is provided to the Australian Institute of Health and Welfare annually.

TABLE 9.1

Birth Notification Requirements in Australian States and Territories (Relevant to Health Professionals)

Jurisdiction	Legislation	Timeframe
Australian Capital Territory	*Births, Deaths and Marriages Registration Act 1997* ss 5–11	7 days (live birth), 48 hours (stillbirth) – s 5
New South Wales	*Births, Deaths and Marriages Registration Act 1995* ss 12–16	7 days (live birth), 48 hours (stillbirth) – s 12
Northern Territory	*Births, Deaths and Marriages Registration Act 1996* ss 13–21	10 days (live birth and stillbirth) – s 12
Queensland	*Births, Deaths and Marriages Registration Act 2003* ss 5–14	2 working days (live birth; stillbirth notified as a death) – s 5
South Australia	*Births, Deaths and Marriages Registration Act 1996* ss 12–17	7 days (live birth), 48 hours (stillbirth) – s 12
Tasmania	*Births, Deaths and Marriages Registration Act 1999* s 11–18	21 days (live birth; stillbirth notified as a perinatal death) – s 11
Victoria	*Births, Deaths and Marriages Registration Act 1996* ss 12–15	21 days (live birth), 48 hours (stillbirth) – s 12
Western Australia	*Births, Deaths and Marriages Registration Act 1998* ss 12–16	1 month (live birth and stillbirth) – s 12

There are also state/territory-based units that monitor births and conduct the above studies, research and investigations. The law may require reporting to such units in addition to the notification made to the Registrar of Births, Deaths and Marriages. For example, sections 44–48 of the *Public Health and Wellbeing Act 2008* (Vic) requires reporting of all births to the Consultative Council on Obstetric and Paediatric Mortality and Morbidity. In Western Australia the *Health Act 1911* requires this data to be reported within 48 hours of the birth to the Maternal and Child Health Unit within the state health department.

Children Born Ex-nuptially

If the child is born outside of marriage, then the father's details must be recorded in accordance with the legislation. In these circumstances, usually information about the father is recorded when there is a joint request of the mother and father of the child, or a request by the father with the mother's consent, or when there is a court order.[8]

Change of Sex

In each jurisdiction of Australia the law allows for a person who has undergone sexual reassignment surgery to apply to the registrar to register a change of his or her sex.[9] Parents may also apply to the registrar to register a change in sex when the sex of a newborn baby is ambiguous and the child later has surgery to give the child the physical appearance of a male or female child.[10]

Definition of Death

Death is a necessary requirement to be formally identified and then confirmed before many activities can occur. For example, death is a necessary condition before certain sections of the human tissue legislation is invoked (see Chapter 13); it is also necessary before a body can be buried or before a criminal charge, such as murder (see Chapter 8), can be made.

A person may be considered legally dead when there is irreversible cessation of all function of the person's brain or irreversible cessation of circulation of blood in the person's body. Such a death may need to be certified by one or more medical practitioners.

When a medical practitioner is not immediately available to verify or certify a death, a person with relevant expertise to competently undertake a clinical assessment of a body may 'verify death'. For example, an appropriately qualified registered nurse or a paramedic may in the course of their work verify death following clinical assessment that finds a minimum of: no palpable carotid pulse; no heart sounds heard for two minutes; no breath sounds heard for two minutes; fixed (non-responsive to light) and dilated pupils; no response to centralised stimulus (e.g. trapezius muscle squeeze, supraorbital pressure, mandibular pressure or the common sternal rub); *and* no motor (withdrawal) response or facial grimace in response to painful stimulus (e.g. pinching the inner aspect of the elbow).[11] Appropriate documentation of the 'verification of death' should include the verifier's name and professional title, the clinical determinants used, the date, the time and where the clinical assessment took place.

Note, legislative definitions of death refer to all brain function, not merely a part or portion of the brain or the patient's absence of response. Therefore, before the decision is made to turn off life-support machines, a clear diagnosis must be made. In this regard it is important to distinguish between altered states of consciousness such as a persistent vegetative state or Guillain-Barré syndrome, where people are not 'brain dead' despite an inability to respond or communicate. People in a permanent vegetative state, for example, may not have a functioning cortex; however, the brain stem continues to function, preserving the cardiac and respiratory systems. People with late-stage Guillain-Barré syndrome have damaged myeloid sheaths, resulting in an absence of conductivity in the nerves, which effectively disconnects the brain from other body parts. The brain continues to function; however, the patient is unable to respond in any way.

All health practitioners involved in the person's treatment should be made aware of the person's condition so as to avoid confusion.

The Registration of Deaths

The registration of deaths provides not only records about people living or deceased but vital statistics about the health and longevity of people. Deaths are registered on the Death Register in the state/territory where the death occurred. This includes where the death occurs in an aircraft in the airspace of a specific jurisdiction. As mentioned above, in some states and the Australian

Capital Territory, 'death' does not include a stillbirth, which is registered separately.

Perinatal Death

Perinatal death occurs when a child is born alive but dies within 28 days after the birth. The certification and notification of a perinatal death are the same as the requirement for notification of death of all people.

Obligation to Notify the Registrar of a Death

There are obligations imposed on certain people to notify the Registrar of Births, Deaths and Marriages of the death. The groups or classes of people with a duty vary between jurisdictions but may include doctors, coroners, funeral directors and the occupier of the premises where the death occurred. The deceased's name, age, sex, marital status, date of birth, parentage and occupation are recorded. In addition the place and time of death and, in some jurisdictions, whether the deceased was of Aboriginal or Torres Strait Islander descent must be completed.[12]

Death certificates in Australia comprise two separate forms: a medical certificate indicating the cause of death and a questionnaire with personal information about the deceased. The medical certificate is completed by the medical practitioner who was either in attendance at the time of death or can certify the cause of death, or the coroner. A questionnaire is completed by the next of kin, usually with the assistance of a funeral director.

THE CORONER

The Coroners Court forms part of the court hierarchy in all Australian jurisdictions (see Chapter 1) and is the most likely court health practitioners will attend at some point in their careers. Traditionally, the role of the coroner in Australia has followed the English model, concentrating on identifying the deceased.

The significance of the coroner lies in the power, inherent in the relevant legislation, to hold public hearings on 'reportable' deaths (inquests) in which public issues can be considered. Since the 1980s the role has expanded to include features from the American equivalent, where the emphasis is on the investigation to determine the cause of death.

Coroners in Australia are usually magistrates who rely on their own legal background and understanding of the issues, in addition to the expertise provided by specialist investigators such as police, scientists, forensic pathologists, aviation investigators, industrial investigators and so on. The courts and the role of the coroner are established by legislation in all jurisdictions and have significant features not seen in other courts. It is for these reasons that the role and function of the coroner requires attention here.

Functions of the Coroner

The coroner's role and functions vary by jurisdiction; however, primarily the office of the coroner is established to provide a means of investigating certain situations where death results to identify impropriety or negligent activity. The coroner's principal task is to investigate deaths that are unexpected, unnatural, accidental or violent. These are called 'reportable deaths' and they must be reported to the coroner.

The coronial process enables the registration of the cause of death, in accordance with state/territory regulation, and the lawful disposal of the body of the deceased person. Moreover, the coroner is to determine whether there are public health or safety issues arising from the death and whether any action is required to prevent deaths in similar circumstances.[13] This is evident in comments or recommendations made by coroners. For example, if a defective product has caused the death, the coroner might make recommendations concerning the availability or manufacture of that product. The outcome of the coronial process enables some explanation concerning the death, and this can provide the bereaved with an opportunity for closure.[14]

Coroners are charged with the authority to investigate the identity of the deceased, the manner the death occurred and the cause of the death.[15] Such wide investigatory power often identifies individuals who have been involved with the death, including health practitioners. Since 2005 Victorian legislation also provides that where there has been a second or subsequent death of a child in a family, this death is termed a 'reviewable death' and must be reported to the state coroner.[16]

One feature that distinguishes the Coroners Court from others is that it is designed to be inquisitorial rather than adversarial. The coroner is not concerned with two or more parties arguing their case, with one party a 'winner' and the other a 'loser'. Instead, the coroner engages in a detailed investigation, drawing together the facts through examining the pertinent scientific data and calling witnesses the coroner considers relevant to the inquiry. The coroner's findings include recommendations about changes in practice or standards, where necessary.

There is also some degree of communication with other agencies. For example, should a health practitioner's conduct be of concern to the coroner, it is likely the professional regulatory authority, such as the Nurses Board or the Medical Board, may be sent the coroner's report. Note, there is no uniform national system that reports whether coronial recommendations have been considered or indeed implemented by responsible government or statutory agencies. In 2009 Victoria was the first state to mandate responses to coronial recommendations. Where a coroner has made recommendations to any minister or public statutory authority or 'entity', they will be required to provide a written response to the coroner's recommendations within three months, specifying any action that has or will be taken.[17]

The Coroners Court is not bound by the rules of evidence, as are other courts, and may conduct the inquiry in any manner it sees fit. This might include admitting evidence that would not be admissible in other courts or asking questions of witnesses whenever the coroner considers it necessary. It is for this reason that a coroner may not make a conclusive finding of guilt; rather the coroner may find that a person has contributed to a death.

Moreover, because of the power to conduct the inquiry in any manner the coroner thinks fit, information used by the coroner cannot automatically be used in another court to 'prove' negligence. However, a coronial inquest might unearth information that could be admissible in another court and may provide relatives of the deceased with some idea of any negligent activity. Therefore, when deaths involving health practitioners occur in healthcare settings, coronial findings may give rise to subsequent legal actions including disciplinary hearings, possible actions in negligence or criminal charges being made once the responsible authorities have undertaken independent investigations to gather evidence.

Reportable Deaths

As mentioned, the category of death that must be conveyed to the coroner is referred to as a 'reportable death'. This varies between jurisdictions but generally includes accidental, unnatural, unexpected, sudden or violent deaths and, in some states, fires, which raise community issues. Reference is made to deaths that take place in certain settings such as deaths that:

- occur while under or as a result of an anaesthetic
- were not reasonably expected to be the outcome of a health procedure
- occur in a prison, in a mental health facility or in state care.[18]

A death is also reportable when the deceased's identity is unknown or where there is no signed death certificate.

There is some discretion for the coroner or state/territory health minister to decide that an investigation is required. In many jurisdictions (except South Australia and Western Australia) relatives of a deceased may request the coroner's involvement.

In some states, when a death is 'reportable' it is the responsibility of *any* person with knowledge of the death to report it. In other situations the attending doctor or, in a hospital setting, the hospital administration is responsible.[19] The coroner's office or the police may be notified of the death. If the deceased is to have organs procured (for transplantation; see Chapter 13) and it is a 'reportable death', the coroner's consent is required.

Health practitioners should be aware of the specific documentation required to certify death and the necessary preparation of the body. Most agencies have guidelines in place for preparing the body when it is reportable. Usually, minimum interference with the body is the guiding principle in these situations. All tubing, including endotracheal tubes, central/intravenous lines, urinary catheters and drain tubes are usually left in situ. They may be cut and tied or the entire tubing placed into appropriate containers and kept with the body.

Coronial Inquests

An inquest provides a public forum to consider issues arising from the death. The coroner has the discretion to hold an inquest in cases where it is not mandatory to do so. Many cases are disposed of without an inquest.

The inquest is a public hearing with the main purpose being to obtain facts and provide a public forum for considering public issues. Thus, if there are no public health and safety issues to consider and there is sufficient uncontested evidence in the witnesses' statements then a public hearing is not necessary.

Should a health practitioner be required to attend and give evidence, preparation and procedure apply as for other court proceedings. It is advisable for health practitioners to seek legal advice from their professional indemnity insurer, their employer or a privately engaged lawyer. Police working at the coroner's office will usually require statements (in writing) regarding the health practitioner's role in the circumstances surrounding the death. Note, many professional organisations have guidelines for preparing statements for members, and these should be consulted. The patient's file may need to be examined to refresh the health practitioner's memory; any notes made independently at the time should be reviewed before a statement is made. The statement contributes to the coroner's investigation and a decision is made as to the need for the health practitioner to attend the court as a witness. If attending court, health practitioners must then decide whether they require legal representation (see Chapter 17).

Postmortem/Autopsy

The phrase 'postmortem examination' is often used interchangeably with the word 'autopsy'. However, a postmortem examination often refers to any analysis of past events or circumstances and is not confined to the scientific examination of a cadaver. All Australian coroners have statutory power to direct a doctor or other qualified person to perform an autopsy. It is only in the Tasmanian, Western Australian and Victorian Acts that reference is made to a 'pathologist'.[20] A pathologist is a medical practitioner who has undertaken a further five years of postgraduate education in the area of disease processes.

There are two categories of autopsy: the hospital autopsy, which is performed with the consent of the relatives; and the medicolegal autopsy, which is performed at the request of the coroner or another authority. The purpose of the procedure is to determine the cause of death and whether there are any pre-existing medical conditions or other relevant information that contributes to an understanding of how the death

occurred. In practice, an autopsy involves a detailed examination of the deceased person's body. However, not every postmortem examination will involve such a detailed examination; taking a small sample of tissue may be all that is requested.

The coroner can direct that the body be taken to a specified place for the postmortem and instruct independent pathologists to undertake the examination. This may be required if the death occurred in a hospital.

Relatives can object to an order for an autopsy, although the extent to which their objections will be considered is unclear. It is important that health practitioners allay anxiety and concern of relatives who do not have an understanding of the process. As many objections are based on religious beliefs, it is essential that qualified professionals are aware of the differing religious and cultural attitudes to autopsy.[21]

Ownership of the Body

When the coroner's office has completed its investigation, the body of the deceased can be released to allow for it to be disposed of properly. A legal claim to a body for the purposes of burial or cremation rests with the executor who has been appointed in the deceased person's will. In cases where no will exists, the deceased is 'intestate' (without a will), and the right vests in the person who is entitled to obtain letters of administration.

Review of the Coroner's Finding Regarding Professional Practice

In terms of the court hierarchy, the Coroners Court is aligned with the Magistrates' Court (also called the Court of Petty Sessions or Local Court) at the lower end of the court spectrum. Nevertheless, decisions of the Coroners Court are important because they frequently highlight healthcare practice issues. Coronial findings relating to professionals, particularly where they have been adverse, have been challenged in superior courts in a bid to have them overturned.

In the case of *Secretary to the Department of Health & Community Services, Schultz and Moreland v Gurvich*,[22] two registered nurses applied for a declaration to overturn the coroner's finding that they had contributed to the death of a mentally ill patient. In this case, the nurses attended the man at a police station at the request of the police. A police surgeon also attended. The police surgeon had administered a sedative to the man and then stayed to examine him. The nurses left the station to return to the hospital in readiness for the imminent admission of the man. During the nurses' time at the police station, one of them had suggested an ambulance be used as transport, but this was dismissed by one of the police officers. At the doctor's direction the man was placed in the back of a divisional wagon to be transported to a psychiatric hospital. By the time the police van reached the hospital, the patient had died.

The coroner found that the man died from a combination of factors including aspiration of gastric contents, therapeutic concentrations of diazepam and a head injury, all of these factors culminating in a cardiopulmonary arrest. In regard to the nurses, the coroner found they had failed to:

- ensure that the deceased was not left alone after the administration of the drugs
- advise of the risks to the man if left in the van alone
- advise of the need for an ambulance
- arrange such transport.

On appeal, Mr Justice Southwell in the Supreme Court of Victoria noted that the doctor, having listened to the nurses' advice regarding appropriate sedation, had referred to his own documents, then telephoned another doctor for advice, given the injections and examined the vital signs of his patient. His Honour stated that the nurses were not duty bound to stay and ensure the doctor's assessment was correct. His Honour observed that neither nurse was trained in cardiopulmonary resuscitation techniques and both were of the opinion that the man required regular monitoring, not continuous monitoring. This, his Honour noted, was also the belief of the doctors involved (a second, more senior doctor arrived later). In addition, the nurses had no access to guidelines on the use of sedation and safe transport. These guidelines were printed by the Victorian health department and given to the doctors but not the nurses.

Mr Justice Southwell said to 'hold the nurses in breach of their professional duty by reason of the fact that they did not volunteer further advice to the doctor is to unreasonably widen their obligations and elevate the appropriate standard of care'.[23] His Honour determined that before a professional person can be found

to have contributed to the cause of another's death, within the course of their professional duties, the coroner must come to a 'comfortable satisfaction that negligence has been established which contributed to the death'.[24] His Honour found that none of the coroner's findings ought to have been made, as they were against the weight of evidence.[25] The nurses' application for a declaration to overturn the coroner's findings that they had contributed to the death of the deceased was granted.

FURTHER READING

Chiarella M. Review of coronial decision involving nurses. *Aust Health Law Bull*. 1995;3(7):77.

Freckelton I, Ranson D. *Death Investigation and the Coroner's Inquest*. Melbourne, VIC: Oxford University Press; 2006.

Lu Oam D, McKenna J. Recent coronial comments on the physical restraint of mental health patients. *Aust Health Law Bull*. 2013;21(5):353–5.

Marino G. NSW coronial inquest into the death of Michael Sutherland – the pitfalls of a lack of empathy. *Aust Health Law Bull*. 2011;19(9):138–41.

Oam A, Harris C. When time is of the essence – inquest into the death of Veronica Campbell. *Aust Health Law Bull*. 2011;19(4):58–61.

Watterson R, Brown P, McKenzie J. Coronial recommendations and prevention of Indigenous death. *Aust Indig Law Rev*. 2008;2,12(2):4–26.

World Health Organization. *Civil registration: why counting births and deaths is important*. Geneva: WHO; 2014. https://www.who.int/news-room/fact-sheets/detail/civil-registration-why-counting-births-and-deaths-is-important. Accessed 22 June 2018.

ENDNOTES

1. World Health Organization. Health Metrics Network and World Health Organization welcome birth registration resolution (23 March 2012). <http://www.who.int/mediacentre/news/statements/2012/HMN_birth_registration/en/>. Accessed 22 June 2018.
2. Ibid.
3. *Births, Deaths and Marriages Registration Act 1997* (ACT); *Births, Deaths and Marriages Registration Act 1995* (NSW) s 43; *Births, Deaths and Marriages Registration Act 1996* (NT) s 38; *Births, Deaths and Marriages Registration Act 2003* (Qld) s 40; *Births, Deaths and Marriages Registration Act 1996* (SA) s 11; *Births, Deaths and Marriages Registration Act 1999* (Tas) s 40; *Births, Deaths and Marriages Registration Act 1996* (Vic) s 41; *Births, Deaths and Marriages Registration Act 1998* (WA) s 49.
4. Stillbirth involves the birth of a stillborn child that exhibits no sign of respiration or heartbeat, or other sign of life, after birth and that is of at least 20 weeks' gestation, or, if it cannot be reliably established whether the period of gestation is more or less than 20 weeks, has a body mass of at least 400 grams at birth.
5. *Births, Deaths and Marriages Registration Act 1997* (ACT) s 5; *Births, Deaths and Marriages Registration Act 1995* (NSW) s 12;

Births, Deaths and Marriages Registration Act 1996 (NT) s 12; *Births, Deaths and Marriages Registration Act 1996* (SA) s 12; *Births, Deaths and Marriages Registration Act 2003* (Qld) s 5; *Births, Deaths and Marriages Registration Act 1999* (Tas) s 11; *Births, Deaths and Marriages Registration Act 1996* (Vic) s 12; *Births, Deaths and Marriages Registration Act 1998* (WA) s 12.

6. *Births, Deaths and Marriages Registration Act 1997* (ACT) s 18; *Births, Deaths and Marriages Registration Act 1995* (NSW) s 12; *Notification of Births Act 1915* (NSW) s 3; *Births, Deaths and Marriages Registration Act 1996* (NT) s 12; *Registration of Births, Deaths and Marriages Act 1962* (Qld) s 23; *Births, Deaths and Marriages Registration Act 1996* (SA) s 12; Births, Deaths and Marriages Registration Regulations 1996 (SA) reg 5; *Births, Deaths and Marriages Registration Act 1999* (Tas) s 11; *Births, Deaths and Marriages Registration Act 1996* (Vic) s 12; *Health Act 1958* (Vic) s 160; *Births, Deaths and Marriages Registration Act 1998* (WA) s 12.

7. *Births, Deaths and Marriages Registration Act 2003* (Qld) s 33.

8. *Births, Deaths and Marriages Registration Act 1997* (ACT) ss 14, 16, 45(2); *Births, Deaths and Marriages Registration Act 1995* (NSW) s 18; *Births, Deaths and Marriages Registration Act 1996* (NT) s 19; *Registration of Births, Deaths and Marriages Act 1962* (Qld) s 25; *Births, Deaths and Marriages Registration Act 1996* (SA) s 18; *Births, Deaths and Marriages Registration Act 1999* (Tas) s 17; *Births, Deaths and Marriages Registration Act 1996* (Vic) s 16; *Births, Deaths and Marriages Registration Act 1998* (WA) s 18.

9. *Births, Deaths and Marriages Registration Act 1996* (ACT) ss 23–29; *Births, Deaths and Marriages Registration Act 1995* (NSW) ss 32A–32J; *Births, Deaths and Marriages Registration Act* (NT) ss 28A–28J; *Births, Deaths and Marriages Registration Act 2003* (Qld) ss 22–24; *Births, Deaths and Marriages Registration Act 1999* (Tas) ss 28A–28J; *Births, Deaths and Marriages Registration Act 1997*; *Births, Deaths and Marriages Registration Act 1996* (Vic) ss 30A–D: persons born in Victoria; ss 30E–30F: Victorian residents born elsewhere; ss 30G–I: other matters; *Sexual Reassignment Act 1988* (SA) ss 7–10; *Gender Reassignment Act 2000* (WA) ss 14–19.

10. Ibid.

11. See, for example: Department of Health. *Guidance Note for the Verification of Death.* Melbourne, VIC: State Government of Victoria; 2010. http://www.health.vic.gov.au/__data/assets/pdf_file/0006/356667/Guidance-Note-for-the-Verification-of-Death-Feb-2010.pdf; NSW Health. *Death – Verification of Death and Medical Certificate of Cause of Death, 22 September 2015.* Sydney, NSW: New South Wales Government; 2015. https://www1.health.nsw.gov.au/pds/ActivePDSDocuments/PD2015_040.pdf. Accessed 22 June 2018.

12. *Births, Deaths and Marriages Registration Act 1997* (ACT) s 38; *Births, Deaths and Marriages Registration Act 1995* (NSW) s 42; *Births, Deaths and Marriages Registration Act 1996* (NT) s 37; *Registration of Births, Deaths and Marriages Act 1962* (Qld) ss 39–40; *Births, Deaths and Marriages Registration Act 1996* (SA) s 39; Births, Deaths and Marriages Registration Regulations 1996 (SA) r 11; *Births, Deaths and Marriages Registration Act 1999* (Tas) s 38; *Births, Deaths and Marriages Registration Act 1996* (Vic) s 40; *Births, Deaths and Marriages Registration Act 1998* (WA) s 48.

13. *Coroners Act 1997* (ACT) s 52; *Coroners Act 1980* (NSW) s 22A; *Coroners Act* (NT) s 34; *Coroners Act 2003* (Qld) s 46; *Coroners Act 2003* (SA) s 25; *Coroners Act 1995* (Tas) s 28; *Coroners Act 2008* (Vic) s 19; *Coroners Act 1996* (WA) s 25.

14. Freckelton I, Ranson D. *Death Investigation and the Coroner's Inquest.* Melbourne, VIC: Oxford University Press; 2006. p. 534.

15. For individual requirements in each jurisdiction see: *Coroners Act 1997* (ACT) s 33(1); *Coroners Act 1980* (NSW) s 22; *Coroners Act 1993* (NT) ss 3, 34; *Coroners Act 2003* (Qld) s 43; *Coroners Act 1995* (Tas) s 12; *Coroners Act 2008* (Vic) s 19(1); *Coroners Act 1996* (WA) ss 3, 25; *Coroners Act 1975* (SA) s 12.

16. *Coroners Act 1985* (Vic) s 15A.

17. *Coroners Act 2009* (Vic) s 72(3)–(5).

18. Note that section 4(2)(b) of the *Coroners Act 2009* (Vic) removed any reference to a death occurring during or following an anaesthetic and refers to a death that was not reasonably expected following a medical procedure.

19. For specific requirements of reportable death and grounds for reporting see: *Coroners Act 1997* (ACT) ss 13, 77; *Coroners Act 1980* (NSW) ss 12A, 13; *Coroners Act* (NT) ss 12(1), 12(3); *Coroners Act 2003* (Qld) s 8(3); *Coroners Act 2003* (SA) s 3; *Coroners Act 1995* (Tas) s 3; *Coroners Act 1985* (Vic) s 3; *Coroners Act 1996* (WA) s 3.

20. *Coroners Act 1995* (Tas) s 35; *Coroners Act 1985* (Vic) s 27; *Coroners Act 1996* (WA) s 34.

21. See *Hunter Area Health Service v Marchlewski* [2000] NSWCA 294.

22. *Secretary to the Department of Health & Community Services, Schultz and Moreland v Gurvich* [1995] 2 VR 69.

23. Ibid. at 79.

24. Ibid. at 74.

25. Ibid. at 81.

REVIEW QUESTIONS AND ACTIVITIES

1. Look up the births, deaths and marriages registration Act in your state or territory. List the legal requirements for (a) notification of and (b) registering a birth in your jurisdiction.

2. Which health practitioners can 'verify' a death?

3. Who has responsibility for 'certifying' a death?

4. List the legal requirements for registering a death in your jurisdiction.

5. What is the role and function of the coroner?

10

ABORTION, WRONGFUL BIRTH, WRONGFUL LIFE AND PRENATAL INJURY

LEARNING OBJECTIVES

Upon completing this chapter you should be able to:

- identify and discuss the legal issues associated with the termination of pregnancy
- explain causes of action in negligence for
  - 'wrongful birth'
  - 'wrongful life'
  - 'prenatal injury'.

INTRODUCTION

This chapter examines laws relevant to the termination of pregnancy as well as legal actions in negligence concerning claims for 'wrongful birth' or 'wrongful life' and 'prenatal injury'. These matters have in common that they raise significant ethical, social and legal challenges and debate and are illustrative of how the law develops over time.

ABORTION

An abortion can be defined as the untimely expulsion (or removal) of a fetus from a uterus. Abortion can be either spontaneous, commonly referred to as a 'miscarriage', or it can be artificially induced, commonly referred to as 'termination of pregnancy'. Active termination of pregnancy in healthcare settings occurs either via medical or surgical means. Medical abortions are only possible within the first nine weeks of pregnancy and involve the use of abortifacient drugs to, first, block the hormone progesterone, which stops the pregnancy from being

viable, and, second, to expel the fetus from the woman's body. The most common drugs used for medical abortions are mifepristone (widely referred to as RU 486) and misoprostol.[1] Surgical abortions are more common and may be performed at any time during the pregnancy, subject to legal restrictions. Although commonly and widely practised, it is the active termination of pregnancy using drugs or surgical instruments that has been the basis of much contention over time.

Early English Law

The law in Australia was traditionally based on the *Miscarriage of Women Act 1803* (UK) and the *Infant Life (Preservation) Act 1929* (UK). Section 1 of the 1803 Act made it a capital offence for a person to unlawfully administer any noxious and destructive substance or thing with the intent to procure the miscarriage of a woman 'quick'[2] with child. It was a felony under section 2 to procure the miscarriage of a woman not being, or not being proved to be, quick with child. The 1929 Act introduced justification for a termination of pregnancy for the purpose of preserving the life of the mother.

At common law, the earliest case that laid down the principles governing abortion is the English case of *R v Bourne*.[3] In that case MacNaghten J considered that the meaning of the word 'unlawful' in the legislation was of vital and decisive significance. He reasoned that an 'unborn child was not to be destroyed unless it was necessary to preserve the yet more precious life of the mother'.[4] His Honour stated that:

[I]f a doctor is of the opinion, on reasonable grounds and with adequate knowledge, that the probable consequence of the continuance of the pregnancy will be to make the woman a physical wreck, the jury are quite entitled to take the view that the doctor who, under those circumstances and in whose honest belief, operates, is operating for the purpose of preserving the life of the mother.[5]

Thus, while it was a criminal act to commit an 'unlawful abortion', a doctor undertaking the abortion would be acting 'lawfully' if there was an honest belief that the intervention was to preserve the life of the mother. Furthermore, the concept of 'life of the mother' included both the mental and physical health of the woman.

The Australian Position

In Australia, laws governing abortion have historically been based in the criminal codes and statutes. Like England, there were then judicial decisions in some states that determined when an abortion was lawful. For example, up until 2008, section 65 of the *Crimes Act 1958* (Vic) provided it was an offence for a woman or other person to procure a miscarriage unlawfully. What constituted 'lawful' or 'unlawful' was determined pursuant to the 'Menhennitt ruling' of 1969.[6] In *R v Davidson*, Menhennitt J said that the basis of determining whether an abortion was lawful is whether the doctor reasonably believed that termination of the pregnancy was (a) 'necessary to preserve the woman from a serious danger to her life or her physical or mental health (not being merely the normal dangers of pregnancy and childbirth) which the continuance of the pregnancy would entail' (necessity);[7] and (b) 'not out of proportion to the danger to be averted' (proportional).[8] The conditions of 'necessity' and 'proportionality' are referred to as the 'Menhennitt rules'. These remain relevant in other states that have applied the Menhennitt rules.

However, in recent years several state/territory governments have amended their laws in a bid to shift the emphasis away from the criminal law and into the realm of health legislation. In the Australian Capital Territory, the Northern Territory, Tasmania, Victoria and Western Australia, abortion has been decriminalised to varying degrees and is largely governed via health legislation, although some states still have criminal law provisions related to 'unlawful' abortion. It remains the case in New South Wales, Queensland and South Australia that abortion is governed under the respective criminal codes. A mixture of legislation[9] and case law in these jurisdictions then determines the circumstances in which a lawful abortion may be performed.

There remains considerable differences among all of the states and territories regarding the criteria required for a lawful abortion ranging from consent, like all other medical treatments, to a requirement for risk to the woman's health and wellbeing. Other criteria include: the time up until which a lawful abortion can be performed, with the only requirement being consent (in some states); what is required after a certain point in the pregnancy has passed (e.g. who needs to agree to the termination and the criteria that must be met); and when an abortion is considered unlawful and the associated penalties. The laws are summarised in Table 10.1.

Conscientious Objection

While performing an abortion is lawful in all jurisdictions of Australia, some jurisdictions permit health practitioners to object to performing or assisting in a termination based on moral grounds of conscientious objection. Legislative provisions exist in the Northern Territory, South Australia, Victoria and Western Australia that permit doctors with moral objections to abortion to refrain from involvement in such procedures.

In the Northern Territory conscientious objection is permitted provided the practitioner refers the woman to another medical practitioner who does not have such objection.[13] Authorised health practitioners, midwives, nurses and pharmacists may also conscientiously object to a direction to assist in a termination, in which case the suitably qualified medical practitioner must direct an alternate authorised practitioner, midwife, nurse or pharmacist who does not have such an objection to assist.[14] Despite any such conscientious objection, the abovementioned health practitioners must perform, or assist, in the termination of pregnancy if necessary to save the life of the woman.[15]

In South Australia medical professionals are not under a duty to participate in abortions unless it is 'necessary to save the life, or prevent grave injury to the physical or mental health, of a pregnant woman'.[16]

TABLE 10.1
Summary of Laws in Australia Relevant to Abortion

Summary of Laws	Applicable Law
Lawful Abortion Governed by Health Legislation (Criminal Law Regarding Unlawful Abortion in Some States)	
Australian Capital Territory	*Health Act 1993* ss 80–84
■ Abortion is governed under health legislation.	
■ Abortion is lawful without reasons and at any stage of pregnancy.	
■ Abortion must be carried out in an approved medical facility.	
■ It remains an offence for an unqualified person to perform an abortion, with a maximum penalty of five years' imprisonment.	
Northern Territory	*Termination of Pregnancy Law Reform Act 2017*
■ Abortion is governed by health legislation.	
■ Abortion is lawful up to 14 weeks' gestation if a medical practitioner considers termination appropriate, taking into account all medical and social circumstances.	
■ The medical practitioner must have regard to: (a) all relevant medical circumstances; (b) the woman's current and future physical, psychological and social circumstances; and (c) professional standards and guidelines.	
■ The 'suitably qualified medical practitioner' may direct an authorised registered health practitioner, midwife, nurse or pharmacist to assist in performing a termination.	
■ Abortion is lawful between 14 and 23 weeks' gestation if two medical practitioners agree that the termination is appropriate, taking into account all medical and social circumstances.	
■ The Act stipulates that a pregnant person's life must be endangered for a pregnancy to be terminated at more than 23 weeks' gestation.	
■ It also removes the possibility for women to be charged for procuring an abortion.	
Tasmania	*The Reproductive Health (Access to Terminations) Act 2013* *Criminal Code Act 1924* ss 178D and 178E
■ Lawful abortion is governed under health legislation.	
■ Abortion is lawful if a woman who is not more than 16 weeks' pregnant consents to the abortion.	
■ After 16 weeks abortion is lawful if two medical practitioners (one an obstetrician or gynaecologist) agree that continuance of pregnancy poses greater risk of injury to the physical or mental health of the woman.	
■ It is a criminal offence if termination occurs intentionally or recklessly without consent, or if an unqualified person performs the termination.	
Victoria	*Abortion Law Reform Act 2008* *Crimes Act 1958* ss 65–66
■ Lawful abortion is governed under health legislation.	
■ Provisions regarding unlawful abortions and penalties remain in the *Crimes Act 1958*.	
■ Abortion is lawful without reason up to 24 weeks' pregnancy.	
■ After 24 weeks a medical practitioner (with a second opinion) must reasonably believe it is appropriate in all the circumstances (includes future physical/psychological and social circumstances).	
■ It is not an offence to procure a woman's miscarriage (s 66); however, pursuant to the criminal law it remains an offence for an 'unqualified person' to perform an abortion, which is subject to a penalty of up to $50,000. (Qualified persons include a registered medical practitioner or, where the abortion is to be performed by administering drugs, a pharmacist or nurse.)	
■ If a person who is not a medical practitioner performs an abortion, that person is guilty of a crime and is liable to imprisonment for five years.	
Western Australia	*Health Act 1911* ss 334–335 *Criminal Code 1913* s 199
■ Abortion is governed under health legislation and the Criminal Code.	
■ It is lawful up to 20 weeks' gestation, subject to consent or other criteria being met.	
■ There are some restrictions for people under 16 years of age (e.g. parental notification); however, a young woman may apply to the Children's Court for an order to proceed with an abortion if it is not considered suitable to involve her parent(s).	
■ After 20 weeks' gestation it is required that two medical practitioners agree it is necessary because the mother or child has a severe medical condition. The abortion must take place in a medical facility.	
■ Unlawful abortion remains a crime – for the doctor but not the patient – and may be subject to a penalty up to $70,000.	

TABLE 10.1	
Summary of Laws in Australia Relevant to Abortion *(Continued)*	
Summary of Laws	Applicable Law

Abortion Governed by Criminal Law; in Some States Common Law Rules Are Also Relevant

New South Wales	*Crimes Act 1900* ss 20, 82–84
■ Unlawful abortion is governed under the *Crimes Act 1900*.	*R v Wald* [1971] 3 DCR (NSW) 25
■ It is an offence for a woman, or someone else, to *unlawfully* procure an abortion using drugs, any noxious thing, an instrument or other means.	*CES v Superclinics Pty Ltd* (1995) 38 NSWLR 47
■ It is also an offence for any person to supply any drug or noxious thing to a woman, or any instrument, to procure an abortion.	(See also the Menhennitt ruling in *R v Davidson* [1969] VR 667)
■ At common law, abortion is 'lawful' when a doctor reasonably believes a woman's physical or mental health is in serious danger. Social, economic and medical factors may be taken into account.	
■ The test regarding reasonable belief is an objective test based on what 'a reasonable person in the position of the accused' would have considered.[10]	
Queensland	*Criminal Code 1899* ss 224–226, 282, 292, 294
■ Abortion is governed under the Criminal Code.	*R v Bayliss & Cullen* (1986) 9 Qld Lawyer Reps 8 (of limited application) in which the Menhennitt rules were applied
■ Unlawful abortion is an offence.	
■ Any person who procures or performs an abortion is guilty of a crime and is liable to imprisonment for 14 years. (Abortion is therefore a crime for women and doctor.)	
■ However, a statutory defence exists in that: A person is not criminally responsible for performing or providing, in good faith and with reasonable care and skill, a surgical operation on or medical treatment of: (a) a person or an unborn child for the patient's benefit; or (b) a person or an unborn child to preserve the mother's life; if performing the operation or providing the medical treatment is reasonable, having regard to the patient's state at the time and to all the circumstances of the case.[11]	
■ The common law principle of necessity has also been held to be a defence to a charge of unlawful abortion.	
South Australia	*Criminal Law Consolidation Act 1935* ss 81–82A
■ Abortion is governed under criminal legislation.	
■ Procuring or performing an unlawful abortion is an offence that carries a maximum liability to be imprisoned for life (or any lesser term).	
■ Section 82A allows for the lawful termination of pregnancy if two doctors agree that a woman's physical or mental health is endangered by the pregnancy, or for serious fetal abnormality. Here, 'account may be taken of the pregnant woman's actual or reasonably foreseeable environment'.	
■ Lawful termination must take place in a hospital.	
■ In emergency situations, the requirement for a second medical opinion is waived, where one doctor considers that 'the termination is immediately necessary to save the life, or to prevent grave injury to the physical or mental health, of the pregnant woman'.[12]	
■ Except for emergency terminations, the Act contains a requirement that the woman must have lived in South Australia for a period of at least two months prior to the abortion.	

In Victoria a practitioner must inform the woman requesting advice regarding or performance of an abortion that they have a conscientious objection and then refer the woman to another medical professional who they know does not have a conscientious objection to abortion.[17] However, Victoria's *Abortion Law Reform Act 2008* also requires doctors to perform an abortion, despite any conscientious objection, 'in an emergency where the abortion is necessary to preserve the life of the pregnant woman'.[18]

In Western Australia the *Health Act 1911* also contains a conscientious objection provision. Unlike its counterparts, the Western Australian legislation does not contain exceptions requiring a doctor to participate in an abortion.

Rights of the Fetus and Father

Customarily, before a fetus is born alive it has no legal rights and is generally considered to be part of the mother's body. Legal recognition is granted when the fetus is 'born alive', which requires some indication of life such as a pulse in the umbilical cord, movement, coughing or breathing. The child can still be attached to the umbilical cord and be considered alive. Equally, the view that a fetus is part of the mother's body assumes that, should the fetus die in utero, the injury is deemed to be an injury to the mother.

If the child is born alive but later dies from a prenatal injury, the criminal law may be invoked against the person who caused the injury. In *R v F*[19] a child was born prematurely and subsequently died after its mother was involved in a car accident caused by the defendant. The court had to decide whether the child was a 'person' within the meaning of the *Crimes Act 1900* (NSW). Justice Grove stated that 'the common law has long recognised that where an unborn child receives injuries, is born alive but dies of those antenatal injuries, the perpetrator may suffer criminal liability for homicide'.[20]

In Paton's case[21] the biological father of a fetus sought to prevent his wife from having an abortion. The judge observed that the 'father can have no rights whatsoever nor can the fetus have any right of its own, at least until it is born and has a separate existence from the mother'.[22]

In the Australian case of *A-G (ex rel Kerr) v T*[23] the biological father sought a restraining injunction to prevent the woman with whom he had conceived a child from seeking an abortion. The court denied the injunction and applied the decision in Paton's case, using the guiding principles that the father and fetus have no identifiable rights.

This reasoning was also applied in *F v F*[24] where the judge considered that to grant the injunction would force the wife to carry and give birth to a baby she clearly did not want. He pointed out that the fact the fetus would grow in the wife's body and not the husband's was a relevant factor and should not be overlooked.[25]

More recently in *Talbot v Norman*[26] a male applied for an injunction to prevent his former partner from leaving Queensland to have an abortion. In keeping with the earlier decisions, Murphy J found that the *Family Law Act 1975* (Cth) applies to children only when they are born.

The law is clear in relation to the rights of the fetus and the father. There is no rule in common law or statute that gives the father the right to be consulted about a termination. Furthermore, the courts distinguish the father's relationship in terms of biological and not marital status.

CLAIMS REGARDING WRONGFUL BIRTH, WRONGFUL LIFE AND PRENATAL INJURY

Wrongful Conception/Birth

In Chapter 6 we examined the civil cause of action known as negligence. Recall that, pursuant to the law of negligence, a health practitioner owes a duty of care to their patients and must act to a reasonable standard of care not to cause them harm or loss. The action known as wrongful birth in Australia (sometimes referred to as 'wrongful conception') is a cause of action in negligence, in which the parent(s) of a child 'claim that the negligent advice or treatment deprived them of the choice of avoiding conception … or … of terminating the pregnancy'.[27] Such claims may include (but are not limited to):

- the negligent performance of a sterilisation operation
- the failure to warn of the risks of failure of sterilisation procedures to prevent contraception
- negligent performance of an abortion (resulting in continued pregnancy)
- supplying defective contraceptives
- failing to advise about the risk of contraceptives not preventing pregnancy
- negligent assisted reproductive treatment that involves implanting multiple embryos, resulting in multiple births, when the parents believed they were only going to have one child
- failure to diagnose a condition in the fetus that, if known, would have allowed the parent(s) to decide to lawfully terminate the pregnancy.[28]

The use of the terms 'wrongful conception' or 'wrongful birth' has arisen on the basis that the child was initially unplanned (wrongful conception) or unwanted (wrongful birth). However, 'wrongful birth' might be a misnomer because, ultimately, it is the negligence that is wrongful and not the birth. Further, parents may have chosen to have the child rather than terminate a pregnancy, as is their right, and so there is nothing wrongful about the 'birth'.

In such claims, the High Court has held that the parent(s) may claim damages for prenatal and postnatal medical expenses, the future economic loss (i.e. costs) of rearing the child, and pain and suffering the parents have experienced during pregnancy and labour. A claim does not rely on a child being born with a disability, although a number of states have introduced statutory provisions to limit liability in cases of a healthy child.

The leading High Court case for wrongful birth, *Cattanach v Melchior*,[29] was decided in 2003. The case concerned a failed sterilisation operation and the failure of the plaintiff's doctor to warn her that pregnancy might occur. Mrs Melchior fell pregnant and gave birth to a healthy baby. The majority of the High Court held the doctor's liability should be based on ordinary negligence principles and, because the costs of raising the child were directly caused by the doctor's negligence (which was conceded), the claim was allowed. They dismissed the argument that the claim should be rejected for reasons of policy/morality, pointing out that the 'wrong' or 'legal harm' for which damages are awarded is not the birth of the child but the negligence of the doctor that leads to identifiable losses by the plaintiff parent(s).

Cattanach v Melchior remains the common law authority in Victoria, Western Australia, the Northern Territory, the Australian Capital Territory and Tasmania, where claims for costs of rearing the child up to the age of 18, as well as costs up to and including the birth such as antenatal, obstetric care, labour care and pain and suffering, are possible. Note, however, that this must be qualified in all states and territories, except the Australian Capital Territory, by reference to the legislative provisions that create thresholds for recovery of damages for non-economic loss.[30]

In New South Wales, South Australia and Queensland legislative provisions exist to qualify what may be recovered in wrongful birth claims.

In New South Wales the *Civil Liability Act 2002* provides that where an action involves a claim for damages for the birth of a child, a court cannot award damages for the costs associated with rearing or maintaining the child that the claimant has incurred or will incur in the future, or for any loss of earnings by the claimant while the claimant rears or maintains the child.[31] However, a person is not precluded from recovering any additional costs associated with rearing or maintaining a child who suffers from a disability that arise by reason of the disability.[32]

In South Australia the *Civil Liability Act 1936* provides that damages are not to be awarded:

- to cover the ordinary costs of raising a child in an action for negligence resulting in the unintended conception of a child, the failure of or an attempted abortion, or in the birth of a child that would have been aborted but for negligence
- in relation to innocent misrepresentation leading to unintended conception or a missed opportunity to abort
- for breach of statutory or implied warranty of merchantable quality or fitness for purpose in a case where a child is conceived as a result of the failure of a contraceptive device.[33]

'Ordinary costs' include all costs associated with the child's care, upbringing, education and advancement in life. Damages are recoverable in the case of a child who has a mental or physical disability, to the extent that those costs would reasonably exceed what would be incurred if the child did not have a disability.[34]

In Queensland the *Civil Liability Act 2003* prevents a court from awarding damages for economic loss arising out of the costs ordinarily associated with rearing or maintaining a child born as a result of failed sterilisation procedures[35] and failed contraceptive procedures or contraceptive advice.[36] The legislation does not address whether there is a right to claim costs for rearing a child with a disability or a child conceived using assisted reproductive technology, which means a common law claim would apply in such instances.

Wrongful Life

In cases of negligence such as those above, courts have also been asked to consider whether a child born with disability may bring a claim for 'wrongful life'. Such cases have focused on the negligent failure of a medical practitioner to diagnose or warn parents of the risk of their child having a disease or disability when, if such a warning had been provided, the parents would have had an abortion or avoided pregnancy.

The questions for determination have been: whether a wrongful life action constitutes a valid cause of action; and, if so, what heads of damages are recoverable.[37] Again, the issue reached the High Court, with the leading authorities in Australia being the cases of *Harriton v Stephens*[38] and *Waller v James*.[39]

In the Harriton case, a child (Alexia Harriton) was born suffering severe congenital disabilities after her mother had contracted the rubella virus during pregnancy. It was agreed that a reasonable medical practitioner would have diagnosed or warned the mother of the consequent risks of her fetus being born with a severe disability, and that if the mother had been so advised she would have aborted the fetus.

In the Waller case, a child (Keedon Waller) was conceived with the assistance of in vitro fertilisation (IVF) treatment.[40] Keedon's father had been found to suffer from anti-thrombin 3 (AT3) deficiency, a genetic condition that results in a propensity of the blood to clot in arteries and veins, prior to Keedon's conception. However, the treating fertility doctor had failed to discuss or follow up on the AT3 condition and had not explained to the parents about the risk of a child inheriting AT3. Keedon was subsequently born with AT3, and the day after he was released from hospital he suffered a cerebral thrombosis[41] that resulted in brain damage, cerebral palsy and uncontrolled seizures. The parents gave evidence that if they had been properly informed about the AT3, they would have: (1) delayed IVF until methods were identified to ensure transfer of only embryos free of the AT3 deficiency; (2) used donor sperm; or (3) terminated the pregnancy.

The High Court denied both claims. The majority held that:

- a duty of care to the children could not be found as such a duty could conflict with the duty of care to the mother[42]
- the children could not properly show that they had suffered legally compensable harm due to an impossible comparison between existence and non-existence[43]
- there are sound policy reasons for rejecting such claims – including that permitting such actions might devalue the lives of people with disabilities[44]

- the disabilities were not the fault of the doctor – he could not have prevented them because he could not compel an abortion.[45]

However, note that Kirby J dissented, referring to examples in which the courts make such comparisons of existence and non-existence on a regular basis, including declaring lawful 'the withdrawal of life-sustaining medical treatment from severely disabled newborns and adults'; and 'separation surgery on conjoined twins in order to preserve the life of one twin, although doing so will result in the death of the other twin'.[46] He was also concerned that finding against such claims would lead to immunity for healthcare providers whose negligence had caused profound and lifelong suffering and that this would fail to encourage proper medical care.[47]

Nevertheless, the result of the High Court judgment is that 'wrongful life' is not currently seen as a plausible cause of action.

Prenatal Injury

There is common law authority in Australia that a child who suffers harm or loss caused by negligence that occurred while it was in utero, or prior to its conception, has a cause of action to recover damages from the person whose negligent action caused the harm or loss, upon being born live and viable.[48] In such cases application of the principles of negligence discussed in Chapter 6 have led to a finding of liability. The difference in such cases to wrongful life is that the negligence directly caused the disability, rather than the birth itself.

FURTHER READING

Burton A. Women, the unborn, the common law and the state. *SCU Law Rev.* 2001;5:159–88.

Lavery J, Linden S. Damages for a healthy but unwanted child – the debate continues. *Aust Health Law Bull.* 2002;10(8):81–4.

ENDNOTES

1. Petersen K. Early medical abortion: legal and medical developments in Australia. *Med J Aust.* 2010;193:26.
2. 'Quickening' is a term understood by those educated in midwifery and obstetrics and equates with the first movements of the fetus felt by the mother (from about 16 weeks' gestation).
3. *R v Bourne* [1938] 1 KB 687.
4. Ibid. at 691.
5. Ibid. at 694.
6. *R v Davidson* [1969] VR 667.

7. *R v Davidson* [1969] VR 667 at 672.
8. *R v Davidson* [1969] VR 667.
9. For all relevant legislative provisions see *Crimes Act 1900* (NSW) ss 20, 82–84; *Crimes Act 1958* (Vic) ss 65–66; *Criminal Law Consolidation Act 1935* (SA) ss 81–82a; *Criminal Code Act 1913* (WA) ss 199, 259, 269, 271; *Health Act 1911* (WA) ss 334, 335; *Acts Amendment (Abortion) Act 1998* (WA) s 8; *Termination of Pregnancy Law Reform Act 2017* (NT); *Criminal Code Act 1899* (Qld) ss 224–226, 282, 292, 294; *Crimes Act 1900* (ACT) ss 10, 40, 42–44; *Health Act 1993* (ACT) ss 30A–30E; *Criminal Code Act 1924* (Tas) ss 51, 134–135.
10. Stewart C. Recent developments in the law: late term abortion conviction in NSW. *J Bioeth Inq.* 2007;4:3–5.
11. *Criminal Code 1899* (Qld) s 282.
12. *Criminal Law Consolidation Act 1935* (SA) s 82A(1)(b).
13. *Termination of Pregnancy Law Reform Act 2017* (NT) s 11.
14. Ibid. s 12.
15. Ibid. s 13.
16. *Criminal Law Consolidation Act 1935* (SA) s 82A(6).
17. *Abortion Law Reform Act 2008* (Vic) s 8(1)(b).
18. Ibid.: sections 8(3) and 8(4) extends this duty to registered nurses.
19. *R v F* (1993) 40 NSWLR 245.
20. Ibid. at 247.
21. *Paton v Trustees of the EPAS* [1978] 2 All ER 987.
22. Ibid. at 989.
23. *A-G (ex rel Kerr) v T* [1982] 1 NSWLR 311.
24. *F v F* (1989) 13 Fam LR 189.
25. Ibid. at 198.
26. *Talbot v Norman* [2012] FamCA 96.
27. *Procanik v Cillo* 478 A2d 755 NJ 1984.
28. Allan S Health Law Central: Wrongful Birth. http://www.healthlawcentral.com/pregnancy-birth/wrongful-birth/. Accessed 11 March 2019.
29. *Cattanach v Melchior* (2003) 199 ALR 131; (2003) 77 ALJR 1312; (2003) Aust Torts Reports 81–704.
30. *Civil Liability Act 2002* (NSW) s 16; *Wrongs Act 1958* (Vic) s 28LF; *Civil Liability Act 1936* (SA) s 52; *Civil Liability Act 1936*

(WA) ss 4, 9–10; *Personal Injuries (Liabilities and Damages) Act 2003* (NT) s 27; *Civil Liability Act 2003* (Qld) ss 61–62; *Civil Liability Act 2002* (Tas) s 27. See Chapter 6 for further discussion.
31. *Civil Liability Act 2002* (NSW) s 70(1).
32. Ibid. s 70(2).
33. *Civil Liability Act 1936* (SA) s 67(3).
34. Ibid. s 67(2).
35. *Civil Liability Act 2003* (Qld) s 49A.
36. Ibid. s 49B.
37. *Harriton v Stephens* (2006) 226 CLR 52 at [33] (Kirby J).
38. *Harriton v Stephens* (2006) 226 CLR 52.
39. *Waller v James; Waller v Hoolahan* (2006) 226 CLR 136.
40. IVF is a method of assisted reproduction in which ovum and sperm are combined in a petri dish (in vitro being Latin for 'in glass'), with the aim of achieving fertilisation. Developing embryos can then be transferred to a woman's uterus with the aim of achieving pregnancy.
41. That is, the formation of a blood clot in an artery that supplies blood to the brain.
42. *Harriton v Stephens* (2006) 226 CLR 52 at [242]–[250] (Crennan J).
43. *Harriton v Stephens* (2006) 226 CLR 52 at [172], [182] (Hayne J); [205]–[206] (Callinan J); [225], [252]–[253] (Crennan J); *Waller v James; Waller v Hoolahan* (2006) 226 CLR 136 at [50] (Hayne J); [64] (Callinan J); [86] (Crennan J).
44. *Harriton v Stephens* (2006) 226 CLR 52 at [258]–[263] (per Crennan J); see note 42 above at [86] (Crennan J).
45. *Harriton v Stephens* (2006) 226 CLR 52 at [176]–[182].
46. *Harriton v Stephens* (2006) 226 CLR 52 at [95] (Kirby J).
47. *Harriton v Stephens* (2006) 226 CLR 52 at [153] (Kirby J).
48. *Watt v Rama* [1972] VR 353; *Lynch v Lynch* (1991) Aust Torts Reports 81–117, 69,091; *X & Y (by her tutor X) v Pal* (1991) Aust Torts Reports 81–098; 23 NSWLR 26.

REVIEW QUESTIONS AND ACTIVITIES

1. Look up the births, deaths and marriages registration Act in your state or territory. List the legal requirements (a) for notification of and (b) registering a birth in your jurisdiction.

2. List the legal requirements for notification of a death in your jurisdiction.

3. Compare the various legislative requirements in each jurisdiction in relation to the law of abortion. Which jurisdiction has addressed the issue, in your opinion, most clearly and effectively?

4. What is the difference between wrongful birth and wrongful life claims? Who are the claimants? What are they claiming? What compensation is or is not available?

5. What is prenatal injury? Who is the claimant? What are they claiming? How would a cause of action proceed?

6. Reflect on the ethical, legal and social issues that the above actions give rise to. How, and to what extent, has the law addressed such issues?

11

ASSISTED REPRODUCTION AND SURROGACY

LEARNING OBJECTIVES

Upon completing this chapter you should be able to:

- describe the differing approaches to regulating assisted reproductive technology taken by the states and territories across Australia
- explain the purpose of the *Ethical Guidelines on the Use of Assisted Reproductive Technology in Clinical Practice and Research*
- discuss key ethical and legal issues raised by assisted reproductive technologies and surrogacy
- describe the necessary requirements for legal surrogacy arrangements in Australia.

INTRODUCTION

This chapter examines assisted reproductive technologies and surrogacy. The primary purpose of assisted reproductive technologies (ART) is to assist people to have children, when otherwise, due to their circumstances, they may not be able to. There are many types of ART including artificial insemination by donor, in vitro fertilisation (IVF) and gamete intrafallopian transfer. While often the woman's egg and the male's sperm are used in ART for heterosexual couples, for some heterosexual couples, as well as singles and same-sex couples, donor sperm, eggs or embryos may be used. ART may also involve preimplantation genetic diagnosis or preimplantation genetic screening, which allow: early embryo screening to avoid a genetic or sex-linked disorder; screening for abnormal chromosomes; and screening for human leukocyte antigen (HLA) typing,

the process used to create 'saviour siblings'. Some people may use ART in surrogacy arrangements.

Advances in ART and surrogacy have raised significant ethical, legal and social issues and questions, including those related to parentage, when life begins, experimentation on embryos, access to information by donor-conceived people, who is entitled to use the technology, record keeping, long-term outcomes for people who undergo ART and the children born as a result. It is not the purpose of this chapter to deal in specific detail with the many complex issues arising in this area but merely to highlight some key issues and the existing legislation and regulation.

REGULATION AND OVERSIGHT OF ART

Both general and specific laws and regulation are relevant to the governance of ART and associated healthcare practice. For example, laws relevant to regulating health practitioners, access to health care and medicines, negligence, trespass to person and crime (to name a few) are all relevant to healthcare treatment and practice in the context of ART. States and territories also have the power to pass specific laws regarding ART. Western Australia and Victoria have comprehensive legislation governing ART; New South Wales and South Australia have laws on certain aspects of ART. The Northern Territory, Australian Capital Territory, Queensland and Tasmania do not have specific ART legislation.

At the Commonwealth level the National Health and Medical Research Council's *Ethical Guidelines on the*

Use of Assisted Reproductive Technology in Clinical Practice and Research (the NHMRC Ethical Guidelines) set out ethical principles that all ART clinics in Australia should follow to the extent that they do not conflict with any state law. There is also a self-regulatory system operated via the Fertility Society of Australia and the Reproductive Technology Accreditation Council (RTAC) that sets certain standards of practice across Australia.

ACCESS TO ART

In most states and territories access to ART is determined by clinical assessment and adherence to NHMRC guidelines and professional standards of practice. In South Australia, Victoria and Western Australia there are legislated provisions that stipulate eligibility criteria.

In Victoria the *Assisted Reproductive Treatment Act 2008* provides that a woman and her partner (if any) may only undergo an ART treatment procedure if:

- she (and her partner if any) has given proper consents[1]
- she (and her partner if any) has undergone counselling[2]
- a doctor is satisfied on reasonable grounds that the woman is
  - unlikely to become pregnant in her circumstances
  - unlikely to be able to carry a pregnancy or give birth to a child, or
  - at risk of transmitting a genetic abnormality or genetic disease to a child born as a result of a pregnancy conceived other than by a treatment procedure *and* a presumption against treatment does not apply to the woman.

Presumptions against treatment apply in Victoria if a criminal record check specifies that charges have been proven against the woman, or her partner (if any), for a sexual or violent offence, or if a child protection order specifies removing a child from the custody or guardianship of the woman or her partner.[3] When such matters exist, the excluded person may apply to a 'patient review panel' for review.[4] Any decision made by the patient review panel may also be reviewed by the Victorian Civil and Administrative Tribunal and subsequently by the courts if necessary.[5]

Section 9 of South Australia's *Assisted Reproductive Treatment Act 1988* requires the health minister to impose conditions on any person registered to provide ART, including a condition preventing the provision of ART except in the following circumstances:

- if it appears to be unlikely that, in the person's circumstances, the person will become pregnant other than by an assisted reproductive treatment[6]
- if there appears to be a risk that a serious genetic defect, serious disease or serious illness would be transmitted to a child conceived naturally[7]
- pursuant to named conditions relevant to the posthumous use of sperm or embryos created with sperm from a deceased person[8]
- for the purposes of a recognised surrogacy agreement[9]
- where there are conditions preventing treatment in the regulations.[10]

The regulations add two further conditions including where a woman or a man living with a woman (on a genuine domestic basis) has an illness that may result in them becoming infertile in the future, and that a registered person must comply with the requirements of the NHMRC Ethical Guidelines.[11] A maximum penalty of $120,000 for failing to comply with a condition may be imposed.[12]

The South Australian Act defines 'artificial reproductive treatment' as 'any medical procedure directed at fertilisation of a human ovum by artificial means and includes an in vitro fertilisation procedure'. It separately defines 'assisted insemination' as being 'assisted reproductive treatment (not being an in vitro fertilisation procedure or a surgical procedure) in which human sperm are introduced, by artificial means, into the human female reproductive system'.[13] The requirement for registration does not apply to *assisted insemination* provided by a health professional 'approved by the Minister'.[14] There are currently no approved health professionals in South Australia providing artificial insemination. In addition, the approval and eligibility requirements do not apply when assisted insemination is provided other than for fee or reward.[15] Such circumstances might include, for example, self-insemination, or the assisted insemination of a friend or partner.

In Western Australia the *Human Reproductive Technology Act 1991* requires that artificial fertilisation procedures be carried out only for the benefit of people eligible under the Act. Participants must be adequately assessed and counselled and their welfare properly promoted. The prospective welfare of any child to be born as a result of the procedure must also be taken into consideration.[16] Section 23 of the Act contains specific access provisions concerning IVF. At the time of writing, the legislation provided that IVF may be conducted for:

- persons who, as a couple, are unable to conceive a child due to medical reasons[17]
- a woman who is unable to conceive a child due to medical reasons[18]
- a couple or a woman whose child would otherwise be likely to be affected by a genetic abnormality or a disease[19]
- a woman who is unable to give birth to a child due to medical reasons and is a party to a surrogacy arrangement (as defined in the *Surrogacy Act 2008* s 3) that is lawful.[20]

The Human Reproductive Technology Act also requires that the reason for infertility must not be age or some other prescribed cause.[21]

Note, at the time of writing, the legislation also required that people seeking to be treated as a couple must be married to each other or in a de facto relationship with each other and be of the opposite sex to each other.[22] However, this provision is contrary to sections 5, 5A, 5B, 5C and 6 of the *Sex Discrimination Act 1984* (Cth), which prohibits discrimination against people on the basis of their relationship status, sexual orientation, gender identity or intersex status. At the time of writing, a review of Western Australia's Human Reproductive Technology Act and Surrogacy Act was being undertaken (by the current author for the Minister for Health) and it was expected, among other things, that such discrimination would be removed. Some further criteria are found in Part 7 of Directions issued in 2004, which were also under review.[23]

PARENTAGE

Laws exist at the state, territory and federal levels in relation to parentage of children born as a result of ART.[24] All jurisdictions recognise that a woman who gives birth to a child as a result of ART procedures is the legal mother of that child, regardless of whether donor gametes were used. The woman's husband or de facto is the legal father/parent, assuming the partner has consented to the treatment.

A donor of sperm, eggs or embryos is not considered to be a legal parent of a resulting child and has no rights or responsibilities. For example, he or she would not be liable to pay child support, nor would a child have a legal right to inherit an estate from the donor (unless the donor provided for the child in his/her will). However, when a 'known donor' is used and the arrangement is one in which she or he is involved in the child's life, it is possible that if the relationship between the adults involved breaks down, the Family Court would support continued visitation with the child on application. There are cases, particularly involving single women and same-sex couples, who appeared initially to have entered into a form of shared parenting with a known donor (a friend) or where visitation with the child from an early age has occurred, where this has been the case.[25]

ACCESS TO INFORMATION BY DONOR-CONCEIVED PEOPLE

Many children born as a result of donated gametes or embryos wish to access information about their donors and donor-siblings. The desire to do so includes wanting to know more about their biological heritage, medical reasons, to avoid forming relationships with first-degree relatives, and a call for openness and honesty and an end to the secrecy and anonymity that has surrounded donor-conception (and infertility generally).

Since 2018, Victorian legislation has provided that all donor-conceived people may have access to identifying information about their donors, regardless of when the donation took place. Those children born as a result of donor-conception since 2010 will also be alerted to their donor-conceived status via an addendum to their birth certificate, which will be provided to them on application for their certificate at age 18.

In Western Australia records have been kept on a central register since 1993. All donor-conceived people may access non-identifying information about their donors. People born after 2004 also have a legislated right to access identifying information about donors when they turn 16. Those born before 2004 may have access to such information only with the donor's consent. There is a voluntary register upon which people may place their names in hope of a 'match' to people related to each other who are also seeking information. At the time of writing, the laws in Western Australia were under review, including consideration of whether all donor-conceived people should be provided with equal access to information.

In New South Wales a central register has operated since 2010. People conceived with sperm donated since that date may access identifying information when they reach the age of 18, or prior with consent. People born before 2010 may also place their name on a 'voluntary register' in the hope that their donor or donor-siblings will also do so, and they will be matched. The success of voluntary registers such as those held by state health departments, although enabling some matches, has not been significant.

In South Australia some donor-conceived people may access information via the clinics from which their mother received treatment. However, this will depend upon when they were born. They will be given non-identifying information if the clinic manages past records, identifying information if the donor consents, or no information if records are located elsewhere and are not under the control of the clinic. This has led to significant distress. A 2017 review of the South Australian legislation recommended that the government establish a donor register as a matter of priority,[26] noting the government has power to do so but has not to date acted due to funding.

In all states and territories since 2004, the NHMRC Ethical Guidelines have also recognised the right to information about genetic heritage and have required that consent be given to releasing identifying information before any donation takes place (or is accepted). Donor-conceived people born in states or territories that do not have legislation must seek such information from the clinics at which their mother received treatment.

In the modern era it is noted that many more donor-conceived people are also finding their donors and siblings, and connecting with them, via DNA testing and ancestry tracing, and that many positive relationships have been forged.

NUMERICAL LIMITS FOR DONATION

In many jurisdictions around the world numerical limits are placed on how many children may be created, or families formed, using a particular donor. Such limits may be set by legislation or guidelines, or are recommended by professional bodies.[27] Limits are generally considered to be required due to the risk of a donor-conceived person forming a consanguineous relationship with another person who shares the same donor, and/or the psychosocial implications of having a large number of donor-conceived siblings/offspring across numerous families.

In Australia, limits vary across jurisdictions. In Victoria the limit is 10 women, including any current or former partner of the donor.[28] The donor may, however, specify a lower number as part of the consent process.[29]

In New South Wales the limit is no more than five women (or such lesser number as may be specified in the donor's consent), including the donor and any current or former spouse of the donor.[30]

In Western Australia the limit is a maximum of five families that may receive gametes from a single donor. This includes families outside of Western Australia.[31]

In Queensland, South Australia, Tasmania, the Northern Territory and the Australian Capital Territory the NHMRC Ethical Guidelines provide that 'clinics must take all reasonable steps to reduce the numbers of genetic relatives created through donor gamete programs'[32] to protect donor-conceived people, and donors, from having too many genetic siblings or too many offspring, respectively. However, although a previous version of the NHMRC Ethical Guidelines stipulated 10 families as the limit, revised editions from 2007 onwards have not stipulated the number of families or women for whom donor gametes may be used, or the number of children that may be created.

The RTAC Code, as reviewed in 2010 and 2014, requires that clinics must provide evidence of review and policy procedures that place 'a limitation on the number of children and families created from one donor'.[33] An RTAC technical bulletin released in 2010 stated that, where state legislation does not apply, the following are advised:

A maximum of ten donor families per sperm donor. This is based on the highest limit in existing state legislation (Victoria). The number of families per donor includes all families wherever the donor's sperm is used, not just the number of families from one unit, in one city, or in one country. This interpretation is based on the definition in existing state legislation.[34]

POSTHUMOUS USE OF GAMETES

Posthumous use of gametes occurs when a person dies and their surviving partner wishes to use their gametes (sperm or ova) to conceive a child. It may also occur when a donor of gametes has died. Laws exist in each state and territory that are relevant to the posthumous use of gametes; the NHMRC Ethical Guidelines are also relevant.

At the state/territory level, generally the issue is addressed in relation to the *removal* of tissue after death (if the gametes of the deceased were not removed and stored prior to death) and the question of whether such gametes may be used to create a pregnancy.

Generally, human tissue and transplantation permits the removal of human tissue after death for transplantation or other therapeutic or medical use in another person, with varying requirements for consent (see Chapter 13).

In New South Wales such consent must have been given prior to death, and not revoked.[35]

In South Australia there must be a reasonable belief that the deceased person had, during their lifetime, expressed the wish for, or consented to, the removal after their death of tissue from their body for the purpose, and had not withdrawn the wish or revoked the consent.[36] Where the designated officer has no reason to believe that the deceased person during their lifetime had neither expressed consent or objection to removing tissue after death, the senior next of kin may give such consent or, if the designated officer is unable to ascertain the existence or whereabouts of the next of kin, the designated officer may authorise the removal of tissue from the body of the deceased person.

In the Australian Capital Territory,[37] the Northern Territory,[38] Tasmania,[39] Queensland[40] and Western Australia,[41] the respective tissue and transplantation Acts permit the removal of tissue posthumously upon similar terms. In Western Australia, in *Re Section 22 of the Human Tissue And Transplant Act 1982 (WA); Ex Parte C* [2013] WASC 3 (2 January 2013), Edleman J held that the hospital should act expediently and not require a court order for such action where the senior next of kin has given consent. In Victoria the removal is subject to written or oral consent (in front of two witnesses for the latter).[42]

The law regarding posthumous use of gametes varies more significantly across states and territories.

In New South Wales the *use* of gametes or embryos is permitted after death if: the gamete donor has consented prior to death; the woman who is to use the gametes has been notified of the death; and the woman consents to use the gametes.[43] New South Wales legislation does not specify that use must be by the partner and therefore may be read to include posthumous use of gametes collected from a donor.

In South Australia the *Assisted Reproductive Technology Act 1988* provides that when semen of a donor was collected or used to fertilise an ova or create an embryo *before* the donor died, and written consent was given to use the semen after the donor's death, the semen (or resultant embryo) may be used after the donor's death for a woman who was living with the donor on a genuine domestic basis.[44] The Act is silent regarding posthumous use of ova and the use of sperm collected *after* death. In *Re H, AE (No 3)* (2013) 118 SASR 259; [2013] SASC 196 where sperm had been collected posthumously, and *written* consent to use the sperm did not exist, the Supreme Court approved an application to transport the sperm to the Australian Capital Territory. There are no laws governing ART or posthumous use of sperm in the Australian Capital Territory, and adherence to the NHRMC Ethical Guidelines is on a self-regulatory basis only.

In Victoria gametes or embryo(s) may be used by the deceased person's partner or, if the deceased is a woman, for use in a surrogate mother, with the deceased's written consent and with the consent of the patient review panel. The person who will undergo treatment must have counselling.[45] Victoria is the only jurisdiction that explicitly provides for the posthumous use of gametes or embryos in a surrogate mother.

In Western Australia the Human Reproductive Technology Act provides that gametes of a person cannot be used without the deceased's consent, and such consent must be in writing.[46] Directions given by the Commissioner of Health pursuant to the Human Reproductive Technology Act further provide that any person to whom a licence applies must not knowingly use or authorise the use of gametes in an artificial fertilisation procedure after the death of the gamete provider.[47] In cases that have permitted the *removal* of sperm under the *Human Tissue and Transplant Act 1982*,[48] the person wishing to use the gametes has to successfully apply for a court order to remove them interstate to a jurisdiction in which their *use* is permissible.[49] Again, it is noted that, at the time of writing, the Western Australian legislation was under review, and the position regarding posthumous use of gametes may change.

The Australian Capital Territory, the Northern Territory, Tasmania and Queensland do not have legislation concerning the posthumous *use* of gametes. In practice, people who cannot use gametes collected posthumously may travel to the Australian Capital Territory to seek treatment.

In all jurisdictions the NHMRC Ethical Guidelines provide guidance on the posthumous use of gametes. The NHMRC Ethical Guidelines state that, where permitted by law, clinics may facilitate such use if:

- the deceased person left clearly expressed directions consenting to such use following their death
- the request to do so has come from the spouse or partner of the deceased person, and not from any other relative
- the gametes are intended for use by the surviving spouse or partner
- sufficient time has passed so that grief and related emotions do not interfere with decision making
- the surviving prospective parent (the spouse or partner) is provided with sufficient information to facilitate an accurate understanding of the potential social, psychological and health implications of the proposed activity for the person who may be born
- the surviving prospective parent (the spouse or partner) has undergone appropriate counselling
- an independent body has reviewed the circumstances and supports the proposed use.[50]

SURROGACY

Surrogacy refers to a situation in which one woman (the surrogate mother) agrees to become pregnant for another woman and her partner, a single person or a same-sex couple (the intending parent(s)). Once the child is born the surrogate mother agrees to hand it over to the intending parent(s). Surrogacy involving assisted reproductive treatment or assisted insemination can involve using the surrogate mother's own eggs, a donor's eggs or the intending mother's eggs.

It may also involve the intending father's sperm or donor sperm.

Surrogacy raises considerable ethical, legal and social issues that are complex and not easy to resolve. From the perspective of ethics and law for health practitioners, it is a practice that requires consideration of the short- and long-term physical and psychological health and wellbeing of multiple parties: the woman who is to undergo ART treatment, become pregnant, birthing and relinquishing the child; the intending parents, who in some instances may themselves have faced significant health issues that have led them to surrogacy; any donor(s) of gametes; and the child(ren) that will be born as a result of such an arrangement.

Although it is beyond the scope of this discussion to detail each jurisdiction's law, it is noted that Australia has seen numerous inquiries into surrogacy over decades that have involved extensive public consultation and debate. All jurisdictions, except the Northern Territory, now have laws regulating surrogacy. While there is variation across states and territories, such laws generally provide for the following:

- the paramountcy of the welfare and best interests of children born as a result of surrogacy or assisted reproduction in a number of states
- acceptance and regulation of **altruistic surrogacy** (intended to account for situations in which family members, close friends or other known parties agree to act as an altruistic surrogate mother – a way of also increasing ongoing connection between the birth mother and child)
- prohibitions on **commercial surrogacy**, including that the Australian Capital Territory, New South Wales and Queensland have extraterritorial prohibitions that mean that it is illegal to enter into such arrangements in other jurisdictions also
- the birth mother is recognised as the legal mother in the first instance
- the reimbursement of costs in altruistic arrangements are permitted but are limited to out-of-pocket expenses related to the agreement, pregnancy and birth (expenses *actually incurred*), noting there are variations among jurisdictions regarding what is actually reimbursed
- the surrogacy agreements are considered void and unenforceable at law other than payment of

reasonable expenses associated with the pregnancy (note: should the parties change their minds, the birth mother could keep the child or it would enter into the foster care system)

- residency requirements in a number of jurisdictions for the commissioning parties and/or surrogate mothers that mean there is a requirement that those engaged in the agreement must live in the state in which the surrogacy arrangement takes place (such requirements are seen as important to avoid people being flown in from overseas to engage in surrogacy)
- requirements for independent legal and counselling advice for both the commissioning parties and the surrogate mother prior to agreement
- prohibitions on acting as an agent/broker to procure a surrogacy agreement
- restrictions on advertising in some jurisdictions
- age requirements for parties to the agreement (noting these vary from jurisdiction to jurisdiction)
- applications for 'substitute' parentage orders to be made before a court (at the state level), with conditions for meeting legal parentage requirements (again these laws vary across jurisdictions).[51]

The laws are intended to support people in creating families in situations in which an altruistic arrangement has been made. However, for those wanting to access surrogacy, the reality that there is not a significant number of women willing to carry and bear a child for others has led some intending parent(s) to seek international commercial surrogacy arrangements.

Questions remain as to what to do from an ethical, social and legal perspective. Only very few countries permit commercial surrogacy. Examples of practices that exploit women or commodify children have been seen. The intended parents may also be vulnerable to financial exploitation. In worse-case scenarios, issues of human trafficking have been raised, and children have been exploited by people who have used surrogacy to access them for abuse. Debates about whether to prosecute intending parents – or the agents, clinics and/or lawyers that lead them into commercial arrangements – are ongoing.

In terms of law, some argue in favour of commercial surrogacy, while many others argue strongly against it. Many argue that altruistic surrogacy is all that should be allowed. Others yet argue against all forms of surrogacy, stating it is never acceptable to use a woman's body to bear children for others. Issues of legal parentage remain for children born as a result of international commercial arrangements, although children who have a genetic connection with the intended parents enter Australia with citizenship by descent and thus are not stateless. Recent government inquiries have rejected calls by those lobbying to see commercial surrogacy introduced here, rather calling for further examination of how to support altruistic arrangements in Australia so that people do not look to engage in commercial arrangements overseas.

This chapter ends by noting that no doubt this topic and the associated issues it raises will continue to challenge people, and be hotly debated, into the future.

FURTHER READING

Allan S. Psycho-social, ethical and legal arguments for and against the retrospective release of information about donors to donor-conceived individuals in Australia. *J Law Med*. 2011;19(1): 354–76.

Allan S. Report on the review of the Assisted Reproductive Technology Act 1988 (SA). Adelaide, SA: South Australian Government; 2017.

National Health and Medical Research Council. Ethical Guidelines on the Use of Assisted Reproductive Technology in Clinical Practice and Research. Canberra: NHMRC; 2017.

Victorian Parliament Law Reform Committee. Report on the Inquiry into Donor Conceived Individuals' Access to Information about Donors. Melbourne, VIC: State Government of Victoria; 2012.

ENDNOTES

1. *Assisted Reproductive Treatment Act 2008* (Vic) ss 10–12.
2. Ibid. s 13.
3. Ibid. s 14.
4. Ibid. s 15.
5. Ibid. s 96(a). An example of the review process may be found in *ABY, ABZ v Patient Review Panel* [2011] VCAT 1382; *Patient Review Panel v ABY & ABZ* (2012) 37 VR 634; [2012] VSCA 264. In that case a prospective patient was denied treatment on the basis of her partner having a previous conviction for three counts of sexual penetration of a person aged 16/17. The patient review panel agreed that the patient should be denied treatment. The patient and her partner appealed to the Victorian Civil and Administrative Tribunal (VCAT), and VCAT held there was no barrier to treatment. The patient review panel appealed to the Supreme Court of Victoria, seeking an interpretation of the relevant sections of the Act. The Supreme Court stated that a broader test should have been applied than that used by VCAT and that they should have considered 'any identifiable and established risk factors', not just those that gave rise to the presumption against treatment. The case was returned to VCAT to be re-heard by a tribunal of different members.

6. *Assisted Reproductive Treatment Act 1988* (SA) s 9(1)(c)(i).
7. Ibid. s 9(1)(c)(iii).
8. Ibid. s 9(1)(c)(iv).
9. Ibid. s 9(1)(c)(iva).
10. Ibid. s 9(1)(c)(v).
11. Ibid. cl 8.
12. Ibid. s 9(3).
13. Ibid. s 3.
14. Ibid. s 5(2).
15. Ibid. s 5(2)(b).
16. *Human Reproductive Technology Act 1991* (WA) s 4.
17. Ibid. s 23(1)(a)(i).
18. Ibid. s 23(1)(a)(ia).
19. Ibid. s 23(1)(a)(ii).
20. Ibid. s 23(1)(a)(iii).
21. No other cause has yet been prescribed.
22. *Human Reproductive Technology Act 1991* (WA) s 23(1)(b)–(d).
23. *Human Reproductive Technology Act Directions 2004* (WA) Pt 7.
24. *Family Law Act 1975* (Cth) s 60H; *Parentage Act 2004* (ACT) s 11; *Status of Children Act 1996* (NSW) s 14; *Status of Children Act 1978* (Qld) ss 15–17; *Family Relationship Act 1975* (SA) s 10C; *Status of Children Act 1974* (Tas) s 10C; *Status of Children Act 1974* (Vic) ss 10C–10F; *Artificial Conception Act 1985* (WA) ss 5–7.
25. See, for example, *Re Patrick* (2002) 28 Fam LR 579.
26. Allan S. Report on the review of the Assisted Reproductive Technology Act 1988 (SA). Adelaide: South Australian Government; 2017.
27. For example, Belgium allows six children per donor; Canada has no set upper limits, but some fertility doctors follow the United States guidance (not law) of 25 children per population of 800,000; Denmark limits donations to 12 children per donor; France, five children; Germany, 15 children; Hong Kong and China, three children; Netherlands, 25 children; New Zealand, 10 children to four families; Norway, eight children; Sweden, 12 children to six families (with two children per family); Switzerland, eight children; the United Kingdom, 10 families worldwide. Note that not all such limits are set by the law; some jurisdictions (e.g. the United States) have guidelines by professional bodies. Adherence to, or enforcement of, such limits is also not consistent.
28. *Assisted Reproductive Treatment Act 2008* (Vic) s 29(1). Note the heading of the section refers to a 10 family limit, but the provision states women.
29. Ibid. s 17(1)(b).
30. Ibid. s 27(1).
31. Western Australian Government. *Government Gazette*, No 201. 30 November 2004, Dir 8.1: Human Reproductive Technology Directions 2004, p. 5434.
32. NHMRC. Ethical Guidelines on the Use of Assisted Reproductive in Clinical Practice and Research. Canberra, ACT: NHMRC; 2017. 5.3.1.
33. Reproductive Technology Accreditation Committee. *Code of Practice for Centres Using Assisted Reproductive Technology*, 2010, Appendix 2. (Note again that the code is currently under revision.)
34. Reproductive Technology Accreditation Committee. *Advice to Units, Technical Bulletin 3* (April 2011). http://www.fertilitysociety.com.au/rtac/technical-bulletins/. Accessed 24 June 2018.
35. *Human Tissue Act 1983* (NSW) Pt 4, ss 23, 24.
36. *Transplantation and Anatomy Act 1983* (Vic) s 21.
37. *Transplantation and Anatomy Act 1978* (ACT).
38. *Transplantation and Anatomy Act* (NT) (as in force at April 2017).
39. *Human Tissue Act 1985* (Tas).
40. *Transplantation and Anatomy Act 1979* (Qld).
41. *Human Tissue and Transplant Act 1982* (NT) s 22.
42. *Human Tissue Act 1982* s 26.
43. *Assisted Reproductive Technology Act 2007* (NSW) ss 17, 23.
44. *Assisted Reproductive Technology Act 2008* (Vic) ss 46–48.
45. *Assisted Reproductive Technology Act 1988* (SA) s 9(1)(iv).
46. *Human Reproductive Technology Act 1991* (WA) s 22.
47. Western Australian Government. *Government Gazette*, No 201. 30 November 2004, Dir 8.9.
48. See, for example, *S v Minister for Health (WA)* [2008] WASC 262; *Re Section 22 of the Human Tissue and Transplant Act (WA); Ex parte M* [2008] WASC 276.
49. See, for example, *GLS v Russell-Weisz* [2018] WASC 79.
50. NHMRC Ethical Guidelines (2017), 8.22–8.23.
51. See further *Parentage Act 2004* (ACT); *Surrogacy Act 2010* (NSW); *Surrogacy Act 2010* (Qld); *Family Relationships Act 1975* (SA); *Surrogacy Act 2012* (Tas); *Assisted Reproductive Treatment Act 2008* (Vic); *Surrogacy Act* (WA).

REVIEW QUESTIONS AND ACTIVITIES

1. Compare and contrast the varying eligibility criteria across Australia for access to ART.

2. Discuss whether and, if so, how the law addresses ethical issues raised by ART and surrogacy.

3. Why is access to information by donor-conceived people about their genetic heritage and siblings important?

4. Are limits on the number of women or families a donor of gametes or embryos may donate appropriate?

5. Fred and his wife Jane had just commenced IVF treatment after six years of infertility. Sadly, Fred was killed in an accident at work. Can Jane legally request Fred's sperm from the hospital where he was taken and continue with IVF without him?

6. What are the ethical and legal issues raised by surrogacy arrangements? What role should the law play?

12

ADVANCE CARE PLANNING AND THE WITHHOLDING AND WITHDRAWAL OF TREATMENT

LEARNING OBJECTIVES

Upon completing this chapter you should be able to:

- identify the statutory requirements and mechanisms that allow people to refuse treatment in all Australian jurisdictions
- describe the terms 'advance care planning' and 'advance care directive'
- outline relevant considerations regarding supported and substitute decision making, including guardianship and the role courts may play
- explain the legal significance of a 'not for resuscitation' order
- discuss the circumstances highlighted in the case law that enable treatment to be withdrawn from incompetent people and neonates.

INTRODUCTION

We have seen in the previous chapters that **consent** is fundamental to any healthcare treatment. Where consent is absent this may give rise to a cause of action in trespass to person or, if consent is not informed (e.g. in relation to material risks of a treatment), a cause of action in negligence. In some circumstances acting without consent can also give rise to criminal issues. In this regard, the law upholds the ethical principles of personal autonomy, self-determination and dignity.

This chapter focuses on when a person wishes to plan for situations where they may lack *some capacity* and therefore may require support to make certain

decisions, and when a person becomes *completely incapacitated* and is therefore unable to make decisions for themselves. In particular, it is concerned with advance care planning and directives and the legal provision to appoint a substitute decision-maker. It then examines the legal significance of 'do not resuscitate' orders, as well as when treatment may be withheld or withdrawn from adults and minors.

ADVANCE CARE PLANNING AND DIRECTIVES

Advance care planning allows people to express their preferences for treatment should illness or disease render them mentally incompetent in the future (either from which a person will recover, and/or for when a person reaches the end of life). Discussing, planning and recording future treatment wishes supports the autonomy and dignity of the person, allowing some control over future care. It is encouraged to be undertaken with the advice and support of health practitioners and family.

A person's wishes may be recorded in an advance care directive (sometimes referred to as a 'living will' or 'advance care plan'). Such directives are provided for by legislation in all Australian jurisdictions except New South Wales and Tasmania, where advance care directives are solely governed by the common law. In most jurisdictions where legislation does exist, legislation does not purport to extinguish the ability to make an advance care directive at common law.[1]

Common Law Advance Care Directives

The common law does not provide for anyone else to consent to medical treatment on behalf of an incompetent adult. However, it does provide that an adult may have, while competent, exercised his or her power to consent to or refuse healthcare treatment. There are no formal requirements for a common law advance care directive to be in writing. Common law advance care directives are valid if:

- the person was competent when making the directive
- at the time of making the advance care directive the person was aware of the nature and purpose of the treatment proposed (but does not need to be 'adequately informed' or to have received information about the risks and benefits of the refusal)
- the person intended and anticipated their decision to apply to the situation that ultimately arose
- no undue influence was exerted on the person in making the directive (i.e. the directive was made voluntarily).

A directive can be made based on religious, social, moral or other grounds and does not need to appear 'rational' to others.

The above was confirmed in *Hunter and New England Area Health Service v A* (2009) 74 NSWLR 88, a case heard in the Supreme Court of New South Wales. In that case, the validity of a document executed by A, who was dependent upon mechanical ventilation and kidney dialysis, was examined. A had purported to appoint two people as his enduring guardians under the New South Wales *Guardianship Act 1987*, but this appointment was invalid. Therefore, the question arose regarding whether the document that directed his guardians to refuse consent to any blood transfusion represented a valid advance care directive at common law.[2] A, a Jehovah Witness, had also completed two worksheets related to his faith in which he indicated his refusal of dialysis. McDougall J stated:

I do not accept the proposition that, in general, a competent adult's clearly expressed advance refusal of specified medical procedures of treatment should be held to be ineffective simply because, at the time

of statement of the refusal, the person was not given adequate information as to the benefits of the procedure or treatment … and the dangers consequent upon refusal. As I have said, a valid refusal may be based upon religious, social or moral grounds or indeed upon no apparent rational grounds …[3]

Statutory Advance Directives

The respective states and territories that have statutory provisions require that an advance care directive be signed and witnessed and be in a 'prescribed form'.[4] The various pieces of legislation then provide for: what is required in terms of mental capacity to execute a valid advance care directive (noting these requirements are not necessarily synonymous with the common law concept of capacity); the making of an advance care directive; and what such a directive may relate to. There is significant variation between the jurisdictions with respect to the scope of advance care directives, particularly in relation to end-of-life treatment decisions.

Australian Capital Territory

In the Australian Capital Territory the legislation requires that the person executing the directive must not have 'impaired decision-making capacity'.[5] Section 7 of the *Medical Treatment (Health Directions) Act 2006* then provides that an adult can make a 'health direction' to 'refuse, or require the withdrawal of, medical treatment generally or a particular kind of medical treatment' ('medical treatment' is not defined). Section 17 provides that a person who has made an advance care directive 'has a right to receive relief from pain and suffering'. A person can refuse any treatment.[6]

Northern Territory

In the Northern Territory a person executing an advance care directive must have 'planning capacity'.[7] Consent decisions can then be made about healthcare actions, which include the withholding or withdrawing of treatment.[8]

Queensland

In Queensland the person executing an advance care directive needs to exhibit their understanding of several matters, including the nature and the likely effects of each direction in the directive.[9] Section 35(2)(b) of the

Powers of Attorney Act 1998 then provides that a principal may, by advance directive, require a life-sustaining measure to be withheld or withdrawn. A life-sustaining measure is defined as 'health care intended to sustain or prolong life and includes CPR, assisted ventilation and artificial nutrition and hydration' but excludes blood transfusions. Section 36(2) provides that an advance care directive cannot operate unless the principal: has a terminal illness or incurable/irreversible condition and is expected to die within a year; is in a persistent vegetative state; is 'permanently unconscious'; or has an illness/injury of such severity that life cannot be sustained without the continued application of life-sustaining measures. The Queensland legislation appears to permit a person to consent in advance to any health care but limits refusals to withholding or withdrawing life-sustaining measures.[10]

South Australia

In South Australia the adult making the advance care directive must be 'competent'.[11] Section 11 of the *Advance Care Directives Act 2013* then provides that a person can give an advance directive relating to future health care. Section 4 states that references to the provision of health care in the Act include the withdrawal or withholding of life-sustaining treatment. A person can make such provision relating to future health care, residential and accommodation matters and personal affairs of the person giving the advance care directive as he or she thinks fit.[12]

The South Australian legislation specifically preserves the validity of an advance care directive even where 'the person giving the advance care directive was not fully informed in relation to each medical condition, or any other circumstance, to which the … directive relates'.[13]

Victoria

In Victoria a person making an advance care directive must have 'decision-making capacity'.[14] The *Medical Treatment Planning and Decisions Act 2016* then provides that a person can make an advance care directive in relation to medical treatment. Section 3 provides that a 'medical treatment decision' means 'a decision to consent to or refuse the commencement or continuation of medical treatment'. In making an advance care directive, a person may consent to or refuse the commencement or continuation of medical treatment or a medical

research procedure; the law does not require the person to be terminally ill.[15]

(Note: As it was seen in Chapter 8 Victoria is the only state to have introduced voluntary assisted dying legislation that, from June 2019, enables a person with full decision-making capacity to access a 'voluntary assisted dying substance' that they intend to take to execute a 'death-causing' act.[16])

Western Australia

In Western Australia the person must have 'full legal capacity' to make an advance care directive.[17] Section 110P of the *Guardianship and Administration Act 1990* provides that a person can make 'an advance health directive containing treatment decisions in respect of the person's future treatment'. Section 3 defines 'treatment decisions' as decisions to 'consent or refuse consent to the commencement or continuation of any treatment'.[18] 'Treatment' is defined to include a life-sustaining measure and palliative care.

When Does an Advance Care Directive Not Need to Be Followed?

Some legislation also details situations in which an advance care directive need not be complied with. In the Australian Capital Territory the legislation does not permit an advance care directive to be followed unless a doctor believes on reasonable grounds that it complies with the legislation.[19] In Victoria a practitioner does not need to comply with an advance care directive when the person's medical condition has changed so that the practical effect of the instructional directive would no longer be consistent with the person's preferences and values.[20] Similar provisions exist in Queensland and Western Australia.[21]

Section 110ZIA of Western Australia's Guardianship and Administration Act also provides that a medical practitioner can disregard an advance care directive when it is suspected that the person has attempted to commit suicide and urgent treatment is needed.

REVOCATION AND LIMITS OF A DECISION REGARDING TREATMENT

It is important to note that, regardless of the legislative or policy frameworks within Australia, an individual can withdraw their refusal to treatment or change their mind at any time. In addition, none of the mechanisms allow for providing care that is unlawful. For example, a person could not provide an advance care directive, or delegate power to an agent, that provided for their suffocation as soon as they became incompetent because this would amount to unlawful homicide (see Chapter 8). People and their agents must operate within the boundaries of what is considered 'reasonable care' and in the person's 'best interests', although this may well include withdrawing life support.

SUPPORT OR SUBSTITUTE DECISION-MAKERS

In Chapter 7 instances in which the law provides for support or substitute decision-makers were noted to include: someone appointed by the person in need of health care; a person assigned by the legislation; or a person appointed by a tribunal or court.[22] The following provides further broad information concerning the relevant law and considerations pertaining to such appointment.

Persons Appointed

The nomenclature of people appointed by a person may vary depending on the state or territory one is in, including 'Enduring Attorney' (Australian Capital Territory), 'Enduring Guardian' (New South Wales), 'Decision Maker' (Northern Territory), 'Attorney' (Queensland), 'Agent' or 'Enduring Guardian' (South Australia), 'Enduring Guardian' (Tasmania), 'Medical decision maker' or 'Support person' (Victoria) and 'Enduring Guardian' (Western Australia).

Reference to substitute decision-makers (or however named as above) indicates *substitute* decision-making power *only* if a person becomes incapacitated. (This differs from a 'power of attorney', which is effective when a person is not incapacitated but wishes for someone to act on their behalf in relation to certain matters.) The roles of such persons may then also differ in terms of the scope of decision making.

Table 12.1 outlines the relevant provisions for substitute decision making for incapacitated adults in the respective jurisdictions of Australia in relation to a person appointed. Note that provision is also made in Victoria for a support person to be appointed to assist in decision making.

Person Recognised/Assigned by Legislation

A 'person responsible' or 'statutory health attorney' is someone recognised by legislation as having the authority to consent to medical, health and dental treatment for an adult who is unable to provide a valid consent to that treatment. Relevant legislation in each jurisdiction assigns such people according to a 'hierarchy', specifically indicating which substitute decision-maker is to take priority. For example, in New South Wales the person responsible is in order: the person's formally appointed guardian; the person's most recent spouse or de facto with whom the person has a close and continuing relationship; an unpaid carer of the person; a relative or friend who has a close personal relationship.[23]

Table 12.2 outlines the relevant provisions for substitute decision making for incapacitated adults in the respective jurisdictions of Australia in relation to a person assigned by legislation.

Person Appointed by a Tribunal, Panel, Board or Court

A tribunal, panel, board or court may make formal guardianship orders in relation to a person over 18 years old to appoint someone to control, manage and make substitute decisions for a person who does not have capacity to do so for themselves. A formal guardianship order may be necessary when:

- a person's own decisions are placing them at risk and are not deemed to be in their own best interests
- a person does not have any family or friends willing and able to support the person and to maintain informal decision-making arrangements
- there is conflict about the person's best interests
- informal decision-making arrangements are proving not to be in the best interests of the person
- a person is being subjected to neglect, harm, abuse or exploitation, or
- a child's parents die.[24]

Table 12.3 notes relative legislative provisions for appointing a guardian by a tribunal.

Decision Making by Substitute Decision-Makers

In exercising their powers, substitute decision-makers are generally required to apply the substituted judgment

TABLE 12.1	
State/Territory Provisions: Substitute Decision-Makers	
Jurisdiction	**Appointed by the Person**
Australian Capital Territory	*Enduring Attorney – Powers of Attorney Act 2006* (ACT). Authority in relation to 'health care matters' (s 12). General principles for decision making are found in Schedule 1.
New South Wales	*Enduring guardian – Guardianship Act 1987* (NSW) s 6. Authority to give consent to 'medical or dental treatment' (s 6E). Principles for decision making are found in s 4.
Northern Territory	*Decision Maker – Advance Personal Planning Act* (NT) s 16 Can make decisions regarding refusal/withdrawal of treatment and give consent for procedures. Cannot give consent for a 'restricted health care action' (e.g. abortion, sterilisation, removal of non-regenerative tissue).
Queensland	*Attorney – Powers of Attorney Act 1998* (Qld). Can be appointed for healthcare decisions under an advance care directive (s 35(1)(c)). Power to decide 'health matters' – s 36(3). Can be appointed by way of an enduring power of attorney (s 32) in relation to personal matters (which includes health matters). Must comply with general principles and healthcare principles (Sch 1).
South Australia	*Agent – Medical Treatment and Palliative Care Act 1995* (SA) s 8. Appointed under a medical power of attorney. Can make decisions about 'medical treatment' (exceptions s 8(7)(b)). Decision-making principles – s 7(8). *Enduring guardian – Guardianship and Administration Act 1993* (SA) s 25. Can make medical or dental treatment decisions. *Substitute decision-maker – Advance Care Directives Act 2013* (SA). Persons can make advance care directives appointing a substitute decision-maker to make 'health care' decisions (Div 2, ss 21, 23). Replaces 'agent' and 'enduring guardian' (i.e. appointment of such people prior to commencement of the Act are valid and considered to be an advance care directive). Decision-making principles – Pt 2, s 10.
Tasmania	*Enduring guardian – Guardianship and Administration Act 1995* (Tas) s 32. Can consent to any health care in the person's best interests – s 25. Decision-making principles are found in s 6.
Victoria	*Medical decision-maker – Medical Treatment Planning and Decisions Act 2016* (Vic). Can make 'medical treatment decisions' to consent to or refuse the commencement of medical treatment – s 26. Must give effect to a values directive in making the decision if this has been completed by the incapacitated person – s 7. If not, the decision must be made on the basis of what he/she reasonably believes is the decision the person would have made – s 61. *A support person* may be appointed to assist in decision making – Part 3, Div 3.
Western Australia	*Enduring guardian – Guardianship and Administration Act 1990* (WA) s 110B. By way of an enduring power of guardianship, can make 'treatment decisions' for a person – ss 100G, 45 ('treatment decisions' defined in s 3).

test, which involves making a decision consistent with what the person would have decided if they had the capacity to do so. Evidence of such wishes may be provided by advance care directives, religious beliefs and/or the previous history of treatment.[25] If such information is not known then the decision-maker must apply a best interests test, which requires a balancing of the benefit to the person who will be treated against the risks of the proposed treatment.

Note that in those jurisdictions (New South Wales and Tasmania) that do not have statutory provisions for advance care directives, the guardianship Acts and common law are relevant regarding what decisions may be made (including refusal of healthcare treatment).

	TABLE 12.2
	State/Territory Provisions: Substitute Decision-Maker Recognised By Legislation
Jurisdiction	**Recognised by Legislation (e.g. Partner, Carer, Friend)**
Australian Capital Territory	*Health attorney – Guardianship and Management of Property Act 1991* (ACT) s 32B (partner, carer, close relative or friend). Decision-making principles are contained in s 4.
New South Wales	*Person responsible – Guardianship Act 1987* (NSW) s 33A (guardian, spouse, carer, close friend or relative). Decision-making principles are found in s 4.
Northern Territory	A default substitute decision-maker is not listed in the NT law. If there is no available consenter (appointed decision-maker or guardian), the healthcare provider or another interested person may apply to the NT Civil and Administrative Tribunal for a decision.
Queensland	*Statutory health attorney – Guardianship and Administration Act 2000* (Qld) s 66. Can consent to health matters. Statutory health attorney defined in the *Powers of Attorney Act 1998* (Qld) s 63(1) (guardian, spouse, carer, close friend, relative). General principles and healthcare principles apply – s 76 PAA.
South Australia	*Person responsible – Guardianship and Administration Act 1993* (SA) s 59 (includes 'prescribed relative') (defined in s 3). Can consent to medical and dental treatment (not prescribed treatment).
Tasmania	*Person responsible – Guardianship and Administration Act 1995* (Tas) s 39. Spouse, carer, close friend or relative (defined in s 4) can consent to medical and dental treatment. Decision-making principles are found in s 6.
Victoria	*Person responsible– Guardianship and Administration Act 1986* (Vic) s 39. Can consent to medical or dental treatment. Person responsible defined in s 37. Decision-making principles are found in s 38.
Western Australia	*Person responsible– Guardianship and Administration Act 1990* (WA) s 100ZD. Can make treatment decisions (spouse, nearest relative, primary carer). Must act in the best interests of the person – s 100ZD(8).

Section 32 of the New South Wales Guardianship Act provides that an enduring guardian 'can only consent to medical or dental treatment that will promote health and well-being'. However, in *FI v Public Guardian* [2008] NSWADT 263, the court said 'the law today recognises that the guardian's functions can properly extend to the making of decisions in connection with health care that include decisions to withdraw life-sustaining treatment'. In Tasmania an enduring guardian appointed under section 2 of the Guardianship and Administration Act may refuse healthcare treatment.

The guardianship legislation in all jurisdictions also specifies certain treatments that cannot be consented to except with the approval of the tribunal or board.[26] These are referred to as 'special' or 'prescribed' procedures or treatments[27] and may include such things as sterilisation, noting variation exists between the jurisdictions as to which treatments or procedures are identified as falling within this category.

COMMONWEALTH LEGISLATION

The *Family Law Act 1975* (Cth) confers on the Family Court the power to make orders authorising a person to carry out medical treatment on an intellectually disabled person who is the 'child of a marriage', even where the treatment is not authorised by the state or territory guardianship Acts. This position is consistent with the Constitution (s 109), which serves to strike down state legislation to the extent that it is inconsistent with federal legislation.

'NOT FOR RESUSCITATION' OR 'DO NOT RESUSCITATE' ORDERS

For health practitioners working in many varied settings, 'not for resuscitation' (NFR) orders are commonplace. Such orders most frequently apply in situations where a person suffers collapse requiring cardiopulmonary resuscitation – the NFR order signifies that the healthcare

TABLE 12.3	
State/Territory Provisions: Substitute Decision-Maker Appointed By A Tribunal	
Jurisdiction	**Appointed by a Tribunal**
Australian Capital Territory	*Guardian* appointed – *Guardianship and Management of Property Act 1991* (ACT) s 7. Decision-making principles are found in s 4.
New South Wales	*Guardian* appointed by tribunal – *Guardianship Act 1987* (NSW) s 14. Under s 36, can give consent to 'medical or dental treatment' and 'special treatment'. Decision-making principles are found in s 4.
Northern Territory	*Guardian* appointed by tribunal – *Guardianship of Adults Act 2016* (NT) s 11. Under s 23, can make decisions regarding healthcare action that is not restricted healthcare action; subject to ss 41 and 42 of the *Advance Personal Planning Act*. Decision-making principles are found in s 4.
Queensland	*Guardian* appointed by tribunal – *Guardianship and Administration Act 2000* (Qld) s 12. Guardian can consent to 'health matters'. Must apply healthcare principles and general principles – s 34.
South Australia	*Guardian* appointed by guardianship board – *Guardianship and Administration Act 1993* (SA) s 29. Guardian as far as reasonably practicable to give effect to advance care directive (s 31A). Can consent to medical and dental treatment (except prescribed treatment) – s 59. Decision-making principles are found in s 5.
Tasmania	*Guardian* appointed by guardianship board – *Guardianship and Administration Act 1995* s 20. Can consent to any health care in person's best interests – s 25 (also s 39 medical or dental treatment). Decision-making principles are found in s 6.
Victoria	*Guardian* appointed by tribunal – *Guardianship and Administration Act 1986* (Vic) s 22. Can consent to medical or other treatment – s 39. Decision-making principles are found in s 38.
Western Australia	*Guardian* appointed by the State Administrative Tribunal – *Guardianship and Administration Act 1990* s 43. Can make 'treatment decisions' – s 45. Requirement to act in best interests of person – s 51.

team will not commence resuscitation. Death will likely ensue.

NFR and 'do not resuscitate' (DNR) orders usually become relevant in situations in which a person's condition is unlikely to improve or is considered hopeless. The practice of NFR should be openly discussed because there are times when a lack of clarity and communication has rendered the practice legally questionable. For example, there may be times when the treating doctor has not conveyed the order to other members in the healthcare team who are placed in a difficult position when the person subsequently collapses. Conversely, there may be confusion about a person's directions and when to follow them.

Several issues need to be addressed to avoid legal problems. The precise criteria and philosophy that underpin an NFR decision should be openly discussed and known to those health practitioners involved. Many hospitals and agencies have criteria clearly listed and incorporated into policies. The method of documenting the order should be clear and concise. The order should be written in the person's healthcare record unambiguously. Covert practices such as abbreviations and symbols used to denote the order can create confusion. The problem with the use of symbols is that the author is anonymous. For example, using self-adhesive coloured dots on a person's healthcare record is an unacceptable method of signifying an NFR order.

NFR can be viewed as a person's decision to refuse treatment or a medical decision not to provide treatment because the resuscitation will be unlikely to succeed due to the person's illness. To comply with the law, whether there is valid refusal of treatment and the relevant law regarding advance care decision making need to be considered. Therefore, the person, or their representative (support or substitute decision-maker), generally should be involved in making the decision.

NFR and DNR orders are not for health practitioners to make alone unless the medical team believe that any further treatment, including resuscitation, is futile. In such circumstances it is always considered good practice to discuss this with the person and/or their representative so they are aware.

Many institutions and employers have developed policies that are intended to guide clinical practice. These should be openly discussed, and staff should have a clear understanding in relation to their professional roles and responsibilities. Health practitioners must balance their duty of care to the person they are caring for and that person's wishes within existing legal parameters. Note, the term 'no cardiopulmonary resuscitation' ('no CPR') has been used in preference to NFR or DNR in some institutions. This is because it unequivocally states which treatment is to be withheld and avoids the implications of decisions not to resuscitate. For a valid 'no CPR' or NFR order, the following criteria are suggested:

- The person or their agent or guardian is involved in the decision, together with key members of the healthcare team.
- The order is clearly written in the person's healthcare record.
- The order is reviewed regularly.

If a person's condition dramatically improves or they change their mind, the order may be revoked. However, while the order is in place and has been consented to by the person to whom it relates, it should be honoured.

This also applies in emergency situations such as prehospital settings in which, for example, paramedics need to make a decision about whether or not to provide treatment/resuscitate. However, while the law is clear, its application in such settings may not be. For example, if a person lacks capacity to communicate their wishes at the time, it may be necessary to establish whether there is anything that *evidences they did not wish to be resuscitated* such as a DNR bracelet, a card stating their wishes or a DNR order signed by them, and then whether the refusal *applies in the circumstances*. The decision will depend on the circumstances and information available to the responder. Note, without clear evidence, and with little time to gather it, it would be unlikely that the responder would be liable for battery if the decision was made to administer resuscitation, even if

it was later found that the person did not wish to be resuscitated. On the other hand, if there is clear evidence supporting a DNR then the responder should not act to treat the person.

EXAMPLES OF GUARDIANSHIP DECISIONS REGARDING WITHHOLDING OR WITHDRAWAL OF TREATMENT

The guardianship boards and appointed guardians do not have the same broad powers as the superior courts, but nonetheless they are more frequently becoming involved in decisions to withdraw or refuse treatment. Examples of cases illustrate the types of situations in which they have confirmed or denied this was warranted.

In Queensland the Civil and Administrative Tribunal has been granted express power to refuse life-sustaining treatments. The tribunal's decision is reliant upon the healthcare provider's opinion that commencement or continuation of treatment is inconsistent with good medical practice. In *Re RWG* [2000][28] the wife of a man with an acquired brain injury made an application for an NFR order and for the power to refuse antibiotics. The Civil and Administrative Tribunal agreed to the NFR order but refused to grant the wife the power to withhold antibiotics, which were not actually required at the time, because the tribunal decided it was premature to examine that issue.

In a more recent case[29] the Queensland tribunal was asked to determine whether a man suffering from Wernicke's encephalopathy and Korsakoff's psychosis, and who had suffered a brain stem stroke, could have artificial hydration and feeding discontinued. The tribunal found that the medical evidence was sufficient to indicate that continuation of the feeding and hydration was inconsistent with good medical practice and that it should cease. The case also highlighted that a finding of good medical practice did not require unanimous support from all medical opinion.

In the New South Wales case of *Re AG* [2007][30] a woman with an intellectual disability who lived alone (with various support services assisting her) had been diagnosed with a renal tumour with lymphadenopathy in the abdomen and pelvis, and possible secondary brain tumours. Her prognosis was very poor, and she had a history of refusing medical treatment. The

Public Guardian, which had previously been appointed to manage her care, was asked to make a decision to refuse resuscitation and dialysis. The Public Guardian approached the Guardianship Tribunal for direction. The tribunal found that the Public Guardian could provide consent or refuse care, provided the care promoted and maintained the woman's health and wellbeing in accordance with the New South Wales Guardianship Act. The tribunal stated that the weight of authority supported the notion that limiting treatment can promote a person's health and wellbeing if it prevents futile treatment. The tribunal also found that guardians involved in healthcare decisions could be involved in advance care planning.

In Victoria, in the case of *Re BWV*,[31] the Public Advocate, appointed by the Victorian Civil and Administrative Tribunal, applied to the Supreme Court seeking clarification of the relevant legislation before making a decision to refuse treatment on behalf of an incompetent person.

In Western Australia, in *BTO* [2004],[32] the Guardianship Board, interpreting section 119 of the Guardianship and Administration Act, allowed the interpretation to be extended to include withdrawal of artificial nutrition and hydration. The board found that consent for withdrawal of treatment could be given, provided it was in the person's best interest. In this case a man had suffered a severe stroke and was in a coma. The board interpreted the legislation to include consent to medical procedures and decisions to withdraw life-sustaining procedures. A guardian was appointed with the power to refuse artificial hydration and feeding.

Summary: Decision Making for Legally Incompetent Adults

When faced with treatment decisions concerning a legally incompetent person, health practitioners must be aware of the order of priority regarding the various alternate decision-making mechanisms and persons responsible. Table 12.4 lists the type of treatment and consent considerations for legally incompetent adults regarding those who can provide consent to (or refuse) treatment.

Withholding and Withdrawal of Treatment From Minors

The issue of withholding or withdrawing life-saving and life-sustaining treatment in relation to minors has

TABLE 12.4
Those Who Can Provide Consent for Legally Incompetent Adults

Type of Treatment	Consent Considerations
Emergency/life-threatening	No consent required.
Routine observation, includes non-intrusive examination	
All other care minor/major	Has the person specified treatment according to the relevant advance care directive common law and/or legislative framework?
	Has an agent or guardian been appointed?
	Are there any guidelines (e.g. from health departments) that should be followed?
	Does the guardianship board have a 'person responsible' list to guide health practitioners?
	If no next of kin, or if relatives are in disagreement and the healthcare team is uncertain, then consult the guardianship board.
Controversial care, special care* or where there is disagreement as to care by family and/or the healthcare team	Guardianship board or court.

*Special or controversial care could include any experimental procedures, sterilisation, termination of pregnancy and any aversive treatment or withdrawal of life support. Disagreement between family or health carers may be in relation to *any* care provided.

been mostly examined in the context of neonates with severe disabilities. Notably, in Australia, there has been little recourse to the courts regarding managing the withdrawal or withholding of life-saving/sustaining treatment from infants and young children, presumably because such issues are most often resolved in the clinical setting by families, the healthcare support team and ethical or religious consultation when required.

However, as discussed in Chapter 7, parental decision-making authority extends only so far as it is in the best interests of the child. Recourse may be had to the courts by the treating health practitioners if there is concern that the parents are not acting in the 'best interests of the child', or by parents if they are concerned about the treatment being provided (or refused) to their child. The recent case of *Re Director Clinical Services, Child and Adolescent Services and Kiszko* [2016] FCWA 19 (*Kiszko*) provides an example regarding these issues.

Six-year-old Oshin Kiszko had been diagnosed with brain cancer in 2015. The court found that 'the focus of Oshin's parents from the outset was upon his suffering and how it could be alleviated while that of the hospital clinicians was upon maximising the prospects of curing him'.[33] The clinical evidence was that it was 'time-critical' that Oshin commence chemotherapy and radiotherapy, but the parents refused such treatment.

The conflict resulted in three court hearings pursuant to the *Family Court Act 1997* (WA) regarding the best interests of the child's welfare. In the first hearing the hospital sought an order that chemotherapy occur in Oshin's best interests; the court agreed. In the second hearing, the treating oncologist gave evidence that Oshin required chemotherapy and radiotherapy to save his life. However, Oshin's parents insisted that natural therapies (herbs, massage) had a higher chance of success. Following expert evidence presented in the court, Oshin's parents agreed to chemotherapy but not radiotherapy. Thackaray CJ took the view that the child's best interests were inextricably linked to the family and that the court should not interfere in parental authority to make decisions unless there was a 'clear justification' for doing so.[34] The impact on the parents of forced treatment was also considered relevant to determining Oshin's best interests.[35]

Oshin showed significant improvement following two cycles of chemotherapy, leading to further chemotherapy and radiotherapy treatment options. However, Oshin's parents refused to consent to this, wanting him to commence palliative care. This led to a third hearing in which O'Brien J concluded that Oshin's chances of long-term survival were now very low. O'Brien J refused to order further treatment, noting:

The importance to Oshin of his relationship with his parents weighs heavily in my decision. That relationship, and the support and love which only his parents can give, are of critical importance to Oshin and to his quality of life over the months to come. I am deeply concerned that the perpetuation of the conflict over Oshin's treatment will continue to diminish the ability of his parents to focus their energies solely on the provision of that support and love directly to him when he needs it most.[36]

Other cases involving parental refusal of potentially life-saving treatment for minors lacking capacity have been less prepared to defer to the parents' views. In the South Australian case of *Women's and Children's Health Network Inc v M, CN* [2013] SASC 16, David J ruled that medical staff had the authority to administer blood transfusions to a three-year-old child with acute lymphoblastic leukaemia, despite the parents' objections to this on the grounds of their religious convictions.[37] In applying the best interests test the court noted that:

Without treatment, the universally accepted prognosis for ALL sufferers is death, probably within a matter of weeks of diagnosis. With treatment, there is an 85 to 90 per cent cure rate … the recommended course of treatment for [congenital mirror movement disorder] cannot be undertaken with any degree of safety without transfusions of blood or blood products.[38]

The efficacy of the treatment and the probability of a successful outcome were regarded as the determining factors. This has been the more consistent feature of the decisions regarding when parents have refused probable life-saving treatment for their children.[39]

Note, the situation in which the parents refuse potentially life-saving or sustaining treatment for their child appears less common than when treating doctors recommend the withholding or withdrawal of treatment from the child, and the parents challenge this. However, these cases have, again, rarely surfaced in Australian courts. Nevertheless, the case law has evolved to focus on the 'best interests' test. In a 2012 Supreme Court of New South Wales case the mother of a nine-month-old baby, 'M', sought to compel medical staff to treat her child, who was suffering from pyruvate dehydrogenase deficiency, a genetic neurodegenerative disorder.[40] The court refused to grant the application, finding that it was not in M's best interests to treat him with mechanical ventilation because it would cause pain and discomfort, with no curative effect or alleviation of his condition.

Although it is beyond the scope of this discussion to explore further cases from abroad, it is noted that there is much more authority on 'best interests' determinations in the United Kingdom.[41] The cases together demonstrate that the determination of best interests is multifaceted and complex: 'susceptible to very different conclusions being drawn by different people of equal compassion, sincerity and integrity'.[42] The cases have also highlighted that there may be a place for mediation or dispute resolution in preference over the court process in some circumstances.[43] Nevertheless, in the most difficult of cases courts have a necessary and important role to play.

FURTHER READING

Butson L, Shircore M, Butson B. A right to refuse: legal aspects of dealing with intoxicated patients who refuse treatment. *J Law Med.* 2013;20:542–559.

Detering KM, Hancock AD, Reade MC, Silvester W. The impact of advance care planning on end of life care in elderly patients: randomised controlled trial. *BMJ.* 2010;23(340):c1345.

Griffiths D. Understanding law in clinical practice: theory or reality? *J Law Med.* 2013;20(4):728–733.

Hafford K. When not to resuscitate a profoundly disabled child – difficult decisions for the courts and practitioners. *Aust Health Law Bull.* 2012;20(10):157–158.

ENDNOTES

1. In Western Australia, Queensland and the Northern Territory the common law is expressly preserved: see *Guardianship and Administration Act 1990* (WA) s 110ZB; *Powers of Attorney Act 1998* (Qld) s 39; and *Advance Personal Planning Act* (NT) (in force from 2016) s 55(2). Impliedly in Victoria and the Australian Capital Territory it is preserved because of the statement in the relevant legislation that other rights to refuse treatment are not affected by the legislation: *Medical Treatment Planning and Decisions Act 2016* (Vic) s 10; *Medical Treatment (Health Directions) Act 2006* (ACT) s 6. There is no mention of the common law being preserved in South Australian legislation.

2. The court accepted that 'to some extent' the *Guardianship Act 1987* (NSW) gives recognition to advance care directives by virtue of section 33(3)(b), but there is no specific vehicle for these under the legislation.

3. *Hunter and New England Area Health Service v A* (2009) 74 NSWLR 88 at [28].

4. *Medical Treatment (Health Directions) Act 2006* (ACT) s 8 (directions can be non-written: s 9); *Medical Treatment Planning and Decisions Act 2016* (Vic) s 16; *Advance Care Directives Act 2013* (SA) s 11(2) (a person must complete an advance care directive form); *Guardianship and Administration Act 1990* (WA) s 110Q(1) (which also contains a requirement that the person be encouraged to seek legal or medical advice); *Advance Personal Planning Act*

(NT) s 9(2) (in force from 2016); *Powers of Attorney Act 1998* (Qld) s 44(3)(a) (although there is no requirement that it be in a prescribed form. Under section 44(6) a doctor must certify that the person appeared to have capacity).

5. See *Medical Treatment (Health Directions) Act 2006* (ACT) s 7(3). It also requires that the person not have a guardian appointed.

6. Or require the withdrawal of any treatment: see *Medical Treatment (Health Directions) Act 2006* (ACT) s 7.

7. *Advance Personal Planning Act* (in force from 2016) (NT) s 8.

8. Ibid. s 38(b).

9. See section 42(1) of the *Powers of Attorney Act 1998* (Qld), which also states that the person needs to understand the effects of capacity and impaired capacity upon the operation of the advance directive.

10. *Powers of Attorney Act 1998* (Qld) s 35. Section 35(20)(c) also allows a person to authorise an attorney to 'physically restrain, move or manage the principal' for the purpose of necessary health care.

11. *Advance Care Directives Act 2013* (SA) s 11.

12. Ibid. s 3.

13. Ibid. s 11(5)(c).

14. *Medical Treatment Planning and Decisions Act 2016* (Vic) s 13(a) (i).

15. Ibid. s 6.

16. *Voluntary Assisted Dying Act 2017* (Vic) s 4.

17. *Guardianship and Administration Act 1990* (WA) s 110P. The section also requires that the person understands the nature of the decision and its consequences.

18. *Guardianship and Administration Act 1990* (WA) Pt 9B s 3. Section 3 defines treatment widely to mean 'medical or surgical treatment' including a life-sustaining measure and palliative care.

19. *Medical Treatment (Health Directions) Act 2006* (ACT) s 12(a).

20. *Medical Treatment Planning and Decisions Act 2016* (Vic) s 51(1).

21. *Powers of Attorney Act 1998* (Qld) s 103(1); *Guardianship and Administration Act 1990* (WA) s 110S(3).

22. South Australia has legislation specific to consent to medical treatment, which provides for medical powers of attorney: *Consent to Medical Treatment and Palliative Care Act 1995* (SA).

23. *Guardianship Act 1987* (NSW) s 33A.

24. Allan S. Health Law Central: Consent-Incapacity (Adults). http://www.healthlawcentral.com/decisions/consent-incapacity/. Accessed 11 March 2019.

25. See, for example, *Hunter and New England Area Health Service v A* (2009) 74 NSWLR 88; [2009] NSWSC 761.

26. Unless there is an advance directive covering the procedure or treatment.

27. *Guardianship and Management of Property Act 1991* (ACT) (prescribed medical procedure in dictionary section); *Guardianship Act 1987* (NSW) s 33 (special treatment); *Guardianship and Administration Act 2000* (Qld) s 68, Sch 2 (6, 7) (special health care); *Guardianship and Administration Act 1993* (SA) s 3(1) (prescribed treatment); *Guardianship and Administration Act 1995* (Tas) s 3(1) (special treatment); *Guardianship and Administration Act 1986* (Vic) (special procedure). The *Guardianship of Adults Act* (NT) refers to restricted health care (s 8(1)). There is no equivalent term in the Western Australian legislation; only

sterilisation is specifically referred to as a procedure that requires the consent of the State Administrative Tribunal.

28. *Re RWG* [2000] QGAAT 2.

29. *Re HG* [2006] QGAAT 26.

30. *Re AG* [2007] NSW GT 1, 5 February 2009.

31. *Re BWV; Ex parte Gardner* (2003) 7 VR 487.

32. *BTO* [2004] WAGAB 2.

33. *Re Director Clinical Services, Child & Adolescent Health Services and Kiszko* at [62].

34. Ibid. at [63].

35. Ibid. at [71].

36. Ian Freckelton QC. Parents' opposition to potentially life-saving treatment for minors: learning from the Oshin Kiszko litigation. *J Law Med.* 2016;24(1):61. Reproduced with permission of Thomson Reuters (Professional) Australia Limited, legal.thomsonreuters.com.au.

37. *Women's and Children's Health Network Inc v M, CN* [2013] SASC 16.

38. Ibid. [2013] SASC 16 at [6]–[7].

39. *Children, Youth & Women's Health Services Inc v YJL, MHL and TL (By His Next Friend)* ('YJL') (2010) 107 SASR 343; *Women's and Children's Health Network Inc v JC, JC, and KC (By Her Litigation Guardian)* ('JC') [2012] SASC 104.

40. 'Mohammed's Case', *TS & DS v Sydney Children's Hospital Network* [2012] NSWSC 1609.

41. See, for example, *Alder Hey Children's NHS Foundation Trust v Evans* [2018] EWHC 953 (Fam) at [3]; *Great Ormond Street Hospital v Yates and others* [2017] EWHC 972; *Portsmouth Hospitals NHS Trust v Wyatt* [2006] 2 FLR 111.

42. *Re Director Clinical Services, Child & Adolescent Health Services and Kiszko* [2016] FCWA 24 at [101].

43. *Great Ormond Street Hospital v Yates* [2017] EWHC 1909 at [20].

REVIEW QUESTIONS AND ACTIVITIES

1. What is meant by the term advance care planning?

2. Is an advance care directive the same as a 'not for resuscitation' order?

3. Identify your state or territory's current legal requirements and compare them with one of the other Australian jurisdictions. How do they differ? Which jurisdiction provides a clearer framework?

4. Who may be a 'person responsible' and what role do they play in patient care?

5. Explain when a 'do not resuscitate' order may be made.

6. What are the legal responsibilities of health practitioners regarding the withholding or withdrawal of treatment from neonates?

Section 4   **FURTHER PRACTICE CONSIDERATIONS**

13

THE REMOVAL AND DONATION OF HUMAN BLOOD, TISSUE AND ORGANS

LEARNING OBJECTIVES

Upon completing this chapter you should be able to:

- explain the circumstances under which regenerative and non-regenerative human tissue may be removed and donated
- discuss the importance of consent to the removal of human tissue and organs
- identify state/territory and Commonwealth powers and participation in regulating and coordinating tissue transplantation and donation
- discuss special considerations relevant to children regarding tissue transplantation
- identify law and guidelines relevant to the removal and donation of human blood, tissue and organs.

INTRODUCTION

Historically, the common law has never permitted the removal of body parts from a living person if it was not considered therapeutic for that person. Removing tissue or an organ from a body constituted the offence of maiming. Even with the person's consent, removal could not be undertaken. The consent did not negate the crime. However, following a historical Australian Law Reform Commission report[1] in 1977, which included draft legislation, all Australian jurisdictions legislated to regulate the donation and removal of tissue from living and dead donors. This chapter considers the current law regarding removing tissue during life and after death.

ETHICAL AND LEGAL ISSUES

Regulation has addressed a wide variety of ethical and legal issues, which include a prohibition on the sale of organs, the donation of tissue after death, requirements for a valid consent, identification of individuals who may provide consent and the legal definition of death. In the Australian context the relevant legislation is based on the presumption that there must be some clear indication that the person intended to donate tissue – that is, a system whereby the person must expressly 'opt in' to be a donor of tissue. This is distinct from the presumption in some European countries that all citizens are potential donors unless they 'opt out'.

Tissue That May Be Removed

The legislation divides human tissue into two categories:

- regenerative tissue, which includes tissue that is capable of replacing itself and includes blood, skin, bone marrow and semen
- non-regenerative tissue, which includes all other tissue that is not capable of replacement due to bodily function – for example, the lungs, heart, kidneys, corneas, blood vessels, bone and cartilage.

Removal of Regenerative Tissue

Blood Donations

All jurisdictions except Queensland require donors to make statements regarding their suitability to give blood. Then, at law, a person over the age of 16 in the Australian Capital Territory, New South Wales, South Australia,

Tasmania and the Northern Territory, or over 18 in Queensland and Western Australia, of sound mind, may consent, either orally or in writing, to the removal (donation) of blood from himself or herself for transfusion into another person or for use of any of its constituents for other therapeutic purposes or for medical or scientific purposes.[2]

In relation to children, all jurisdictions except the Northern Territory also make provision for the donation of blood by a child for transfusion into another person with the consent of a parent.[3] Before a donation can proceed, a medical practitioner must advise the parties concerned that removing the blood is not likely to be prejudicial to the health of the child and the child must agree to such removal (if able to do so).

Note, in 2018 the Australian Red Cross Blood Service implemented a policy to only accept donations from people over the age of 18 due to evidence that donation prior to this age may negatively affect the health and wellbeing of the child.

Blood Transfusions

In relation to transfusion, when an adult patient's competence to consent to, or refuse, such treatment is in doubt a court may be called upon to decide.[4]

The giving of a blood transfusion to a child, particularly when the parents refuse consent, has been specifically addressed in various state and territory legislation. Some jurisdictions require that one or two doctors may provide consent when the parents refuse consent, provided the transfusion is 'necessary for the child's health' or the 'child is in danger of dying'.

Other Regenerative Tissue

Legislation in all jurisdictions allows donation of regenerative tissue by competent consenting adults for: the purposes of transplantation into the body of another living person; other therapeutic purposes; medical purposes; and other scientific purposes.[5] For the consent to be effective, the donor must consider and specify the tissue to be removed and the purpose of the removal.[6] There is a general requirement in all jurisdictions that the adult's consent must be verbal and in writing, ensuring that the common law principles of consent are fulfilled. In South Australia and Western Australia consent cannot be given in the presence of the person's family. This presumably serves to avoid the risk of

coercion or undue pressure being placed on a person considering live donation during the consent process.

In all jurisdictions except South Australia and Western Australia there is the additional requirement that the consent is given in the presence of a doctor, who certifies the patient's consent in writing. The notion of a 'certified' person refers to a medical practitioner who must ensure that the requirements of the consent have been properly addressed. In addition, the certified person is usually not the same person as the one removing the tissue.

In the case of children, written parental consent is required, and many jurisdictions specify which types of regenerative tissue may be taken. The New South Wales Act expressly states that the competent child must also agree.[7]

Three states, New South Wales, Queensland and Victoria, specify conditions relating to taking tissue from young and incompetent children, and there is a requirement that medical practitioners certify that certain conditions or factors have been addressed. In Queensland three medical practitioners must certify that:

- due to the child's age obtaining consent from the child is not possible
- the family member receiving the tissue is likely to die without the transplant
- the risk to the child is minimal.

New South Wales requires two medical practitioners to certify the same three factors as in Queensland, plus several factors associated with the parent's consent including that: the procedure and its effects have been explained; the parent is of sound mind; the parent understands the nature and effects of the removal and transplantation; and that consent was freely given.

In Victoria when the child is too young to understand, removal can only occur when it is necessary to save the life of a sibling.

In most state and territory legislation the person for whom the tissue is intended is also identified and usually refers to 'a parent or sibling' (New South Wales, Queensland, Victoria) or 'for another living person' (South Australia) or 'another member of the family or relative' (the Australian Capital Territory, Tasmania, Western Australia), and this can include adoptive and step-siblings.

The Family Court also has the power to consent to removing regenerative tissue, provided it is in the child's best interests. For example, in *GWW and CMW*[8] a 10-year-old boy and his parents consented to donating the boy's bone marrow to treat his aunt's leukaemia. The Family Court found that the child was not competent to provide consent and the parents did not have the power to consent to the procedure. The court, however, did find that removing the bone marrow was in the child's best interests after balancing the relationship between the child and the aunt, the value of a continued relationship with her and the risks associated with the donation.

In New South Wales a designated person is responsible for making decisions to remove tissue when there is no next of kin. The Northern Territory makes no provision for removing any tissue, either regenerative or non-regenerative, from a child.

Non-Regenerative Tissue

Adults may consent to the removal of non-regenerative tissue. The most common provision in the legislation across the state and territory jurisdictions is the stipulation of a suitable lapse of time from the point at which consent, usually written, is obtained until the tissue is removed. This can be likened to a 'cooling off' period to allow the donor time to change their mind. In the case of children, the South Australian, Western Australian and Victorian Acts expressly refer to children and do not permit removal of non-regenerative tissue from a minor. There is no provision for removing such tissue from children in the New South Wales, Northern Territory, Queensland or Tasmanian Acts.

The Australian Capital Territory is the only jurisdiction that allows specified non-regenerative tissue to be removed from a child.[9] The legislation in that jurisdiction states that the transplantation of tissue must be to the body of 'another member of the family of the child' and when a 'family member' is in danger of dying. The provisions that outline the required procedure of obtaining consent are set out in section 14 of the Act. Both parents must provide written consent 24 hours after the verbal consent is given. The time the consent was given is recorded and a doctor must certify in writing that, prior to obtaining the written consent, the parents were advised that the family member was in danger of dying. Additional requirements include an explanation of both the nature and effect of removing the tissue from the child, together with the nature of the tissue

transplantation. Prior to certifying the consent, the doctor must be satisfied that, at the time consent was given, the child understood the nature and effect of removing the tissue, understood the transplantation procedure and agreed with that procedure.

The certifying doctor must give the written consent and the certification documents to a formal committee appointed by the Minister for Health. It is the role of the committee to review the application and, if of the opinion that the tissue transplantation is desirable in the circumstances, authorise the removal of that tissue.

Revocation of Consent

In the jurisdictions that permit the removal of non-regenerative and/or regenerative tissue, the donor may change their mind at any time. Should this be the case, there is a general onus on the health practitioners involved to inform the 'designated officer' or equivalent individual of the withdrawal of consent. Designated officers are specifically appointed under each Act and are usually senior medical staff or the medical staff in charge of the hospital. To ensure the revocation of consent is made clear to all involved, documentation and, in some jurisdictions, specific requirements such as the return of the consent form to the donor are required.[10] In Victoria, for example, the revocation of a donor's consent for non-regenerative tissue must be recorded and kept for three years and the designated officer must be informed by the health practitioners.[11]

Removing Tissue From an Incompetent Adult

When patients are deemed incompetent the general rule is that medical procedures require the consent of a substitute decision-maker such as a guardian, medical attorney or persons responsible (see Chapters 7 and 12). The guiding principle is that the procedure or intervention is in the patient's best interests and represents, wherever possible, what the person would have decided themselves.

The law generally does not allow for substitute decision-makers to provide consent for removing non-regenerative tissue from someone lacking competency to decide for themselves because it is not generally arguable to be in their 'best interests'. Any removal of tissue is considered a 'special procedure' in Victoria and 'special healthcare' in Queensland, requiring consent from the Victorian Civil and Administrative Tribunal or the Queensland Civil and Administrative Tribunal respectively. In Tasmania and the Australian Capital Territory the removal of non-regenerative tissue requires guardianship authority. In New South Wales no substitute decision-maker, including the Guardianship Tribunal, can provide consent to remove tissue. Instead consent must be sought by the New South Wales Supreme Court. Indeed, the Supreme Court in each jurisdiction has the *parens patriae* jurisdiction to consent to removing tissue if the donation serves the incompetent patient's best interests.

An example of such a case is that of *Northern Sydney and Central Coast Area Health Service v CT*[12] in which the New South Wales Supreme Court gave consent for bone marrow to be removed from an adult with an intellectual disability (CT) to be given to his brother (NT), who had non-Hodgkin's lymphoma. The donation of the bone marrow served CT no therapeutic purpose and the court was asked to use its *parens patriae* power to assess CT's best interests in light of him being the best suitable donor for his brother. The court found that, having regard to all the circumstances (e.g. NT was CT's co-guardian) and the minimal risks involved in the procedure, the overwhelming evidence favoured a benefit to CT if NT's life was saved. The court ordered that CT should participate as a donor.

Removing Tissue After Death

If a person dies in hospital, in all jurisdictions except Queensland, tissue can be removed from a body if a designated officer of the hospital, after making reasonable enquiries, concludes that the person had, during their lifetime, expressed the wish for, or consented to, the removal after death of tissue from that person's body and had not withdrawn the wish or consent.[13] For example, an individual's consent (or refusal) to donation may have been lodged on the Australian Organ Donor Register or expressed in his or her will.

If the designated officer cannot establish the deceased's prior consent, tissue can be removed if the designated officer, after making reasonable enquiries, concludes the person had not, during his or her lifetime, expressed an objection to tissue being removed from his or her body *and* that the person's next of kin has consented to, or not objected to, removing tissue from the person's body.[14]

In all jurisdictions except Victoria, if there is more than one available next of kin, an objection by any one of the next of kin will be sufficient to prevent the removal of tissue.

In the Australian Capital Territory, Victoria, South Australia and the Northern Territory the respective legislation provides that when a designated officer is unable to ascertain the existence or whereabouts of a next of kin, he or she may authorise the removal of tissue.[15] The other jurisdictions are silent on this issue.

If there is an evident disagreement between the wishes of the donor and the next of kin, the general rule is that the donor's wishes are to be respected. The Victorian legislation is the exception in that it appears to allow the senior available next of kin to consent, even when the donor objected. Nevertheless, in practice when relatives express their objections to tissue removal clearly and consistently, health practitioners often do not proceed, even when the donor's wishes were to donate tissue. One reason argued is that the potential harm done to the deceased's relatives by removing tissue against their express wishes outweighs the harm done in not proceeding with the deceased's wishes.[16]

If the deceased person is not in a hospital (e.g. dies at home), in all jurisdictions except Western Australia the senior available next of kin may make written authorisation for tissue removal for the purposes of transplantation. The senior available next of kin must make reasonable enquiries as to whether the deceased ever expressed a consent or objection to tissue removal and to establish whether another senior available next of kin objects. In the absence of an expressed refusal by the deceased or an objection by another senior available next of kin, tissue removal may be authorised by the senior available next of kin.[17] In Victoria medical practitioners may authorise removal if they are unable to ascertain the whereabouts or existence of the next of kin and if they have no reason to believe that the deceased expressed an objection to tissue removal.[18] (Note, Western Australian legislation addresses only donation of tissue on the death of a person who died in a hospital or whose body has been brought to a hospital.[19])

Removing tissue from deceased people is prohibited when a coroner has jurisdiction to hold an inquest[20] or, in the Australian Capital Territory and the Northern Territory, when there is no death certificate.[21] In such cases the consent of the coroner is required before invoking the provisions of the legislation for the purpose of tissue donation.[22] See Chapter 9 for more information about the coroner's role.

The Australian Organ and Tissue Donation and Transplantation Authority

The Australian Organ and Tissue Donation and Transplantation Authority (the OTA) is an independent statutory agency established in 2009 following enactment of the *Australian Organ and Tissue Donation and Transplantation Authority Act 2008* (Cth). While the states and territories regulate tissue donation and transplantation (as described above), the OTA works with states/territories, clinicians and the community to deliver the Australian Government's national program to improve organ and tissue donation and transplantation outcomes. In June 2017 the OTA released the *Best Practice Guideline for Offering Organ and Tissue Donation in Australia*.[23]

National Health and Medical Research Council Guidelines

Organ and tissue donation raise complex ethical issues. As such, the National Health and Medical Research Council has also developed recommendations and guidelines that provide health practitioners with clear ethical foundations for practice. These guidelines include:

- *Organ and Tissue Donation by Living Donors: Guidelines for Ethical Practice for Health Professionals* (2007) (currently under review)
- *Organ and Tissue Donation after Death, for Transplantation: Guidelines for Ethical Practice for Health Professionals* (2007) (currently under review)
- *Ethical Guidelines for Organ Transplantation from Deceased Donors* (2016).[24]

Clinical Guidelines

In addition the Transplant Society of Australia and New Zealand has developed clinical guidelines regarding inclusion and exclusion criteria for eligibility for transplantation of each organ and general conditions that apply across the organ types.[25]

FURTHER READING

Allan S. Psycho-social, ethical and legal arguments for and against the retrospective release of information about donors to donor-conceived individuals in Australia. *J Law Med*. 2011;19(1):354–76.

International Summit on Transplant Tourism and Organ Trafficking. The Declaration of Istanbul on Organ Trafficking and Transplant Tourism. Istanbul: The Transplantation Society and International Society of Nephrology; 2008. http://multivu.prnewswire.com/mnr/transplantationsociety/33914/docs/33914-Declaration_of_Istanbul-Lancet.pdf. Accessed 13 March 2019.

Naffine N, Richards B, Rogers W. Scaring us all to death: the need for responsible legal scholarship on post-mortem organ donation. *J Law Med*. 2009;16(4):696–707.

World Health Organization. WHO Guiding Principles on Cell, Tissue and Organ Transplantation. Geneva: WHO; 2010. https://www.who.int/transplantation/Guiding_PrinciplesTransplantation_WHA63.22en.pdf. Accessed 13 March 2019.

ENDNOTES

1. Australian Law Reform Commission. *Human tissue transplants*. Canberra, ACT: AGPS; 1977. Report No. 7.
2. *Transplantation and Anatomy Act 1978* (ACT) s 20; *Human Tissue Act* (NSW) s 19; *Transplantation and Anatomy Act 2014* (NT) s 14; *Transplantation and Anatomy Act 1979* (Qld) s 17; *Transplantation and Anatomy Act 1983* (SA) s 18; *Human Tissue Act 1985* (Tas) s 18; *Human Tissue Act 1982* (Vic) s 21; *Human Tissue and Transplant Act* (WA) s 18.
3. *Transplantation and Anatomy Act 1978* (ACT) s 21; *Human Tissue Act 1983* (NSW) s 19; *Transplantation and Anatomy Act 1979* (Qld) s 17; *Transplantation and Anatomy Act 1983* (SA) s 18; *Human Tissue Act 1985* (Tas) s 18; *Human Tissue Act 1982* (Vic) s 21; *Human Tissue and Transplant Act 1982* (WA) s 21.
4. *Qumsieh v Guardianship and Administration Board* [1998] VSCA 45, unreported, 17 September 1998.
5. *Transplantation and Anatomy Act 1978* (ACT) s 8; *Human Tissue Act 1983* (NSW) s 7; *Transplantation and Anatomy Act 2014* (NT) ss 4, 8; *Transplantation and Anatomy Act 1979* (Qld) s 10; *Human Tissue Act 1982* (Vic) s 7; *Transplantation and Anatomy Act 1983* (SA) s 9(1); *Human Tissue Act 1985* (Tas) s 7; *Human Tissue and Transplant Act 1982* (WA) s 8(1).
6. *Transplantation and Anatomy Act 1978* (ACT) s 15; *Human Tissue Act 1983* (NSW) s 12; *Transplantation and Anatomy Act 2014* (NT) 10(2)(b); *Transplantation and Anatomy Act 1979* (Qld) s 13; *Transplantation and Anatomy Act 1983* (SA) 15; *Human Tissue Act 1985* (Tas) s 14; *Human Tissue Act 1982* (Vic) s 10; *Human Tissue and Transplant Act 1982* (WA) s 15.
7. *Children (Care and Protection) Act 1987* (NSW) s 11.
8. *GWW and CMW* (1997) FLC 92-748.
9. *Transplantation and Anatomy Act 1978* (ACT).
10. *Human Tissue Act 1983* (NSW) s 16.
11. *Human Tissue Act 1982* (Vic) s 18.
12. *Northern Sydney and Central Coast Area Health Service v CT* [2005] NSWSC 551.
13. *Transplantation and Anatomy Act 1978* (ACT) s 27(1); *Human Tissue Act 1983* (NSW) s 23(1); *Transplantation and Anatomy*

Act 2014 (NT) s 18(1)(a); *Transplantation and Anatomy Act 1983* (SA) s 21(2); *Human Tissue Act 1985* (Tas) s 23(1); *Human Tissue Act 1982* (Vic) s 26(1)(c); *Human Tissue and Transplant Act 1982* (WA) s 22(2)(a). In Queensland a person may give written consent to the removal of tissue after his or her death: *Transplantation and Anatomy Act 1979* (Qld) s 22(5).

14. *Transplantation and Anatomy Act 1978* (ACT) s 27(2); *Human Tissue Act 1983* (NSW) s 23(3); *Transplantation and Anatomy Act 2014* (NT) s 18(1)(b); *Transplantation and Anatomy Act 1979* (Qld) ss 22(1), 22(2); *Transplantation and Anatomy Act 1983* (SA) s 21(3); *Human Tissue Act 1985* (Tas) s 23(2); *Human Tissue Act 1982* (Vic) s 26(1); *Human Tissue and Transplant Act 1982* (WA) s 22(2)(b).

15. *Transplantation and Anatomy Act 1978* (ACT) s 27(3); *Transplantation and Anatomy Act 2014* (NT) s 18(1)(b); *Transplantation and Anatomy Act 1983* (SA) s 21(3); *Human Tissue Act 1982* (Vic) s 26(1).

16. Stewart C, Kerridge I, Parker M. *The Australian Medico-legal Handbook.* Sydney, NSW: Elsevier; 2008.

17. *Transplantation and Anatomy Act 1978* (ACT) s 28; *Human Tissue Act 1983* (NSW) s 24; *Transplantation and Anatomy Act 2014* (NT) s 19(a); *Transplantation and Anatomy Act 1979* (Qld) s 23; *Transplantation and Anatomy Act 1983* (SA) s 22; *Human Tissue Act 1985* (Tas) s 24; *Human Tissue Act 1982* (Vic) s 26(2). Western Australia has no equivalent provision.

18. *Human Tissue Act 1982* (Vic) s 26(2)(e), 26(3).

19. *Human Tissue and Transplant Act 1982* (WA) s 22(1), (2).

20. *Human Tissue Act 1983* (NSW) s 25; *Transplantation and Anatomy Act 1979* (Qld) s 24; *Transplantation and Anatomy Act 1983* (SA) s 23; *Human Tissue Act 1985* (Tas) s 28A; *Human Tissue Act 1982* (Vic) s 27; *Human Tissue and Transplant Act 1982* (WA) s 23.

21. *Transplantation and Anatomy Act 1978* (ACT) s 28; *Transplantation and Anatomy Act 2014* (NT) s 20.

22. *Transplantation and Anatomy Act 1978* (ACT) s 29(2); *Human Tissue Act 1983* (NSW) s 25(2); *Transplantation and Anatomy Act 2014* (NT) s 20(1)(b); *Transplantation and Anatomy Act 1979* (Qld) s 24(2); *Transplantation and Anatomy Act 1983* (SA) s 23(1); *Human Tissue Act 1985* (Tas) s 28(A)(1); *Human Tissue Act 1982* (Vic) s 27(1); *Human Tissue and Transplant Act 1982* (WA) s 23(1).

23. Organ and Tissue Authority. *Best practice guideline for offering organ and tissue donation in Australia.* Canberra, ACT: Australian Government; 2017.

24. National Health and Medical Research Council. *Ethical guidelines for organ transplantation from deceased donors.* Canberra, ACT: NHMRC; 2016.

25. Transplantation Society of Australia and New Zealand. *Organ transplantation from deceased donors: consensus statement on eligibility criteria and allocation protocols.* Sydney, NSW: TSANZ; 2014.

REVIEW QUESTIONS AND ACTIVITIES

1. Maya is eight years old and her parents want to take blood and possibly some non-regenerative tissue from her for her younger sister, who has a life-threatening disease. What advice can you provide?

2. Explain the circumstances under which regenerative and non-regenerative human tissue may be removed and donated from (a) a living adult and (b) a deceased adult.

3. Summarise the state/territory and Commonwealth powers and participation in regulating and coordinating tissue transplantation and donation.

4. Find and examine relevant ethical and clinical guidelines concerning the removal and donation of human tissue and organs.

14 THE REGULATION OF DRUGS AND POISONS

LEARNING OBJECTIVES

Upon completing this chapter you should be able to:

- outline the purpose of federal legislative provisions regarding medicines
- list the state and territory Acts relevant to the management of medication
- discuss the legal responsibility of health practitioners in relation to drugs and poisons
- explain what is meant by a 'drug schedule'
- describe factors relevant to prescribing and administering drugs in a variety of healthcare settings.

INTRODUCTION

Many health practitioners may have responsibilities that require them to store, prescribe and/or supply a variety of medicines and chemicals. This includes, but is not limited to, dentists, dental hygienists, oral health therapists, nurses, midwives, nurse practitioners (and other endorsed nurses), pharmacists, podiatrists, medical practitioners, optometrists and orthoptists. Practitioners may have different legislative requirements and responsibilities, and different lists of approved medicines, depending on their profession and scope of practice. This chapter introduces key issues regarding regulation, policy and practice matters related to drugs and poisons.

FEDERAL REGULATION

Therapeutic Goods Act

The *Therapeutic Goods Act 1989* (Cth) regulates the licensing, manufacture and distribution of therapeutic substances. 'Therapeutic substances' include any product used in the prevention, diagnosis, cure and alleviation of disease.

The Act establishes the Therapeutic Goods Administration (TGA) authority, which is responsible for regulating such things as prescription medicines, vaccines, sunscreens, vitamins/minerals, medical devices, blood and blood products. The role of the TGA includes:

- evaluating therapeutic goods before they are marketed
- monitoring products once they are on the market
- assessing the suitability of medicines and medical devices for export from Australia
- regulating manufacturers of therapeutic goods to ensure they meet acceptable standards of manufacturing quality.[1]

Manufacturing inspectors audit manufacturing facilities worldwide to ensure products supplied in Australia are of high quality.

The Act also provides for the Australian Register of Therapeutic Goods (ARTG), upon which any product for which therapeutic claims are made must be 'listed' or 'registered' before it can be supplied in Australia. High-risk medicines are 'registered' on the ARTG, while lower risk medicines are 'listed'. To register higher risk medicines, the quality, safety and effectiveness of the product is evaluated. Lower risk medicines containing preapproved, low-risk ingredients that make limited claims are assessed by the TGA for quality and safety but not efficacy (e.g. some over-the-counter medicines and most complementary medicines).

The Therapeutic Goods Act imposes standards, by way of licences, on corporations manufacturing therapeutic goods including those that export, import and manufacture therapeutic goods. Licensed companies are monitored to ensure their operations comply with international standards in the manufacture of products; the premises and actual process of manufacture are strictly regulated.

Customs Import and Export Regulations

The Customs (Prohibited Imports) Regulations 1956 and the Customs (Prohibited Exports) Regulations 1958 allow respectively for the import and export of otherwise prohibited substances with the permission of the administering agencies. The Office of Drug Control administers the following regulations:

- Regulation 5: Narcotic, psychotropic drugs and precursor chemicals
- Regulation 5A: Antibiotics
- Regulation 5G: Various substances which include hormones
- Regulation 5H: Various substances which include anabolic and androgenic substances.

Narcotic Drugs

Under the *Narcotic Drugs Act 1967* the Commonwealth also has powers to meet certain obligations under the *Single Convention on Narcotic Drugs 1961*, which include regulating narcotic drug manufacture and cannabis cultivation for medicinal and related scientific purposes. The Narcotic Drugs Regulation 2016 gives effect to the regulatory framework for manufacturing drugs under the Narcotic Drugs Act and for licensing the cultivation and production of cannabis and cannabis resins for medicinal and scientific purposes. The Narcotic Drugs Regulation also specifies: the information and documentation an applicant must provide for a licence or permit; requirements for any variation of a licence or permit; and arrangements for suspending and revoking licences and permits.

National Drugs and Poisons Schedule Committee

The Australian Government established the National Drugs and Poisons Schedule Committee in 1999. The committee's function is to classify and schedule substances and to provide advice to governments about policies affecting the advertising, labelling and packaging of substances. Factors the committee must consider when classifying and scheduling substances include the potential danger, toxicity and the risks or benefits of each substance. The committee comprises a member who is nominated from the federal government and one from each state and territory government.

Pharmaceutical Benefits Scheme

As discussed in Chapter 2, the Pharmaceutical Benefits Scheme (PBS) is a significant federally funded scheme to enable patients to access low-priced medication. The Pharmaceutical Benefits Advisory Committee advises the federal Minister for Health and Ageing about which medications should be subsidised by the PBS. If a medication is not listed on the PBS, patients bear the total cost of the drug.

STATE AND TERRITORY REGULATION

Legislation exists in all states and territories in relation to medication management. The legislation in each state and territory varies; however, there are some basic similarities. Table 14.1 lists the relevant legislation in each jurisdiction, the common law requirements of drug administration and the potential policies that affect health practitioners.

The Acts tend to set out broad expectations including labelling requirements, who may prescribe, the professional groups that may legally supply and administer specified drugs, wholesaling requirements and the criminal aspects of drug misuse.

Regulations generally deal in more detail with the day-to-day requirements of drug control such as administration, requirements of a valid prescription, storage requirements and record keeping.

Definitions appear in both the Acts and the regulations.

Common Law

The legislation in Australian states and territories does not address the details of *administering* medication to patients. The common law cases provide the basis for many of the principles expected in clinical practice. For example, many health practitioners are familiar with the phrase 'the five rights'; this phrase provides

TABLE 14.1

Drug and Poisons Legislation By Jurisdiction

Jurisdiction	Legislation
Commonwealth	*Therapeutic Goods Act 1989* Therapeutic Goods Regulations 1990 *Narcotic Drugs Act 1967*
Australian Capital Territory	*Medicines, Poisons and Therapeutic Goods Act 2008* Medicines, Poisons and Therapeutic Goods Regulation 2008 *Drugs of Dependence Act 1989* Drugs of Dependence Regulation 2009
New South Wales	*Poisons and Therapeutic Goods Act 1966* Poisons and Therapeutic Goods Regulation 2008
Northern Territory	*Medicines, Poisons and Therapeutic Goods Act* Medicines, Poisons and Therapeutic Goods Regulation
Queensland	*Health Act 1937* Health (Drugs and Poisons) Regulation 1996 Health Regulation 1996
South Australia	*Controlled Substances Act 1984* Controlled Substances (Poisons) Regulations 2011 Controlled Substances (Controlled Drugs, Precursors and Plants) Regulations 2000
Tasmania	*Poisons Act 1971* Poisons Regulations 2008
Victoria	*Drugs, Poisons and Controlled Substances Act 1981* Drugs, Poisons and Controlled Substances Regulations 2006
Western Australia	*Poisons Act 1964* Poisons Regulations 1965

the underpinning for routine administration practice (see 'Administration of drugs' on page 157). An action in negligence might arise and be considered a breach of a duty of care if there has been a failure to administer:

- the 'right' drug
- the 'right' dose
- to the 'right' patient
- at the 'right' time and/or
- via the 'right' route.

An action in trespass might occur where a health practitioner fails to obtain patient consent before administering medications.

Drug Schedules

States and territories have their own laws regarding where medicines or poisons can be bought and how they must be packaged and labelled. However, to achieve a uniform approach to the scheduling of substances and to labelling and packaging requirements, most medicines and poisons are classified by state and territory governments in line with the *Standard for the Uniform Scheduling of Medicines and Poisons* (SUSMP) (the 'Poisons Standard').[2] The classification of drugs into schedules incorporates all poisonous substances including therapeutic, industrial and agricultural poisons, based on recommendations made by the National Drugs and Poisons Schedule Committee.

Grouping or classifying of poisonous substances regulates those individuals who may access them or the availability of the drug, as each schedule has defined regulatory requirements. The overriding aim is to maintain public health and safety. Thus, drugs can be rescheduled from one category to another. When practising, health practitioners must therefore locate the state and territory legislation that details the schedule or category to which a drug belongs. For example, it is accepted that a prescription is required before Schedule 4 and Schedule 8 drugs are administered to patients.

The schedules of the Poisons Standard set out decisions about the classification of drugs and poisons. These are then included in the relevant state and territory legislation. The schedules most commonly referred to are set out in Table 14.2.

POLICY

Many employers and professional entities formulate written guidelines or policies for health practitioners regarding medication administration:

- Health departments – federal, state and territory – appoint various committees such as the National Drugs and Poisons Schedule Committee.
- Most employers have medication protocols that are specifically formulated for their patient cohorts.
- Regulatory authorities such as the National Boards (see Chapter 4) provide such guidelines.
- Professional organisations such as the Australian Medical Association also provide guidelines.

TABLE 14.2
Most Commonly Referred to Schedules of the Poisons Standard

Schedule 1	Poisons of plant origin of such danger to life as to warrant supply only from medical practitioners, pharmacists, dentists or veterinary surgeons. There are no longer any scheduled poisons in this category.
Schedule 2	Substances or poisons for therapeutic use that should be available to the public from pharmacies or from people licensed to sell or supply them. These drugs do not require a prescription and are often sold directly to the public. Examples include paracetamol and aspirin.
Schedule 3	Substances or poisons for therapeutic use that are dangerous or are so liable to abuse as to warrant restriction of the right of supply to doctors, dentists, pharmacists and veterinary surgeons. This group of poisons may be required for urgent use so their supply only on prescription from doctors, dentists or veterinary surgeons may cause hardship. Hence, pharmacists can supply these poisons without a prescription. Examples include salbutamol aerosol inhalers and insulin.
Schedule 4	Substances or poisons and substances intended for therapeutic use that require professional management, monitoring and further evaluation. These substances require a prescription from an authorised prescriber such as a doctor, dentist or veterinary surgeon. Most medications administered to patients in the healthcare arena belong to this schedule and include antibiotics, anaesthetics, some antidepressants, anticonvulsants, antihypertensives and chemotherapeutic drugs.
Schedule 5	Substances and poisons of a hazardous nature that are available to the public but are potentially dangerous and require caution in handling, storage and use. This group includes many domestic poisons such as kerosene, methylated spirits and ammonia.
Schedule 6	Substances and poisons that are available to the public but are more hazardous or poisonous than those in Schedule 5. Poisons in this schedule are generally used for agricultural and industrial purposes and include formaldehyde and cyanide.
Schedule 7	Substances and poisons that require special precautions in their manufacture, handling, storage or use, or require special individual regulations regarding labelling or availability. Substances such as arsenic, strychnine and thalidomide are included in this group.
Schedule 8	Substances and poisons to which the restrictions recommended for drugs of dependence by the 1980 Australian Royal Commission of Inquiry into Drugs should apply. This group includes drugs that are addictive or potentially addictive. The more common drugs include cocaine, codeine (except when it is in a different form and included in another schedule such as Schedule 2 or Schedule 4), methadone, morphine and pethidine.
Schedule 9	Poisons that are drugs of abuse for which the manufacture, possession, sale or use should be prohibited by law except for amounts that may be necessary for medical or scientific research conducted with the approval of the Commonwealth or state/territory authorities. Heroin is one example.

At the federal level, two important committees were set up in the early 1990s to advise the federal Minister for Health in relation to the national medicinal drug policy. The Australian Pharmaceutical Advisory Council (APAC) comprises representatives of peak health professions including pharmacy, medicine and nursing. There are also representatives from the pharmaceutical industry, consumer organisations and government members with an interest in implementing Australia's national medicines policy. APAC identifies and considers issues and needs in health care with reference to pharmaceuticals. Effectively, APAC comments on, reviews or endorses guidelines, standards and practices.

The Pharmaceutical Health and Rational Use of Medicines Committee's agenda has been to develop a national 'quality use of medicines' policy. This has included developing education strategies, assisting with funding research projects and evaluating issues associated with the way drugs are used.[3] This committee has representatives from: pharmacy, nursing and general practice; health education and promotion; community development; consumers; and teaching. The vision for quality use of medicines involves a partnership between those who prescribe, those who dispense, those who manufacture and those who take drugs, and the government, which monitors safety, efficacy and quality.

In addition to policy initiatives at the federal level, the requirements of practice are sometimes guided by the respective state and territory health departments that administer the legislation. Policies will be considered should a health practitioner injure a patient as a result of adverse drug use.

Most professional organisations and regulatory authorities also have guiding policy statements in relation to drug administration. It is the responsibility of health practitioners to be aware of the guiding policies, noting that, at times, the policies, particularly employer policies, are more prescriptively written than the law demands. For example, in many jurisdictions Schedule 2 medicines do not require a written prescription, although many hospital policies will require all drugs to be ordered by a doctor and a record kept. This provides a clear record of all drugs given to the patient while in hospital. By recording all Schedule 2 medicines, the hospital can keep track of where the Schedule 2 medicines are used.

COMPLEMENTARY MEDICINES

Health practitioners will have access to medicines, including vitamins, herbal and homoeopathic preparations, lotions and creams that are not included in the standard scheduling scheme. It is necessary to highlight that while the medication may not be subject to the various state and territory poisons legislation, health practitioners should work within their employer's policies or guidelines to avoid potential problems.

The Therapeutic Goods Act established the Complementary Medicines Evaluation Committee to provide scientific and policy advice relating to the supply and control of complementary medicines. Health practitioners using complementary medicines should be careful to acknowledge the requirements and any restrictions on the use of specific complementary medicines. The TGA website provides further useful guidance.[4]

DEFINITIONS

The legislation in all jurisdictions provides definitions to help interpret the obligations of health practitioners. The definitions vary in each jurisdiction, although the focus tends to be associated with the criminal aspects of the legislation as well as the healthcare aspects. Hence the words 'possession' and 'supply' have particular meaning:

- ■ 'Possession' of a substance includes custody or control over the substance.
- ■ 'Supply' means to provide, give or deliver, whether or not for payment or reward.

However, 'supplying' a substance in the Australian Capital Territory, Queensland, Victoria and Western Australia does not include the administration of the substance, while in New South Wales, the Northern Territory and Tasmania it does. The South Australian legislative definition of 'supply' includes to provide, distribute, barter or exchange a substance.

The legislation authorises certain practitioners to possess, administer and, in some situations, provide a supply of a drug.

STORAGE

The legislative requirements relating to storage vary. In some jurisdictions there is a requirement to store Schedule 4 drugs in a locked cupboard or equivalent, while in other jurisdictions no such requirement exists. There are, however, clear directions in relation to Schedule 8 and Schedule 9 drugs. In all jurisdictions they are to be stored in a locked cupboard and remain separate from other drugs. The legislation in some Acts nominates the precise specifications of the cupboard, including the thickness of the steel plate. The keys of the drug cupboard are to be kept on the person of the individual in charge of the unit or facility. Infringing the requirements in relation to Schedule 8 drugs often leads to criminal penalties.

All agencies with or without pharmacies are obliged to keep a register to record the details of Schedule 8 and Schedule 4D drugs. The information recorded includes the patient's name, the prescribed drug and dose, the doctor's name, the date and time of administration and the balance of the ampoules or tablets. Usually a witness checks this information with the practitioner who is to administer the drug. The health practitioner giving the drug must be authorised to administer it; this includes a registered nurse or doctor in the hospital environment. The witness may be another health practitioner.

The balance of the Schedule 8 drugs remaining in the drug cupboard is recorded at regular intervals. The regularity of the record keeping depends on the practice setting and the frequency of use of the Schedule 8 medication. For example, the acute care environment will require checking and recording at the completion of each shift, whereas an aged care facility may check the balance only once every 24 hours. When a discrepancy in the record is identified, there is a responsibility to report it, normally to the pharmacist, the director of nursing or a senior medical officer. The police drug squad may become involved if there is tampering with Schedule 8 drugs, which is a reminder of the criminal focus of the legislation. This situation may suggest a staff member with an addictive illness.

Whenever ampoules are damaged or destroyed, this must also be reported. If the drug is discarded or destroyed, policy often dictates that it is done in the presence of a witness.

PRESCRIBING

Prescribing refers to the writing of a drug order in either a prescription notepad or on a medication chart. To authorise the use of many scheduled substances, the health practitioner must belong to a particular professional group. The legislation in each jurisdiction identifies which professional groups may prescribe and the legal requirements for a valid prescription. Medical practitioners, dentists and veterinary surgeons are the most commonly identified professional groups in all jurisdictions, with the widest prescribing authority. They may prescribe a variety of drugs including those commonly used in healthcare settings – Schedule 2, 3, 4 and 8 drugs.

Other professional groups with limited prescribing rights include nurse practitioners, optometrists, Chinese medicine practitioners (in Victoria) and dental therapists. The drugs they are authorised to prescribe relate specifically to their areas of expertise.

From 1 September 2010 nurse practitioners endorsed to prescribe under state or territory legislation have been able to apply for approval as PBS prescribers (authorised nurse practitioners), which means patients can access the benefits of the PBS system. Information for nurse practitioners to become authorised PBS prescribers is available from the Commonwealth Department of Human Services. PBS prescribing is limited by a nurse practitioner's scope of practice and by state and territory prescribing rights. Prescribing of PBS medicines is also contingent on a prescriber being an authorised nurse practitioner and having collaborative arrangements in place, as required by the *National Health Act 1953*.

Elements of a Valid Prescription

The requirements of a valid prescription are specified in most jurisdictions and generally include:

- identifying prescriber information including name and address (the prescriber's address is not always included in the hospital setting)
- the patient's name and address (usually the patient's address is modified to an identifying number when a drug chart is used in an institution)
- the date of the prescription
- the drug, either as a generic or trade name (the PBS authorises pharmacists to dispense a cheaper version of a drug when the trade name is used)
- other drug details including the dose, route and frequency (in some jurisdictions, where an unusual dose is ordered, it should be underlined and initialled)
- legibility (in some jurisdictions computer-generated prescriptions are valid but a handwritten signature is required).

ADMINISTRATION OF DRUGS

In practice the groups authorised to prescribe may either administer the drugs themselves or provide a written or verbal order to other professionals to administer. Registered nurses comprise the largest number of health practitioners who administer drugs on the written or verbal orders of doctors. In many jurisdictions, including the Australian Capital Territory, New South Wales, Queensland, Tasmania and Victoria, enrolled nurses are permitted to administer some scheduled drugs under registered nurse supervision and after completing an approved course. Paramedics are authorised to administer drugs in specified practice settings for the purposes of their profession. Aboriginal health workers may also administer in some jurisdictions.

The precise requirements of administration are generally not dealt with in legislation; instead, the legislation tends to specify the form a medication order will take – for example, a written order or a verbal order. As noted above, the common law cases provide the guiding principles, ordinarily referred to as the 'five rights' (the right patient, the right drug, the right dose, the right route and the right time). These principles form the basis of all drug administration.

There are no definitions of what administration actually entails. At first instance, the concept of administration would seem obvious; however, those groups without prescribing rights who administer medication have found themselves in varying degrees of uncertainty in many practice settings. For example, can one administer certain drugs from a standing order or protocol? What are the requirements of administering drugs according to verbal orders, and what is the legal significance of nurse-initiated drugs? It is also important to note that all groups that administer drugs take legal responsibility for their actions, even if they did not actually prescribe the drug. When a patient suffers harm following the incorrect administration of a medication, it provides an opportunity to review clinical practice; it may also lead to litigation.

VERBAL ORDERS

All jurisdictions allow verbal orders. The notion of a verbal order includes oral orders, be it in person or by telephone. In some jurisdictions, the verbal order is specifically contextualised and refers to telephone orders, orders by facsimile or by any 'approved' manner. 'Approval' must come from an authorised person; for example, in New South Wales it is the Director General.

In four jurisdictions, the Australian Capital Territory, New South Wales, Tasmania and Victoria, a verbal order must relate to an emergency. It is relevant to note that an emergency is not defined in the statutes or regulations. Presumably it remains the decision of the prescriber whether any given situation is an emergency.

In some jurisdictions, including the Australian Capital Territory, New South Wales, Queensland and Tasmania, the medical practitioner must record the verbal order within 24 hours. In Western Australia, if the patient is in a hospital, the doctor is required to endorse the patient's medication chart within 24 hours.

In the Australian Capital Territory, New South Wales and Queensland responsibility rests with the registered nurse to report or follow up if the written order is not

forthcoming. In Victoria and the Northern Territory the order must be written up 'as soon as practicable' after the verbal order has been given. This allows for more realistic timeframes and attendances on the part of the prescriber. Moreover, the Australian Capital Territory's legislation requires the prescriber to inform the nurse or pharmacist that a particular verbal order is an unusual dose.

The New South Wales regulation does not permit the verbal order to be ongoing but rather a 'one off' dose. The South Australian and Tasmanian legislation allows for the registered practitioner to continue to administer the drug – for 10 days in South Australia and, in Tasmania, if in the opinion of the registered practitioner it is necessary for the patient's wellbeing.

In Queensland several categories exist. A registered nurse or midwife may possess and administer Schedule 4 and 8 medications on a verbal order. Both a registered nurse and midwife in isolated practice can supply medication on an oral instruction to an outpatient or discharged patient. Isolated practice is defined as more than 25 kilometres from a pharmacy. In rural areas (defined according to specific location) a director of nursing or nominee can supply medication to an outpatient or discharged patient where there is no employed pharmacist or the pharmacist is not on duty.

In Western Australia a registered nurse working in a designated remote area can supply Schedule 4 medications for up to three days to treat an acute medical condition on the instructions of a doctor.

NURSE-INITIATED DRUGS

Not all scheduled medication requires a written or verbal order from someone who is authorised to prescribe. The requirement of a prescription for Schedule 2 drugs is absent from the legislation, and these drugs may therefore be administered by a registered nurse. A pharmacist may dispense Schedule 3 drugs without a prescription. Some first-aid environments keep Schedule 3 drugs, such as Ventolin inhalers, for emergency use. The fact the legislation is silent in some jurisdictions does not endorse the practice of unauthorised prescribers making decisions regarding all Schedule 3 drugs. For example, it would be highly irregular to administer insulin to a patient without a proper order from a prescriber. The jurisdictions in which the legislation is silent in relation to the administration of Schedule 2 and/or 3 drugs are South Australia, Victoria, Western Australia, Tasmania and the Australian Capital Territory.

In practice, employers often provide a policy that identifies the requirements for initiating and administering Schedule 2 medication. However, this may vary considerably between jurisdictions, state health departments, institutions and employers.[5]

It is noted that the Nursing and Midwifery Boards of Australia and the Australian and New Zealand Council of Chief Nursing and Midwifery Officers have been working together to develop potential future models of prescribing by registered nurses and midwives and quality use of medicines, with a focus on promoting 'safe and improved access to medicines for communities' and 'workforce flexibility'.[6]

STANDING ORDERS

Generally, standing orders provide a legal written instruction for an authorised person to administer medicines in situations where a prompt response using a standard procedure will improve care and where a medicine is part of this procedure. Note, a standing order is *not* a 'when required' prescription for an individual consumer. Commonwealth guiding principles note that:

> … *where standing orders are required, for example in rural and remote areas and some immunisation programs, service providers should develop policies and procedures describing the development, authorisation, use and routine monitoring of the standing order. They must be in accordance with Australian, state and territory legislation and policy, and promote the quality use of medicines.*[7]

Due to considerable differences across jurisdictions and professions, practitioners are encouraged to check their respective state and territory legislation and investigate situations where the relevant health department has granted authorisation for standing orders. If health practitioners are working with standing orders, ideally, they should identify the drug or list of drugs to be given, the clinical circumstances in which the medication is to be administered and the acceptable environment. The order must have the approval of the relevant institution or authority employing the health practitioner.

MEDICATION ERROR

Regardless of the environment in which individuals practise, medication error is a reality. Courts, employers, regulatory authorities and health practitioners have historically blamed individual practitioners for errors. While a punitive response may appear reasonable, the research demonstrates that such action is unlikely to change the actual error rate occurring in the clinical environment.[8] In addition it has been suggested that any system of reporting that leads to punishment risks that the reporting of errors will not occur.[9] This is not to condone nor disregard drug errors but rather to recognise that merely punishing the individual is unlikely to address problems of medication error. Alternative responses are also required.

The most commonly used definition of medication error was formulated by the American Society of Hospital Pharmacists in 1993. The definition emphasises the practice of the 'five rights' mentioned above, highlighting mistakes where a wrong dose, patient, route, drug or time occurs. The definition has been construed to largely focus on incidents or errors at the end-point – the patient.[10] Errors made at the prescribing or dispensing stage discovered before they reach the patient have traditionally not been considered medication errors. However, this interpretation has been recognised as problematic because the focus rests with those practitioners who are largely responsible for drug administration.

Over time it was recognised that it is useful to take a broader focus and include all stages of the medication process – from prescribing and dispensing to administration. All medication incidents can be regarded as potential errors, having their origin in the system, so that incidents or errors are grouped with other adverse events. Effectively, this results in a shift from focusing on a failure of the individual to examining a failure of the system. Leape argues that the delivery of a single drug to a patient is the result of a long and complicated process, and all elements of the process should be examined.[11]

This has several effects on health practitioners. First, they are encouraged to report events, not from the perspective of the 'defective' practitioner but as a source of information to be used for improving the system. Second, when the entire system is addressed, errors that are discovered at the point of administration can be traced back to the point in the system where the failure began. Third, to remove a punitive approach is to encourage self-reporting. Moreover, many institutions are encouraging maximum patient involvement where possible. Patients are encouraged to self-medicate and, in many healthcare environments, medication is stored in lockable drawers beside the patient's bed.

Research in Australia demonstrates that medication incidents in acute care settings remain the second most frequent incident reported, with falls being the predominant incident. Omission and overdose are the most common type of medication incident, with failure to read, or misreading of the medication chart and failing to follow protocol or guidelines, the most commonly cited causes. One study in Queensland examining prescribing errors by hospital interns found that many factors were identified.[12] The study highlighted four key areas of causation:

- environmental factors including the level of staffing, workloads and managerial support
- team factors including issues such as communication and supervision
- individual factors including knowledge, skills, motivation and individual health
- task factors including issues related to medication chart design, protocols and availability of tests.

In a 2016 literature review of studies of medication errors in hospitals, Roughead et al suggested that 'on admission to hospital … there may be an overall rate of two errors for every three patients at the time of admission to hospital'.[13] They also found that large studies examining the rates of prescribing errors in major Australian teaching hospitals suggest prescription error rates of up to one error per patient. The best available evidence suggests that errors occur in around 9% of medication administrations in hospital (excluding errors of timing). The review also indicated that 'errors in medication documentation in discharge summaries may occur at a rate of up to two errors per patient'.[14] The authors concluded that medication safety in the various stages of the patient journey through acute care in Australia continues to be a significant problem, the cost of adverse medication-related admissions at around $1.2 billion per year.[15] Clearly, in relation to this issue, law alone does not suffice. Continued work on patient safety and practice review is necessary.

FURTHER READING

Department of Health and Ageing. The Regulation of Complementary Medicines in Australia – An Overview. Canberra, ACT: Australian Government; 2006.

Dragon N. A new prescription needed for nurse practitioners. Aust Nurs J. 2008;16(3):21–3.

Roughead E, Semple S, Rosenfeld E. The extent of medication errors and adverse drug reactions throughout the patient journey in acute care in Australia. Int J Evid Based Healthc. 2016;14(3):113–22.

Therapeutic Goods Administration. The Poisons Standard. Canberra, ACT: Australian Government Department of Health; 2018. http://www.tga.gov.au/industry/scheduling-poisons-standard.htm#susmp. Accessed 13 December 2018.

ENDNOTES

1. Therapeutic Goods Administration. TGA Basics. http://www.tga.gov.au/about/tga.htm. Accessed 24 June 2018.
2. Therapeutic Goods Administration. Medicines and TGA Classifications. https://www.tga.gov.au/node/4043. Accessed 24 June 2018.
3. Murray M. What is QUM? In: Hunt S, Parkes R, eds. Nursing and the Quality Use of Medicines. Sydney, NSW: Allen and Unwin; 1999. p. 15.
4. Useful information in relation to the regulation of complementary medicines can be accessed from the Department of Health's Therapeutic Goods Administration website. See https://www.tga.gov.au/complementary-medicines. Accessed 24 June 2018.
5. Griffiths D, Baker H. An Analysis of the Australian State and Territory Drugs and Poisons Legislation in Relation to Nursing Practice. Melbourne, VIC: Monash University Printing Service; 1998. p. 22.
6. Nursing and Midwifery Board of Australia and Australian and New Zealand Council of Chief Nursing and Midwifery Officers. Registered Nurse and Midwife Prescribing – Discussion Paper; 2017.
7. Department of Health. Guiding Principles for Medication Management in the Community – July 2006: Guiding Principle 11 – Standing orders. Canberra, ACT: Australian Government; 2006. http://www.health.gov.au/internet/publications/publishing.nsf/Content/nmp-guide-medmgt-jul06-contents~nmp-guide-medmgt-jul06-guidepr11. Accessed 24 June 2018.
8. Baker H. Nurses, Medications and Medication Errors: An Ethnomethodological Study. Unpublished PhD Thesis. Brisbane, QLD: Central Queensland University; 1994.
9. Ibid.

10. Baker H. Medication error – Where does the fault lie? In: Hunt S, Parkes R, eds. *Nursing and the Quality Use of Medicines*. Sydney, NSW: Allen and Unwin; 1999. p. 73.

11. Leape L. Out of the darkness: hospitals begin to take mistakes seriously. *Health Syst Rev*. 1996;26(6):21–4.

12. Roughead L, Semple S. *Literature Review: Medication Safety in Acute Care in Australia*. Canberra, ACT: Australian Commission on Safety and Healthcare; 2008.

13. Roughead E, Semple S, Rosenfeld E. The extent of medication errors and adverse drug reactions throughout the patient journey in acute care in Australia. *Int J Evid Based Healthc*. 2016;14(3):113–22.

14. Ibid.

15. Ibid.

REVIEW QUESTIONS AND ACTIVITIES

1. Identify the areas of law that regulate the daily practice of drug storage, prescription and administration.

2. Discuss the legal responsibility of health practitioners in relation to drugs and poisons.

3. What is meant by a drug schedule? Describe the main schedules referred to in Australia.

4. Discuss your professional group's administration of medication requirements.

15

MENTAL HEALTH LEGISLATION

LEARNING OBJECTIVES

Upon completing this chapter you should be able to:

- identify the prevalence of mental health conditions and illness in Australia

- describe the provisions of influential international law instruments relevant to mental health and illness

- outline key Australian policies regarding mental health and illness

- explain the ambit and effect of state and territory mental health legislation.

INTRODUCTION

Mental illness or (or 'mental disorder') includes a wide range of short- and long-term conditions. Illness and disorder may vary in severity, be episodic or persistent in nature, and may be indicated by a variety of symptoms. The National Survey of Mental Health and Wellbeing has estimated that 45% of people aged between 16 and 85 years will experience a common mental health-related condition such as depression, anxiety or a substance-use disorder in their lifetime.[1] An estimated 2–3% of Australians have a severe mental disorder including psychotic disorder and severe and disabling forms of depression and anxiety.[2] Another 4–6% of the population are estimated to have a moderate disorder and 9–12% a mild disorder.[3] Mental disorder affects all age groups and genders across Australian society.[4]

Historically, people experiencing a mental illness have received less than optimal treatment and care. In part, this was related to the stigma and lack of understanding of psychiatric disorders. Although there is now recognition of this, and fewer people end up institutionalised, improvements have been slow to come and there is still much to resolve. For example, in Australia the National Mental Health Commission 2014 *Report of the National Review of Mental Health Programmes and Services* said:

> *In many places we have ended up with what is effectively a new 'institutionalisation in the community', where people experiencing mental illness live in the community but do not live well. They receive fragmented help or no help at all and become stuck in a vicious cycle of poor health and limited life chances. They are moved between disconnected silos of intervention, including hospital wards, patchy support systems in housing, education and employment, and overstretched community and nongovernment services.*[5]

The commission emphasised the need to: improve the lives of people living with a mental illness; realign mental health systems and services; and engage in evidence-based practices.

INTERNATIONAL LAW AND POLICY

International law is calling for the protection of the rights of people who experience disability and/or mental illness and demanding that they are respected, not discriminated against, accepted and protected. Two instruments, the United Nations *Convention on the Rights of Persons with Disabilities* (CRPD)[6] and the United Nations *Principles for the Protection of Persons with Mental Illness and the Improvement of Mental Health Care* (MI Principles), have had particular impact in Australia.

In 2008 Australia signed and ratified the CRPD[7] and in 2009 its Optional Protocol. The CRPD aims to promote, protect and ensure the full and equal enjoyment of all human rights and fundamental freedoms by all people with disabilities. It also has the objective of promoting respect for their inherent dignity.[8] Pursuant to Article 1, 'persons with disabilities include those who have long-term physical, *mental*, intellectual or sensory impairments which in interaction with various barriers may hinder their full and effective participation in society on an equal basis with others'[9] (italics added). The eight guiding principles of the CRPD further require:

- respect for inherent dignity, individual autonomy (including the freedom to make one's own choices) and independence
- non-discrimination
- full and effective participation and inclusion in society
- respect for difference and acceptance of people with disabilities as part of human diversity and humanity
- equality of opportunity
- accessibility
- equality between men and women
- respect for the evolving capacities of children with disabilities and respect for the right of children with disabilities to preserve their identities.[10]

Specific rights recognised in the Convention include:

- right to life (Article 10)
- protection in situations of risk and humanitarian emergencies (Article 11)
- equal recognition before the law and legal capacity (Article 12)
- access to justice (Article 13)
- liberty and security of the person (Article 14)
- freedom from torture or cruel, inhuman or degrading treatment or punishment (Article 15)
- freedom from exploitation, violence and abuse (Article 16)

- right to respect physical and mental integrity (Article 17)
- freedom of movement and nationality (Article 18)
- right to live in the community (Article 19)
- freedom of expression and opinion and access to information (Article 21)
- respect for privacy (Article 22)
- respect for home and the family (Article 23)
- right to education (Article 24)
- right to health (Article 25)
- right to habilitation and rehabilitation (Article 26)
- right to work and employment (Article 27)
- right to an adequate standard of living and social protection (Article 28)
- right to participate in political and public life (Article 29)
- right to participate in cultural life, recreation, leisure and sport (Article 30).

While it is beyond the scope of this discussion to detail the articles further,[11] it is noted that Articles 12, 14, 17 and 26 are of particular relevance to mental illness in respectively emphasising: legal capacity and supported decision making (which has often been restricted by mental health law in certain circumstances); liberty and security (thus raising questions about involuntary detention and deprivation of liberty); the right to respect for physical and mental integrity on an equal basis with others (prohibiting, for example, any form of intervention, including, for example, medical intervention or physical restraint that is imposed against the will of the person); and a requirement for countries to take effective and appropriate measures to enable people with a disability to develop, attain and maintain maximum ability, independence and participation through providing habilitation and rehabilitation services and programs.

The CRPD also has an 'Optional Protocol', which can be signed and ratified separately. The Optional Protocol allows the CRPD Committee to 'receive and consider communications from or on behalf of individuals or groups of individuals subject to its jurisdiction who claim to be victims of a violation by that State Party of the provisions of the Convention'.

The MI Principles were very influential on the early development of Australian state and territory laws regarding the treatment of people with mental illness. The principles recognise fundamental freedoms and basic rights including: the right to the best available mental health care; treatment with humanity and respect for the inherent dignity of the human person; the right to protection from economic, sexual and other forms of exploitation, physical or other abuse or degrading treatment; non-discrimination; and the right to exercise all civil, political, economic, social and cultural rights as recognised in other international instruments.[12]

Of note is they require the delivery of services in the least restrictive manner, using individualised planning, and under the independent and impartial authority of mental health tribunals. They also emphasise autonomy, require that the administration of medication be restricted to therapeutic use, require that no treatment shall be given to a patient without his or her informed consent, and require notification to a person of their human rights upon admission to a mental health facility. In addition, they require that medical examinations cannot take place by compulsion except in accordance with domestic laws, that patient rights of confidentiality shall be respected and that treatment be delivered in the least restrictive environment with the preservation of personal integrity and autonomy.

The MI Principles should be read in light of the CRPD; the latter being a binding treaty. The International Disability Alliance[13] states that the CRPD supersedes the MI Principles when clauses or principles contained in the two documents cannot be reconciled.

Also of note at the international level are the World Health Organization's *Mental Action Plan 2013–2020*, which has the goal to promote mental wellbeing, prevent mental disorders, provide care, enhance recovery, promote human rights and reduce the mortality, morbidity and disability for people with mental disorders,[14] and the World Health Organization's Quality Rights Program directed at improving mental health and related services worldwide.[15] Further, in September 2017 the United Nations Human Rights Council approved the *Resolution on Mental Health and Human Rights*,[16] which called for changes to mental health policies and practices. The resolution called for nations to take active steps to fully integrate a human rights perspective into mental health and community services, to eliminate all forms of violence and discrimination

within that context, and to promote the right of everyone to full inclusion and effective participation in society. It also emphasised community-based, people-centred services and supports that do not lead to over-medicalisation and inappropriate treatments.

AUSTRALIAN POLICIES AND STANDARDS

The Australian Health Minister's Advisory Council named mental health as a national health priority in 1996. The Australian Government and all state and territory governments share responsibility for mental health policy and for providing support services for Australians living with a mental illness. State and territory governments are responsible for funding and delivering state and territory public specialised mental health services and associated support services. The Australian Government leads in national mental health reform initiatives and funds a range of services for people living with mental health difficulties. The following policies, strategies, statements and plans form the overall National Government Strategy on Mental Health that has driven mental health reform in Australia for 25 years.[17]

The National Mental Health Policy

The *National Mental Health Policy* coordinates government efforts in mental health reform and service delivery. It is guided by a strategic framework that provides a foundation for developing national, state and territory mental health plans. The policy emphasises that to achieve improvements in mental health outcomes across the community, there must be collaboration across sectors, levels of government and government agencies.

The National Standards for Mental Health Services

The Australian Mental Health Commission introduced the *National Standards for Mental Health Services* in 2010. They apply to all mental health services across Australia, although they are not mandatory. They have been implemented at varying levels, the most common being standards related to rights and responsibilities and safety, the least being promotion and prevention and integration of services.[18]

The Mental Health Statement of Rights and Responsibilities

The revised *Mental Health Statement of Rights and Responsibilities* 'seeks to ensure that consumers, carers, support persons, service providers and the community are aware of relevant rights and responsibilities and can be confident in exercising them'.[19] The updated statement (revised in 2012) is consistent with Australia's international obligations, particularly the CRPD, the *Convention on the Rights of the Child* and state and territory human rights instruments.

The Fifth National Mental Health and Suicide Prevention Plan

The *Fifth National Mental Health and Suicide Prevention Plan*, endorsed in 2017, spans the years 2017 to 2022. The fifth plan identifies eight priority areas for action:

- 'achieving integrated regional planning and service delivery.
- effective suicide prevention.
- coordinating treatment and supports for people with severe and complex mental illness.
- improving Aboriginal and Torres Strait Islander mental health and suicide prevention.
- improving the physical health of people living with mental illness and reducing early mortality.
- reducing stigma and discrimination.
- making safety and quality central to mental health service delivery.
- ensuring that the enablers of effective system performance and system improvement are in place.'[20]

National Framework for Recovery-Oriented Mental Health Services

The *National recovery-oriented mental health practice framework* is a policy direction that has been adopted to enhance and improve mental health service delivery in Australia. It brings together a range of recovery-oriented approaches developed in Australia's states and territories and draws on national and international research to provide a national understanding about what constitutes recovery-oriented practice and service delivery, and how recovery-oriented models can be translated into practice.[21] The framework uses nine domains to structure guidance for specialist mental health services: promoting a culture of hope; promoting autonomy and self-determination; collaborative partnerships and meaningful engagement; focus on strengths; holistic and personalised care; family, carers, support people and significant others; community participation and citizenship; responsiveness to diversity; and reflection and learning.

The primary intention of recovery-oriented mental health services is that specialist mental health practitioners work together with a person who has a mental illness towards that person's self-defined and self-determined life regardless of whether there are any ongoing symptoms. This is based on the view that people with lived experience are experts on their lives and experiences, while mental health professionals are experts on available treatment services.

STATE AND TERRITORY LEGISLATION

The power to legislate on issues pertaining to mental health falls to the states and territories. Legislation concerned with mental health varies across jurisdictions. Most states and territories have separate, but complementary, legislation in relation to people with intellectual or other disabilities, as distinct from mental illness. However, South Australia addresses intellectual disability and psychiatric illness together in its mental health legislation; and in the Australian Capital Territory, the distinction is not made. Legislation in each of the states and territories has provisions (to a greater or lesser degree) that define who falls within the ambits of the respective Acts for the purpose of care, treatment and control issues. Legislation in operation at the time of writing is listed in Table 15.1.

DEFINITIONS OF MENTAL ILLNESS

There is no uniformly accepted legal definition of mental illness across Australia.

The Australian Capital Territory,[22] New South Wales[23] and the Northern Territory[24] define 'mental illness' as:

… a condition that seriously impairs, either temporarily or permanently, the mental functioning of a person and is characterised by the presence in the person of any one or more of the following symptoms: delusions, hallucinations, serious

TABLE 15.1

Mental Health Legislation by Jurisdiction

Jurisdiction	Legislation
Australian Capital Territory	*Mental Health Act 2015*
New South Wales	*Mental Health Act 2007*
Northern Territory	*Mental Health and Related Services Act 1998*
Queensland	*Mental Health Act 2016*
South Australia	*Mental Health Act 2009*
Tasmania	*Mental Health Act 2013*
Victoria	*Mental Health Act 2014*
Western Australia	*Mental Health Act 2014*

disorder of thought form, a severe disturbance of mood, sustained or repeated irrational behaviour indicating the presence of any one or more of the above symptoms.

In Queensland[25] and Victoria[26] mental illness is 'a condition characterised by a clinically significant disturbance of thought, mood, perception or memory', while in South Australia 'mental illness' is defined as 'any illness or disorder of the mind'.[27] In Tasmania the legislation provides that a person has a mental illness if he or she 'experiences, temporarily, repeatedly or continually: (a) a serious impairment of thought (which may include delusions); or (b) a serious impairment of mood, volition, perception or cognition'.[28]

In Western Australia section 6(1) of the *Mental Health Act 2014* provides that 'a person has a mental illness if the person has a condition that is characterised by a disturbance of thought, mood, volition, perception, orientation or memory; and where that condition temporarily or permanently significantly impairs the person's judgment or behaviour'.

A number of Acts also have similar provisions about when a person is not considered to have a mental illness – for example, if he or she: holds, or refuses or fails to hold, a particular religious, cultural, political or philosophical belief or opinion; engages, or refuses or fails to engage, in a particular religious, cultural or political activity; is not a member of a particular religious, cultural or racial group; has or does not have a particular political, economic or social status; is sexually promiscuous, or has a particular sexual preference or orientation;

engages in immoral or illegal conduct; has an intellectual disability; uses drugs or alcohol; is or has been involved in personal or professional conflict; demonstrates antisocial behaviour; or has been treated for a mental illness, admitted by or detained at a hospital for the purpose of such treatment.[29]

ADMISSION TO HOSPITAL AND CARE ORDERS

Voluntary Admission

In New South Wales,[30] South Australia,[31] the Northern Territory,[32] Western Australia[33] and Tasmania[34] there is provision for patients seeking treatment for a mental health condition to be admitted to a psychiatric hospital on their own request as a voluntary patient. The permissible age for voluntary admission varies across states and territories.[35]

In the Australian Capital Territory a person may seek assessment of their mental condition by the ACT Civil and Administrative Tribunal under section 33 of the *Mental Health Act 2015*, but this does not constitute voluntary admission in the conventional sense. In Queensland the *Mental Health Act 2016* does not provide for voluntary admission.

In New South Wales[36] and the Northern Territory[37] the relevant authorised medical practitioner may refuse to admit a voluntary patient unless satisfied that the patient is likely to benefit from being admitted.

Involuntary Admission and Treatment at a Healthcare Facility

In all jurisdictions there is provision for involuntary admissions for treatment in a healthcare facility for people who fall under the auspices of the respective Acts.[38] Involuntary admission is generally permitted by the legislation if a person is suffering from a mental illness or mental disorder, is in need of treatment, and either refuses to or is unable to accept treatment voluntarily and poses a threat to himself or herself or others.[39] The legislation and recent case law requires the least restrictive alternative in considering the involuntary detention of persons with a mental illness.[40] Review by a mental health tribunal or administrative appeals tribunal within a set time is required by the legislation.

In Queensland, Tasmania and Western Australia a person cannot be admitted involuntarily for treatment if they have the capacity to refuse the treatment and do refuse it. In Victoria, when a person has the capacity to give informed consent to treatment this must be sought, although treatment can be given even where that is not obtained.[41]

Involuntary Treatment in the Community

Each of the states and territories provides for an alternative to an involuntary treatment order in a healthcare facility, which instead involves an order that authorises compulsory treatment in the community.[42] Community treatment orders may require a person to accept medication, therapy, counselling, management, rehabilitation or any other appropriate treatment either at home or at a mental health facility.[43] Generally, such orders may be made by a tribunal[44] or an authorised psychiatrist.[45] The treatment order may relate to a person who is in a mental health facility (voluntarily or otherwise) or a person who is not in a mental health facility.

In the Australian Capital Territory, Queensland, Victoria and Western Australia consideration must be given to whether compulsory treatment in the community provides the least restrictive option for treatment.

TREATMENT WITHOUT THE PATIENT'S CONSENT

In recent years, several Australian jurisdictions have introduced new mental health legislation which is more aligned with international human rights law. For example, in Western Australia, Tasmania and Queensland a person may no longer be the subject of involuntary detention or treatment if they have the capacity to refuse.

In Tasmania, while the requirement for evaluation of whether, without treatment, the mental illness will or is likely to seriously harm a person's 'health or safety' or the 'safety of others' remains, other considerations must also be had – this includes that: the person 'does not have decision-making capacity'; treatment will be appropriate and effective; and treatment cannot be given adequately except under a treatment order.[46] This indicates movement away from involuntary detention and/or treatment based on an assessment of there being a risk of harm to the person or to others.

In the new Victorian and Australian Capital Territory legislation there is reference to the need to seek the informed consent of the person in relation to proposed involuntary treatment.[47] However, all jurisdictions continue to provide in their legislation that treatment may occur without a person's consent, subject to restrictions on the type of treatment that can be administered.

In the Australian Capital Territory, emergency treatment, care or support may be administered to a patient subject to emergency involuntary detention, provided that it is the minimum necessary to prevent any immediate and substantial risk of the patient causing harm to himself or herself or to another person.[48] A psychiatric treatment order made by the ACT Civil and Administrative Tribunal may require a patient to either undergo psychiatric treatment (other than electroconvulsive therapy (ECT) or psychosurgery) or to undertake a counselling, training, therapeutic or rehabilitation program.[49] The chief psychiatrist is responsible for decisions about the treatment, care or support of patients subject to psychiatric treatment orders and for determining the nature and extent of psychiatric treatment to be given to a patient after taking all reasonable steps to consult him or her and any other relevant person listed under section 62(5).[50] The chief psychiatrist must not determine treatment that has, or is likely to have, the effect of subjecting the patient to undue stress or deprivation, having regard to the likely benefit of the treatment.[51] Before any treatment, care or support is provided, the chief psychiatrist must explain its nature and effects (including side effects) to the patient in a way that he or she is most likely to understand.[52]

In New South Wales an authorised medical officer may give, or authorise the giving of, any treatment to a person, without their consent, if they are detained in accordance with the legislation.[53] A medical practitioner must not, in relation to any mental illness or condition or suspected mental illness or condition, 'administer, or cause to be administered to a person a drug or drugs in a dosage that, having regard to professional standards, is excessive or inappropriate'.[54] If a person who falls under the ambit of the Act requires surgery, an authorised medical officer must apply to the mental health tribunal or the Secretary to the Ministry of Health for consent for the surgery to be performed.[55] In the case of an emergency, an authorised medical officer or the Secretary may consent to the surgery if the patient is incapable of giving consent or is capable but either refuses or does not give that consent and the surgical operation is urgently required to save the life or prevent serious damage to the health of the person or to prevent the patient from suffering significant pain or distress.[56] In such circumstances notice is to be given to the Mental Health Review Tribunal.[57]

In the Northern Territory treatment may be given without the consent of a person for whom a recommendation for psychiatric examination is made or who is detained or admitted as an involuntary patient on the order of the Mental Health Review Tribunal.[58] If treatment is not authorised by the tribunal it must not be administered to the person unless it is either: necessary to prevent the person causing (or likely to cause) serious harm to himself/herself or to someone else; to prevent further physical or mental deterioration of the person; or to relieve acute symptomatology.[59] In such circumstances treatment must be authorised by a registered psychiatric practitioner.[60]

The Northern Territory also permits non-psychiatric treatment of involuntary patients or people on community orders that does not have the primary purpose of treating a mental illness or mental disturbance or their effects, if approval has been given by the Mental Health Review Tribunal, a registered psychiatrist, a court or a guardian.[61] The person must be incapable of giving informed consent. Such treatment may include: surgical operations or procedures; anaesthetic for the purposes of medical investigation; or a course of treatment or medication requiring a prescription or medical supervision. Non-psychiatric treatment may be performed without approval if it is: immediately necessary to save the life of the person or to prevent irreparable harm to the person; to remove a threat of permanent disability to the person; or to remove a life-threatening risk to, or to relieve acute pain of, the person.[62]

In Queensland a patient about whom a treatment authority has been made aware may receive treatment and care without their consent.[63] An authorised doctor making a treatment authority must decide the nature and extent of treatment and care to be provided in consultation with the patient, the patient's family, carers and other support people (subject to the patient's right to privacy).[64] Treatment includes anything done, or to be done, with the intention of having a therapeutic effect on a person's mental illness, and care includes providing rehabilitation, developing living skills and giving support, assistance, information and other services to a person with an intellectual disability.[65] ECT and

neurosurgery are further regulated in other parts of the Act.[66]

In Tasmania if an approved medical practitioner authorises the treatment as being urgently needed in the patient's best interests, an involuntary patient may be given treatment ('urgent circumstances treatment') without informed consent or Mental Health Tribunal authorisation.[67] An approved medical practitioner may make such an authorisation only if they believe that achieving the necessary treatment outcome would be compromised by waiting for the treatment to be authorised by the tribunal (or by a member thereof on an interim basis).[68] Treatment orders made by the Mental Health Tribunal constitute authority for the patient to be given treatment without his or her informed consent. They must specify the treatment, or types of treatment, that may be administered to the patient.[69] A medical practitioner involved in the treatment or care of an involuntary patient subject to a treatment order must make a treatment plan for that patient. The medical practitioner must consult the patient and may subsequently consult anyone else they see fit to.[70] Treatment in urgent circumstances or pursuant to a treatment order includes only such professional intervention as necessary to: prevent or remedy mental illness; manage and alleviate the ill effects of mental illness; reduce the risks that people with mental illness may, on that account, pose to themselves or others; or monitor or evaluate a person's mental state. It does not include psychosurgery, termination of pregnancy, sterilisation, the removal of non-regenerative tissue for transplantation, general health care, seclusion or chemical, mechanical or physical restraint.

In South Australia treatment may be given, despite the absence or refusal of consent, to a patient to whom an inpatient treatment order applies for his or her mental illness, or for any other illness that may be causing or contributing to the mental illness, when treatment is authorised by a medical practitioner who has examined the patient.[71] Certain prescribed medical or surgical treatment may only be performed on a detained person who is incapable of giving consent with the authorisation of the Prescribed Psychiatric Treatments Panel[72] or the South Australian Civil and Administrative Tribunal.[73]

In Victoria a person admitted as an involuntary patient may be given treatment for his or her mental illness if the person does not have capacity to give informed consent or has refused to consent to such treatment pursuant to the decision of an authorised psychiatrist. An authorised psychiatrist may make a treatment decision only when satisfied that there is no less restrictive way for the patient to be treated having regard to the views and preferences of the patient, including as expressed in an advance care directive (see Chapter 12) and/or the patient's nominated person, guardian and carer (if the decision will directly affect the carer and the care relationship).[74] Different provisions and procedures apply for ECT or neurosurgery and to treatment that is not intended to either remedy the person's mental illness or alleviate the symptoms and reduce the ill effects of the person's mental illness.[75] In Western Australia a medical practitioner may provide emergency psychiatric treatment to a person without that person's consent if the treatment is needed to save the person's life or to prevent the person from behaving in a way that is likely to result in serious physical injury to the person or another person.[76] An involuntary patient, or a mentally impaired defendant in an authorised hospital, may be given psychiatric, medical, psychological or psychosocial treatment without his or her consent, but this requires the patient's psychiatrist to ensure that a medical practitioner making treatment decisions has regard to the patient's wishes.[77] The treatment must be intended to alleviate or prevent the deterioration of a mental illness or a condition that is a consequence of a mental illness.[78] ECT, psychosurgery and prohibited treatments are dealt with separately in the Act and cannot be provided pursuant to these provisions.[79]

SECLUSION AND RESTRAINT

Seclusion, in a mental health context, includes confinement at any time of the day or night alone in a room or area from which free exit is prevented. **Restraint** includes physical restraint (e.g. where force is used to control a person's freedom of movement), chemical restraint (e.g. where medication is used to control a person's behaviour, as opposed to treating a mental or physical condition) and mechanical restraint (where a device such as straps, safety vests or mittens is used to restrict/control a person's freedom of movement).

While all Australian jurisdictions have legislation (or guidelines) permitting restraint and seclusion in certain circumstances, reducing the use of such methods has been a national priority for mental health since the *National Safety Priorities in Mental Health: A National Plan for Reducing Harm*[80] implemented initiatives through Australian mental health pilot sites to progress this priority from 2007.[81] Where the use of restraint is regulated, it is done so by reference to requirements of 'necessity' and 'reasonableness', although these terms are often not further defined.

While each jurisdiction's laws vary and should be examined closely by health professionals working in mental health facilities and hospitals, some common elements exist. This includes that law or guidelines provide that seclusion and restraint should be kept to a minimum and used to manage the risk of serious imminent harm only when appropriate, safe alternative options have been considered and trialled, and for the briefest period required to allow the consumer to regain control of their behaviour and maintain their safety.[82] The need for continuous observation, monitoring and timely review is emphasised in state and territory legislation.[83] A person who is restrained or secluded must be supplied with suitable bedding, clothing, food and drink at appropriate times, adequate toilet arrangements, and any other psychological and physical care appropriate to the patient's needs.[84] Emphasis regarding human rights, dignity and self-respect is also given.

Approval for seclusion and restraint is required by an authorised person, such as a psychiatrist, registered medical practitioner or the senior nurse on duty, although the definition of who an authorised person is varies across jurisdictions.[85] In an emergency, an alternative person, such as a registered nurse, may approve the use of restraint in some states if it is necessary as a matter of urgency to prevent imminent and serious harm to the person or another person.[86]

It is also a requirement that records must be kept regarding any mechanical restraint or seclusion of a person.[87]

Note, the South Australian *Mental Health Act 2009* provides that 'medication should be used only for therapeutic purposes or safety reasons' – as such, chemical restraint is not generally permitted.[88]

RESTRICTED TREATMENT

'Restricted treatment' is treatment that is only permitted in certain circumstances, subject to certain criteria being met. This includes treatment such as ECT, psychosurgery and sterilisation.

ELECTROCONVULSIVE THERAPY

ECT is a procedure in which electric currents are passed through the brain, intentionally triggering a brief seizure. ECT is said to cause changes in brain chemistry that may reverse symptoms of certain mental illnesses such as major depression, mania and acute psychosis. It has been found at times to work when other treatments are unsuccessful. However, it has also been a controversial treatment due to risks and side effects; for example, memory declines with ECT, and although it usually returns to normal within a few weeks, this does not occur for all patients and in all respects.[89]

Specific provision exists in every jurisdiction except Tasmania regarding the administration of ECT for both voluntary and involuntary patients. Health practitioners working in mental health facilities would need to be familiar with the exact provisions in their state or territory. Some general similarities are found across jurisdictions that have legislation. In each respective jurisdiction informed consent to the treatment must be given[90] or approved for involuntary patients by the requisite state mental health or civil and administrative tribunal.[91] There may also be stipulations requiring where ECT may be given (such as a mental health facility) and who must be present during the treatment. For example, in New South Wales no fewer than two medical practitioners must be present, one of whom is experienced in the administration of ECT and another of whom is experienced in administering the anaesthesia.[92] Minimum age limits generally also apply; however, they vary among jurisdictions.

Some jurisdictions provide for emergency ECT. For example, Western Australia allows emergency ECT if the patient needs to be provided with ECT to either save his or her life or because there is an imminent risk of the patient behaving in a way that is likely to result in serious physical injury to himself or herself or to another person.[93]

PSYCHOSURGERY

Psychosurgery, or neurosurgery for mental illness (NMI), involves the neurosurgical 'treatment' of psychiatric disorders.[94] During the operation, which is carried out under a general anaesthetic, a small piece of brain is destroyed or removed. This surgery may be used in relation to severe depressive disorder, obsessive compulsive disorder or severe anxiety that does not respond to other treatments. Approximately a third of patients show improvement in their symptoms after surgery,[95] but risks still exist.[96] More recent forms of psychosurgery include 'deep brain stimulation', which is a technique used to modulate basal ganglia and thalamic function to attenuate the symptoms of Parkinson's disease. It has been found to yield positive results regarding bradykinesia (slowness of movement), tremor, rigidity and postural and gait abnormalities.[97] There is some evidence that deep brain stimulation has potential use in psychiatric disorders.

In Australia the use of psychosurgery is limited or banned. Legislation in each jurisdiction controls the use of psychosurgery.[98] In Queensland,[99] New South Wales[100] and the Northern Territory[101] psychosurgery is a prohibited treatment. In jurisdictions in which it is permitted, it appears to be used infrequently. For example, in Victoria, where NMI may be lawfully performed with the informed consent of a person and consideration of an application by the Mental Health Tribunal,[102] there were only 11 applications for NMI between 2014 and 2017 (all for deep brain stimulation).[103]

ILL-TREATMENT AND NEGLECT

It is an offence for the employees of a psychiatric service to ill-treat or wilfully neglect mentally ill people undergoing treatment in a psychiatric facility.[104]

MENTAL HEALTH REVIEW BOARDS/TRIBUNALS

The mental health legislation in most jurisdictions establishes boards or tribunals to carry out a number of functions. The functions of each are set out in legislation. There is some variation; however, the general review process in relation to detained patients is consistent. The boards and tribunals have the responsibility of hearing and determining appeals from a magistrate and periodically review all patients who have been detained – for example, informal patients who have been detained for a period of 12 months or longer. They also make determinations in relation to detained patients when there is disagreement between the patient and the treating doctor as to treatment, category of admission or detention. Moreover, appeals against community treatment orders and counselling orders made by a magistrate can be heard and determined by the boards and tribunals. They may hear reports relating to restraint and seclusion and the non-psychiatric treatment of a patient.

In South Australia there is a close relationship between mental health legislation and the Guardianship Board, which has the power to review consent issues and detention orders.[105]

FURTHER READING

Australian Government. The National Mental Health Statement of Rights and Responsibilities. Canberra, ACT: Australian Government; 2012.

Department of Health. Fifth National Mental Health and Suicide Prevention Plan and Implementation Plan. Canberra, ACT: Australian Government; 2017.

Gooding P. *A New Era for Mental Health Law and Policy*. Cambridge, UK: Cambridge University Press; 2017.

International Disability Alliance. Position Paper on the Convention on the Rights of Persons with Disabilities (CRPD) and Other Instruments. Geneva: IDA; 2008. Available from: http://www.internationaldisabilityalliance.org/resources/position-paper-convention-rights-persons-disabilities-crpd-and-other-instruments. Accessed 13 March 2019.

McSherry B, Maker Y. International human rights and mental health: challenges for law and practice. *J Law Med*. 2018;25:315.

United Nations General Assembly. A/HRC/22/53, Report of the Special Rapporteur on Torture and Other Cruel, Inhuman or Degrading Treatment or Punishment, Juan E Méndez, 1 February 2013. Available from: https://www.ohchr.org/documents/hrbodies/hrcouncil/regularsession/session22/a.hrc.22.53_english.pdf. Accessed 13 March 2019.

United Nations General Assembly. The Convention on the Rights of Persons with Disabilities, adopted on 13 December 2006 during the 61st session of the General Assembly by resolution A/RES/61/106. Available from: http://www.un.org/en/development/desa/population/migration/generalassembly/docs/globalcompact/A_RES_61_106.pdf. Accessed 13 March 2019.

World Health Organization. *Mental health action plan 2013–2020*. Geneva: WHO; 2013.

ENDNOTES

1. Australian Bureau of Statistics. National Survey of Mental Health and Wellbeing, Summary of Results 2007. Canberra, ACT: ABS; 2007.
2. Department of Health and Ageing. National Mental Health Report 2013: Tracking Progress of Mental Health Reform in Australia 1993–2011. Canberra, ACT: Commonwealth of Australia; 2013.
3. Australian Institute of Health and Welfare. Mental Health Services in Australia. https://www.aihw.gov.au/reports/mental-health-services/mental-health-services-in-australia/report-contents/summary/prevalence-and-policies. Accessed 18 February 2018.
4. Although mental health problems are equally common in men and women, the types of problems differ. Women are more than twice as likely to be affected by depression, while men suffer more from substance abuse (e.g. 80% of those dependent on alcohol are men). Men are also more prone to suicide – see Australian Bureau of Statistics. *National Survey of Mental Health and Wellbeing, Summary of Results 2007*. Canberra, ACT: Commonwealth of Australia; 2007.
5. National Mental Health Commission. The National Review of Mental Health Programmes and Services. Sydney, NSW: NMHC; 2014. p. 14.
6. United Nations General Assembly. *The Convention on the Rights of Persons with Disabilities*, adopted on 13 December 2006 during the sixty-first session of the General Assembly by resolution A/RES/61/106. Entered into force 3 May 2008 (CRPD). The Convention has 158 signatories, with 137 ratifications/accessions; the optional protocol has 92 signatories, with 78 ratifications/accessions. Australia has signed and ratified the CRPD, and the Optional Protocol.
7. United Nations General Assembly. The Convention on the Rights of Persons with Disabilities.
8. CRPD Article 1. Note one of the main impetuses to the CRPD was that people with disabilities were marginalised from the substance of human rights, sometimes specifically being excluded. Shifts in recognising the human rights of people with disabilities began to occur when the UN announced that 1981 would be the International Year of Disabled Persons. This was followed by the World Programme of Action Concerning Disabled Persons and the Decade of Rights of People with Disability, culminating in 1993 with the publication of the *Standard Rules on the Equalization of Opportunities for Persons with Disabilities*.
9. CRPD Article 1.
10. CRPD Article 3.
11. Gooding P. *A New Era for Mental Health Law and Policy*. Cambridge: Cambridge University Press; 2017. For a more detailed discussion of the CRPD as it relates to mental illness see: Allan S, Blake M. *Australian Health Law*. Sydney, NSW: LexisNexis Butterworths; 2018.
12. MI Principle 1.
13. The International Disability Alliance member organisations include Disabled Peoples International; Inclusion International; International Federation of Hard of Hearing People; Rehabilitation International; World Blind Union; World Federation of the Deaf; World Federation of the DeafBlind; World Network of Users and Survivors of Psychiatry; European Disability Forum; and Arab Organization of Disabled People.
14. World Health Organization. Mental Health Action Plan 2013–2020. Geneva: WHO; 2013.
15. See World Health Organization. QualityRights Initiative – Improving Quality, Promoting Rights. https://www.who.int/

mental_health/policy/quality_rights/en/. Accessed 13 March 2019.

16. Human Rights Council (HRC) Resolution on Mental Health and Human Rights (A/HRC/36/L.25). Australia was one of the co-sponsors of the resolution.

17. Australian Government. The Fifth National Mental Health and Suicide Prevention Plan. Canberra, ACT: Australian Government; 2017. p. 4.

18. Australian Commission on Safety and Quality in Health Care. Scoping Study on the Implementation of National Standards in Mental Health Services. Sydney, NSW: ACSQHC; 2014. https://www.safetyandquality.gov.au/wp-content/uploads/2014/11/Scoping-Study-on-the-Implementation-of-National-Standards-in-Mental-Health-Services.pdf. Accessed 18 February 2018.

19. Australian Government. The National Mental Health Statement of Rights and Responsibilities. Canberra, ACT: Australian Government; 2012. p. 3.

20. Department of Health. The Fifth National Mental Health and Suicide Prevention Plan. Canberra, ACT: Commonwealth of Australia; 2017. p. 4.

21. See: Australian Health Ministers Advisory Council. *A National Framework for Recovery-Oriented Mental Health Services: Guide for Practitioners and Providers*. Canberra, ACT: Commonwealth of Australia; 2013, and Australian Health Ministers Advisory Council. *A National Framework for Recovery-Oriented Mental Health Services: Policy and Theory*. Canberra, ACT: Commonwealth of Australia; 2013.

22. *Mental Health Act 2015* (ACT) ss 10, 11.

23. *Mental Health Act 2007* (NSW) s 4.

24. *Mental Health and Related Services Act 1998* (NT) s 6.

25. *Mental Health Act 2016* (Qld) s 10(1).

26. *Mental Health Act 2014* (Vic) s 4(1).

27. *Mental Health Act 2009* (SA) s 3.

28. *Mental Health Act 2013* (Tas) s 4(1)(a).

29. For example, see *Mental Health Act 2007* (NSW) s 15; *Mental Health Act 2013* (Tas) s 4(2); *Mental Health Act 2014* (Vic) s 4(2); *Mental Health Act 2014* (WA) s 6(2).

30. *Mental Health Act 2007* (NSW) s 5.

31. *Mental Health Act 2009* (SA) s 8.

32. *Mental Health and Related Services Act 1998* (NT) s 25.

33. *Mental Health Act 2014* (WA) s 175.

34. *Mental Health Act 2013* (Tas) s 16(1).

35. See, for example, *Mental Health Act 2007* (NSW) s 6(1); *Mental Health Act 2009* (SA) s 4(1)(a); *Mental Health and Related Services Act 1998* (NT) ss 25(1), 25(2).

36. *Mental Health Act 2007* (NSW) s 5(2).

37. *Mental Health and Related Services Act 1998* (NT) s 25(8).

38. *Mental Health Act 2007* (NSW) ss 12–13, 18–33; *Mental Health Act 2016* (Qld) Ch 2 Pt 4; *Mental Health Act 2009* (SA) Pt 5; *Mental Health Act 2013* (Tas) Pt 3; *Mental Health Act 2014* (Vic) Pt 4; *Mental Health Act 2014* (WA) Pt 6; *Mental Health and Related Services Act 1998* (NT) Pt 6.

39. *Mental Health Act 2015* (ACT) Ch 6; *Mental Health Act 2007* (NSW) s 12; *Mental Health and Related Services Act 1998* (NT) ss 14, 15; *Mental Health Act 2016* (Qld) s 39; *Mental Health Act*

2009 (SA) ss 21(1), 25(1); *Mental Health Act 2014* (Vic) s 5; *Mental Health Act 2014* (WA) s 26.

40. *Hunter and New England Local Health District v McKenna, Hunter and New England Local Health District v Simon* [2014] HCA 44.

41. *Mental Health Act 2014* (Vic) ss 68, 70.

42. *Mental Health Act 2007* (NSW) Pt 3; *Mental Health Act 2016* (Qld) s 52; *Mental Health Act 2009* (SA) Pt 7; *Mental Health Act 2013* (Tas) ss 39, 40; *Mental Health Act 2014* (Vic) s 52; *Mental Health Act 2014* (WA) s 23; *Mental Health Act 2015* (ACT) Pt 5.5 (in the ACT the order is referred to as a 'community care order'); *Mental Health and Related Services Act 1998* (NT) s 16 (referred to in the NT as a 'community management order').

43. For example, see *Mental Health Act 2007* (NSW) ss 51, 53, 57; *Mental Health Act 2015* (ACT) s 67 (in the ACT the order may also limit a person's communication with other people).

44. For example, *Mental Health Act 2007* (NSW) s 51(1).

45. For example, *Mental Health Act 2009* (SA) s 10.

46. *Mental Health Act 2013* (Tas) s 40.

47. Although a refusal can be overridden in limited circumstances – see *Mental Health Act 2014* (Vic) s 70; *Mental Health Act 2015* (ACT) s 58(2)(b)(ii).

48. *Mental Health Act 2015* (ACT) s 88.

49. Ibid. s 59(1).

50. Ibid. s 62.

51. Ibid. s 62(4).

52. Ibid. s 63.

53. *Mental Health Act 2007* (NSW) s 84.

54. Ibid. s 85.

55. Ibid. ss 100–101.

56. Ibid. s 99(1).

57. Ibid. s 99(4).

58. *Mental Health and Related Services Act 1998* (NT) s 55(1).

59. Ibid. s 55(2).

60. Ibid. s 55(3).

61. Ibid. s 63(1).

62. Ibid. s 63(4).

63. *Mental Health Act 2016* (Qld) s 18(1). Recall that the Queensland Act only authorises a treatment authority to be made for a person who does not have capacity to consent.

64. *Mental Health Act 2016* (Qld) ss 23(5) and 53.

65. Ibid. Sch 3.

66. Ibid. s 23(5).

67. Ibid. s 55(1).

68. Ibid. s 55(2). Note: see s 55 (3) for the full urgent circumstances treatment criteria.

69. Ibid. ss 41, 42.

70. Ibid. ss 51, 53.

71. *Mental Health Act 2009* (SA) ss 24(1), 28(1), 31(1).

72. Ibid. Pt 7. Prescribed treatment under the *Mental Health Act 2009* (SA) includes ECT and neurosurgery.

73. *Guardianship and Administration Act 1993* (SA) s 61. Prescribed treatment under the *Guardianship and Administration Act 1993* (SA) includes sterilisation and termination of pregnancy.

74. *Mental Health Act 2014* (Vic) s 71.

75. Ibid. Pt 5 Divs 3, 5, 6.

76. *Mental Health Act 2014* (WA) ss 202, 203.

77. Ibid. ss 178–180.

78. Ibid. s 4. Note: treatment does not include bodily restraint, seclusion or sterilisation.

79. Ibid. ss 178(2), 202(2).

80. Australian Government Health Department. National Safety Priorities in Mental Health: A National Plan for Reducing Harm. Canberra, ACT: Commonwealth Government; 2005.

81. As part of the National Mental Health Seclusion and Restraint (Beacon Site) Project 2007–2009.

82. See, for example, *Mental Health and Related Services Act 1998* (NT) s 61(3); *Mental Health Act 2016* (Qld) ss 268–270; *Mental Health Act 2009* (SA) s 7; *Mental Health Act 2013* (Tas) ss 56, 57; *Mental Health Act 2014* (Vic) ss 3, 105. Note: New South Wales Health has guidelines: *Aggression, Seclusion & Restraint in Mental Health Facilities in NSW*, GL2012_005, 26 June 2012, p. 15. http://www.health.nsw.gov.au/policies. Accessed 25 April 2018. Note: Some jurisdictions stipulate a maximum time period.

83. See *Mental Health Act 2016* (Qld) s 256; *Mental Health Act 2009* (SA) s 90; *Mental Health Act 2014* (Vic) s 115; *Mental Health Act 2014* (WA) ss 222, 238.

84. See, for example, *Mental Health and Related Services Act 1998* (NT) s 61(8).

85. *Mental Health and Related Services Act 1998* (NT) s 61(4); *Mental Health Act 2016* (Qld) ss 244–253 (mechanical restraint) ss 254–262 (seclusion); *Mental Health Act 2014* (Vic) s 114; *Mental Health Act 2014* (WA) ss 213, 214, 229, 230.

86. *Mental Health Act 2014* (Vic) s 115.

87. See, for example, *Mental Health and Related Services Act 1998* (NT) ss 61(12), 62(12).

88. *Mental Health Act 2009* (SA) s 7(1)(g), but note ss 56(3)(d) and s 56(6) in relation to the powers of authorised officers to use chemical restraint in certain circumstances.

89. Rose D, Wykes T, Leese M, et al. Patients' perspectives on electroconvulsive therapy: systematic review. *BMJ.* 2003;326:1363–5.

90. *Mental Health Act 2015* (ACT) s 148; *Mental Health Act 2007* (NSW) s 91; *Mental Health and Related Services Act 1998* (NT) ss 66(1), 66(1A); *Mental Health Act 2016* (Qld) s 236; *Mental Health Act 2009* (SA) s 42(1); *Mental Health Act 2014* (Vic) s 9; *Mental Health Act 2014* (WA) s 197.

91. *Mental Health Act 2015* (ACT) s 149; *Mental Health Act 2007* (NSW) s 89; *Mental Health and Related Services Act 1998* (NT) s 66(2); *Mental Health Act 2016* (Qld) s 507; *Mental Health Act 2009* (SA) s 42(1); *Mental Health Act 2014* (Vic) s 92; *Mental Health Act 2014* (WA) s 198.

92. *Mental Health Act 2007* (NSW) ss 88(2)–(3); *Mental Health and Related Services Act 1998* (NT) ss 66(6)–(7).

93. *Mental Health Act 2014* (WA) s 199(2). See also, for example, *Mental Health Act 2015* (ACT) s 162; *Mental Health and Related Services Act 1998* (NT) s 66(3); *Mental Health Act 2016* (Qld) s 237.

94. Mashour GA, Walker EE, Martuza RL. Psychosurgery: past, present, and future. *Brain Res Rev.* 2005;48:409–19.

95. Ibid.

96. Ibid.

97. Ibid. p. 415.

98. *Mental Health Act 2007* (NSW) s 83; *Mental Health Act 2014* (Vic) ss 100–104; *Mental Health Act 2009* (SA) s 43; *Mental Health Act 2014* (WA) ss 205–209, 416–421; *Mental Health Act 2016* (Qld) s 241; *Mental Health Act 2015* (ACT) ss 167–175; *Mental Health and Related Services Act 1998* (NT) s 58; *Mental Health Act 2013* (Tas) ss 122–128.

99. *Mental Health Act 2016* (Qld) s 241.

100. *Mental Health Act 2007* (NSW) ss 83(1)(c), 83(2).

101. *Mental Health and Related Services Act 1998* (NT) s 58(2).

102. *Mental Health Act 2014* (Vic) ss 100–104.

103. Mental Health Tribunal. 2016/2017 Annual Report. Melbourne, VIC: State Government of Victoria; 2017, p. 17. Note: The tribunal granted 10 of the 11 applications from 2014 to 2017. All granted applications were for patients with a diagnosis of depression. The application not granted was for a patient with a diagnosis of obsessive compulsive disorder.

104. For example, *Mental Health Act 2007* (NSW) s 69 (offence to ill-treat patients); *Mental Health Act 2009* (SA) s 49 (neglect or ill-treatment); *Mental Health Act 2014* (WA) s 253 (duty not to ill-treat or wilfully neglect patients); *Mental Health Act 2016* (Qld) s 621 (offence relating to ill-treatment); *Mental Health Act 2013* (Tas) s 214 (person must not neglect or ill-treat person with mental illness).

105. *Mental Health Act 2009* (SA) s 10.

REVIEW QUESTIONS AND ACTIVITIES

1. Identify the types of mental health conditions faced in Australia and their prevalence.

2. What is the relevance of international law to mental health legislation and practice?

3. Outline the key Australian policies regarding mental health and illness.

4. Discuss when a person with mental health issues can be treated without their consent.

5. Describe the general legal requirements relevant to restraint and seclusion, psychosurgery and electroconvulsive therapy.

6. Explain the mechanisms that are in place to ensure adequate transparency and the maintenance of patient rights for those experiencing a mental illness.

16 CHILD AND ELDER ABUSE

LEARNING OBJECTIVES

Upon completing this chapter you should be able to:

- identify and discuss the different types of child abuse
- describe the law regarding voluntary and mandatory reporting of child abuse
- identify who has mandatory reporting obligations regarding child abuse and when reporting must occur
- explain what is meant by the term 'elder abuse'
- explain the law regarding elder abuse.

INTRODUCTION

Abuse, neglect and exploitation have serious physical and mental health effects that necessitate treatment and prevention strategies. Health practitioners are often in a position where they are able to identify and address abuse, neglect and exploitation due to the unique relationship they have with people within families and the community. They are often the most knowledgeable about a person's physical and mental health needs and how well these needs are being met. They are also well positioned to detect health changes that are the result of intentional or unintentional mistreatment. Often health practitioners are not only required to assess whether there exists some form of abuse but they may also be required to involve protective services when indicated. This chapter focuses on child abuse and elder abuse to illustrate principles about which health practitioners should be aware of abuse, noting that all health practitioners have a professional and ethical obligation to protect and promote public health and safe health care.

CHILD ABUSE

The World Health Organization defines child abuse as:

> … *physical and/or emotional ill-treatment, sexual abuse, neglect, negligence and commercial or other exploitation, which results in actual or potential harm to the child's health, survival, development or dignity in the context of a relationship of responsibility, trust or power.*[1]

In addition, child abuse is now recognised to include exposure to domestic violence, which may cause long-term damage on children due to experiencing or witnessing such violence.

The Australian Royal College of Physicians explains further the wide range of behaviours that constitute child abuse:[2]

- **Physical abuse** – intentional use of physical force or objects against a child that results in, or has the potential to result in, physical injury which includes hitting, kicking, punching, beating, stabbing, biting, pushing, shoving, throwing, pulling, dragging, shaking, strangling, smothering, burning, scalding and poisoning.
- **Emotional/psychological abuse** – intentional behaviour that conveys to a child that he/she is worthless, flawed, unloved, unwanted, endangered or valued only in meeting another's needs, which can include blaming, belittling, degrading, intimidating, terrorising, isolating or otherwise behaving in a manner that is harmful,

potentially harmful or insensitive to the child's developmental needs, or can potentially damage the child psychologically or emotionally. This includes threatening, yelling, taunting, debasing (e.g. 'you're worthless', 'you're dumb', 'no-one likes you'). Witnessing intimate partner abuse can also be classified as exposure to emotional/psychological abuse.

- **Sexual abuse** – any completed or attempted sexual act, sexual contact or non-contact sexual interaction which includes penetration, touching a child inappropriately and exposure to sexual activity, filming or prostitution.
- **Neglect** – failure to meet a child's basic physical, emotional, medical/dental or educational needs; failure to provide adequate nutrition, hygiene or shelter, or failure to ensure a child's safety which can include: failure to provide adequate food, clothing or accommodation; not seeking medical attention when needed; allowing a child to miss long periods of school; and failure to protect a child from violence in the home or neighbourhood or from avoidable hazards.
- **Exposure to intimate partner abuse** – children living in families where intimate partner abuse (any incident of threatening behaviour, violence or abuse (psychological, physical, sexual, financial or emotional) between adults who are, or have been, intimate partners or family members) occurs are considered to be victims of child abuse, whether directly or indirectly abused.

The role of a health practitioner in relation to such abuse may include to: prevent child abuse; detect the problem and respond to it when it occurs; and minimise the long-term negative effects of child abuse.[3]

Government policy to protect children from abuse focuses on safe environments, aims to consider risk factors for child abuse and neglect, and promotes support and care for those who have been exploited.[4] The *National Framework for Protecting Australia's Children 2009–2020* represents the current policy approach across Australia and is relevant to the Commonwealth, state/territory governments, non-government organisations, service providers and individuals with an interest in ensuring Australia's children are safe and well. Its focus is on:

- children living in safe and supportive families and communities
- children and families accessing adequate support to promote safety and intervene early
- risk factors for child abuse and neglect
- children who have been abused or neglected receiving the support and care they need for their safety and wellbeing
- Indigenous children being supported and safe in their families and communities
- child sexual abuse and exploitation being prevented and survivors receiving adequate support.

Government policy and legislation come together to provide protection for children from abuse and maltreatment through voluntary and mandatory reporting systems. The legislative definitions of what conduct or circumstance constitutes 'abuse' or 'maltreatment' or identifies children who are in 'need of care' differ between jurisdictions. It is therefore important that, in addition to understanding the general definitions provided above, health practitioners familiarise themselves with the particular legislative criteria applicable in their own state or territory. The principal legislation is noted in Table 16.1.

Reporting of Child Abuse

Voluntary Reporting

In all states and territories other than Western Australia and South Australia the legislation provides for the voluntary reporting of child abuse.

TABLE 16.1
Child Protection Legislation – Principal Acts

Jurisdiction	Legislation
Australian Capital Territory	*Children and Young People Act 2008*
New South Wales	*Children and Young Persons (Care and Protection) Act 1998*
Northern Territory	*Care and Protection of Children Act 2007*
Queensland	*Child Protection Act 1999*
South Australia	*Children's Protection Act 1993*
Tasmania	*Children, Young Persons and Their Families Act 1997*
Victoria	*Children Youth and Families Act 2005*
Western Australia	*Children and Community Services Act 2004*

Section 24 of the New South Wales *Children and Young Persons (Care and Protection) Act 1998* provides that where a person on reasonable grounds believes that a child is at risk of harm they may notify the Director-General of the Department of Child Safety.

In Queensland, under section 22 of the *Child Protection Act 1999*, a person may notify the Chief Executive if they suspect a child is being, or is likely to be at risk of harm.

In Tasmania, pursuant to section 13 of the *Children, Young Persons and Their Families Act 1997*, an adult who knows, believes or suspects on reasonable grounds that a child is suffering, has suffered or is likely to suffer abuse or neglect has a responsibility to take steps to prevent the abuse. This may include notifying the Secretary to the Department of Health and Human Services of their knowledge, belief or suspicion.

Section 64 of Victoria's *Children, Youth and Families Act 2005* provides that any person who believes a child needs protection may notify a protective intervener, who is identified under the legislation as the Director-General of Community Services or the police.

In the above jurisdictions the legislation protects reporters from actions in defamation, breach of privacy laws or professional disciplinary proceedings, provided such reporting is done in good faith. In South Australia, where there is no legislative provision for voluntary notification, a person who on reasonable grounds and in good faith does report their suspicions or beliefs will not be liable in civil, criminal or other legal proceedings.[5]

Mandatory Reporting

In addition to voluntary reporting provisions, it is an offence in all Australian jurisdictions for a nominated professional to fail to notify the appropriate authorities such as child protection departments or police when child abuse is suspected. As with voluntary reporting, there is legislative protection from legal action and disciplinary proceedings where notifications are based on reasonable grounds and carried out in good faith to the correct authority.

The legislation contains lists of occupations that are mandated to report. The occupations most commonly named as mandated reporters are those that deal frequently with children during their work, including teachers, doctors, nurses and police. The lists then vary regarding who else has mandatory reporting obligations. There are also differences in the types of abuse and neglect that must be reported. In some jurisdictions it is mandatory to report physical and sexual abuse (Australian Capital Territory, Queensland, Victoria); in South Australia, physical, sexual and emotional/psychological abuse and neglect must be reported. The remaining jurisdictions are like South Australia but also require reports of exposure to domestic violence (New South Wales, Northern Territory, Tasmania, Western Australia).

Details of each jurisdiction's requirements are summarised in Table 16.2.

In addition to the state and territory laws above, at the Commonwealth level, there is a mandatory reporting duty for particular personnel from the Family Court

---

TABLE 16.2
State and Territory Laws Regarding Mandatory Reporting of Child Abuse

State/Territory Law	Mandated Reporter		Abuse Type to be Reported	What Must Be Reported?
Australian Capital Territory *Children and Young People Act 2008* s 356	■ Doctor ■ Dentist ■ Nurse ■ Enrolled nurse ■ Midwife ■ Psychologist ■ Teacher ■ Inspector of home education programs ■ Police officer ■ School counsellor ■ Childcare worker	■ Person monitoring family day care ■ Public servant working with children, young people or families ■ The Public Advocate ■ Person working with children, young people or families prescribed by regulations	■ Physical ■ Sexual	A belief, on reasonable grounds, that a child or young person has experienced or is experiencing sexual abuse or non-accidental physical injury, and the belief arises from information obtained by the person during or because of the person's work (whether paid or unpaid)

TABLE 16.2

State and Territory Laws Regarding Mandatory Reporting of Child Abuse *(Continued)*

State/Territory Law	Mandated Reporter	Abuse Type to be Reported	What Must Be Reported?
New South Wales *Children and Young Persons (Care and Protection) Act 1998* ss 23, 27	A person who, during his or her professional work or other paid employment, delivers: ■ health care ■ welfare ■ education ■ children's services ■ residential services, or ■ law enforcement wholly or partly to children A person who holds a management position in an organisation, the duties of which include direct responsibility for, or direct supervision of, the provision of the above services wholly or partly to children	■ Physical ■ Sexual ■ Emotional/psychological ■ Neglect ■ Exposure to domestic violence	Reasonable grounds to suspect that a child is at risk of significant harm, and those grounds arise during or from the person's work
Northern Territory *The Care and Protection of Children Act 2007* ss 15, 16, 26	■ Any person ■ A health practitioner or someone who performs work of a kind that is prescribed by regulation	■ Physical ■ Sexual or other exploitation ■ Emotional/psychological ■ Neglect ■ Exposure to physical violence (e.g. domestic)	■ Any person: A belief on reasonable grounds that a child has suffered or is likely to suffer harm or exploitation ■ Health practitioner: Reasonable grounds to believe child aged 14 or 15 years has been/is likely to be a victim of a sexual offence and the age difference between the child and offender is greater than 2 years (s 26(2))
Queensland *Child Protection Act 1999* s 13 *Education (General Provisions) Act 2006* ss 364, 365, 365A, 366, 366A	■ An authorised officer, a public service employee employed in the department, a person employed in a departmental care service or licensed care service ■ Relevant persons: doctors; registered nurses; teachers; a police officer who is responsible for reporting; a person engaged to perform a child advocate function under the *Public Guardian Act 2014*; early childhood education and care professionals ■ School staff (sexual abuse only)	■ Physical ■ Sexual	■ Reasonable suspicion that a child in care has suffered, is suffering, or is at unacceptable risk of, significant harm caused by physical/sexual abuse ■ Reasonable suspicion that a child has suffered, is suffering or is at an unacceptable risk of suffering, significant harm caused by physical/sexual abuse and may not have a parent able/willing to protect the child from the harm ■ Awareness or reasonable suspicion that a child has been, or is likely to be, sexually abused; the suspicion is formed during the person's employment

Continued on following page

TABLE 16.2			
State and Territory Laws Regarding Mandatory Reporting of Child Abuse *(Continued)*			
State/Territory Law	Mandated Reporter	Abuse Type to be Reported	What Must Be Reported?
South Australia *Children's Protection Act 1993* ss 6, 10, 11	■ Medical practitioners ■ Dentists ■ Pharmacists ■ Registered or enrolled nurses ■ Psychologists ■ Police and community corrections officers ■ Social workers ■ Ministers of religion/employees or volunteers in a religious or spiritual organisation ■ Teachers ■ Family day care providers ■ Any other person managing/employed/volunteering in a government/non-government organisation who provides health, welfare, education, sporting or recreational, childcare or residential services wholly or partly for children	■ Physical ■ Sexual ■ Emotional/psychological ■ Neglect	■ Reasonable grounds to suspect that a child has been or is being abused or neglected, and the suspicion is formed during the person's work (whether paid or voluntary) or carrying out official duties
Tasmania *Children, Young Persons and Their Families Act 1997* ss 3, 4, 14	■ Medical practitioners ■ Registered or enrolled nurses ■ Persons registered under the Health Practitioner Regulation National Law (Tas) in midwifery, dental or psychology professions ■ Police officers ■ Probation officers ■ Principals and teachers ■ Persons who provide childcare or a childcare service for fee or reward ■ Persons concerned in the management of an approved education and care service ■ Any other person who is employed or engaged as an employee for, of, or in, or who is a volunteer in, a government agency that provides health, welfare, education, childcare or residential services wholly or partly for children, and an organisation that receives any funding from the Crown for the provision of such services ■ Any other person of a class determined by the Minister by notice in the Gazette to be prescribed persons	■ Physical ■ Sexual ■ Emotional/psychological ■ Neglect ■ Exposure to family violence	■ A belief, or suspicion on reasonable grounds, or knowledge that a child has been or is being abused or neglected or is a child whose safety, psychological wellbeing or interests are affected or likely to be affected by family violence ■ There is a reasonable likelihood of a child being killed or abused or neglected by a person with whom the child resides ■ While a woman is pregnant there is a reasonable likelihood that after the birth of the child the child will suffer abuse or neglect, or may be killed by a person with whom the child is likely to reside, or that the child will require medical treatment or another intervention because of the behaviour of the woman or another person with whom the woman resides, or is likely to reside, before the birth of the child

TABLE 16.2

State and Territory Laws Regarding Mandatory Reporting of Child Abuse (Continued)

State/Territory Law	Mandated Reporter	Abuse Type to be Reported	What Must Be Reported?
Victoria *Children, Youth and Families Act 2005* ss 182(1)(a)–(e), 184, 162(c)–(d) *Crimes Act 1958* s 327	▪ Registered medical practitioners ▪ Nurses ▪ Midwives ▪ A person registered as a teacher or an early childhood teacher or granted permission to teach ▪ Principals of government/non-government schools within the meaning of the *Education and Training Reform Act 2006* Police officers ▪ Any person (regarding a sexual offence)	▪ Physical ▪ Sexual	▪ Belief on reasonable grounds that a child needs protection formed during practising his or her profession or carrying out the duties of his or her office, position or employment as soon as practicable after forming the belief and after each occasion on which he or she becomes aware of any further reasonable grounds for the belief ▪ A reasonable belief that a sexual offence has been committed against a child under the age of 16 years by another person of or over the age of 18 years must be reported to a police officer as soon as practicable, unless the person has a reasonable excuse for not doing so; failure to disclose the information to police is a criminal offence
Western Australia *Children and Community Services Act 2004* ss 124A, 124B *Family Court Act 1997* ss 5, 160	▪ Doctors; nurses and midwives; teachers or boarding supervisors; and police officers ▪ The Principal Registrar, a registrar or a deputy registrar; family counsellors; family consultants; family dispute resolution practitioners, arbitrators or legal practitioners independently representing the child's interests	▪ Physical ▪ Sexual ▪ Neglect ▪ Psychological harm including but not limited to being exposed to domestic violence	▪ Belief on reasonable grounds that child sexual abuse has occurred or is occurring and forms this belief during the person's work, whether paid or unpaid ▪ Reasonable grounds for suspecting that a child has been: abused, or is at risk of being abused; ill-treated, or is at risk of being ill-treated; or exposed or subjected to behaviour that psychologically harms the child

Information included in this table was drawn from the relevant legislation and quoted from: Australian Institute of Family Studies. *Mandatory Reporting of Child Abuse and Neglect: CFCA Resource Sheet – September 2017.* See: https://aifs.gov.au/cfca/publications/mandatory-reporting-child-abuse-and-neglect.

of Australia, the Federal Circuit Court of Australia and the Family Court of Western Australia pursuant to the *Family Law Act 1975* (Cth). This includes, among other people, family consultants and counsellors. If such people have reasonable grounds for suspecting that a child has been abused, or is at risk of being abused, the person must, as soon as practicable, notify a prescribed child welfare authority of the suspicion and the basis for the suspicion.[6]

ELDER ABUSE

Elder abuse has been defined as the 'wilful or intentional harm caused to older adults by other people with whom they have a relationship implying trust'.[7] Most often the abuser will be a spouse or adult children; however, the abuse may also be perpetrated by other family members or a paid or unpaid carer. While there are many types of abuse, those most commonly reported include physical abuse (sexual abuse, shaking, striking, restraining), psychological abuse (threatening, intimidating, creating dependence, isolation and ignoring), neglect (failing to provide the necessaries of life) and financial abuse.

Abuse of the elderly is frequently difficult to detect. This may be due to reluctance on the part of the elderly person to disclose the abuse, a lack of capacity to seek assistance or an inability to access assistance due to social isolation. Abuse may take many different forms and this also hinders identification and detection. For example, the abuse may not be physically evident or not identifiable through financial irregularities.

Issues Relevant to Elder Abuse

Unlike the child protection provisions in each of the states and territories there is no similar protective framework to either identify or notify about elder abuse once the abuse has been suspected or confirmed. Other than recent provisions applicable to the aged care sector through Commonwealth legislative reforms (discussed below), reports of elder abuse would be dealt with by the police as a criminal matter.

The Commonwealth report *Older Persons and the Law*[8] identified the difficulties that an elderly person has in accessing appropriate legal assistance in response to abuse. The report indicated that, apart from the considerable hurdle posed by financial limitations, the problems experienced by elderly people are comprehensive, diverse and require multidisciplinary responses.

The report also recognised that there is a paucity of reliable data on the incidence of elder abuse, thought to be due to an inability or unwillingness of the elderly to report when they are, or have been, the victim of an abusive episode. Elderly people's failure to report abuse was said also to be partly due to their inability to recognise that the abuse, in whatever form, is a legal problem necessitating a legal response. This leads to a failure to seek appropriate legal and other assistance or services.

Even when an allegation of abuse is made, there may be large barriers to carrying out an investigation of the allegation. This is particularly relevant to the aged care sector where a significant proportion of residents are extremely frail and vulnerable. In addition, many aged care residents have multiple and complex health problems including conditions such as severe dementia, stroke and arthritis. These individuals are frequently maintained on polypharmacy regimens including medications that potentially interfere with their cognitive capacity, memory and communication ability. This can create enormous difficulties for health practitioners who may attempt to investigate complaints of elder abuse. While it is not a complete solution, some international jurisdictions have attempted to address this later problem by expediting criminal matters where the witnesses are older,[9] creating statutory exceptions to the rule against hearsay and permitting the elderly person to give evidence in their ordinary surroundings.[10]

Relevant Law

The law applies equally to the elderly as it does to other members of the community – for example, the law of trespass against person (assault, battery and false imprisonment), negligence, and regarding guardianship issues. Notably, elder abuse is also a form of family violence. The legal protections available to people who experience family violence also equally apply to older people. This includes the right to apply for an intervention order to protect someone from further abuse.

The *Aged Care Act 1997* (Cth) also addresses several of the issues surrounding identification and notification of elder abuse in the aged care sector. The Act enables the relevant minister to formulate rules to regulate the care to be provided and the responsibilities owed by aged care providers.

The Aged Care Act requires mandatory reporting of 'reportable assaults' of residents in aged care facilities by 'approved providers', imposing the obligation on the 'approved providers' to report all allegations or incidents of an assault to the police and the Commonwealth Department of Health and Ageing within 24 hours.[11]

Operators of aged care services that receive Australian Government subsidies are also required to ensure staff, volunteers and contractors who are having, or are likely to have, unsupervised contact with residents undergo a national criminal history check.

The Aged Care Act also establishes the Aged Care Complaints Scheme[12] and the offices of the Aged Care Commissioner[13] and Aged Care Pricing Commissioner.[14] The Aged Care Complaints Scheme enables any person to make a complaint about the quality of the care or service provided by an aged care service that is funded or subsidised by the Commonwealth. Complaints are resolved in accordance with complaint guidelines and the *Complaints Principles 2014*. This involves consideration of whether the approved provider is meeting their responsibilities under all principles covered by the Aged Care Act.

Numerous Commonwealth Aged Care Principles guiding service provision have also been made under the Aged Care Act. These include:

- the *Quality of Care Principles 2014*, which specify the Accreditation Standards and the Home Care Common Standards to be met by residential care providers and home care providers respectively, as well as the care and services to be provided
- the *Users Rights Principles 2014*, which set out the responsibilities of approved providers in providing residential or home care services, including describing the required content of agreements between approved providers and care recipients, and the information that approved providers are required to provide to care recipients
- information about fees and charges, which are governed by the *Fees and Payments Principles 2014* and the *Aged Care (Transitional Provisions) Principles 2014*.[15]

There is also a *Charter of Care Recipients' Rights and Responsibilities – Residential Care* and the *Charter of Recipients' Rights and Responsibilities – Home Care*.

Beyond this, most state and territory governments have policies that also attempt to address elder abuse,[16] noting it has been argued that such policies/guidelines still have scope for improvement.[17]

Limitations

While the Aged Care Act imposes on the 'approved provider' the obligation to report abuse, this obligation does not apply to medical practitioners, nursing staff or allied health professionals. Unless the approved provider is made aware of elder abuse, there are no provisions compelling disclosure by any member of the healthcare team. It is also noteworthy that protection for disclosing a reportable assault is predominantly limited to staff members and approved contractors of the aged care provider. As the aged care sector is staffed by both regulated health practitioners and unregulated health workers, there remain issues when the carer is the perpetrator of the abuse.

Disciplinary Responses

There have been few reported cases of elder abuse involving health practitioners. However, in *Gabrielsen v Nurses Board of South Australia*[18] a registered nurse was found to have physically and sexually assaulted an elderly patient who suffered from dementia; and in *HCCC v Gabrielsen*[19] the same nurse was held to have physically abused another elderly patient. In relation to the first case, the court heard how the registered nurse had entered a bathroom where the woman was being bathed by an enrolled nurse and attempted to pick her up by the nipples. He had also, while drying the patient in a passageway, slapped her bottom with a towel wrapped around his hand. The second incident also involved an elderly patient who was suffering from dementia. After the registered nurse had finished drying the patient he threw her roughly onto a chair. The enrolled nurse who witnessed the incidents lodged a complaint with the hospital's director of nursing, who notified the then South Australian Nurses Board.

In reviewing the allegations, both the South Australian Nurses Board and the New South Wales Health Care Complaints Commission found Gabrielsen guilty of unprofessional conduct and professional misconduct. He had demonstrated a level of knowledge and judgment in his practice of nursing that was significantly below the standard reasonably expected of a nurse of an equivalent level of training or experience and he had engaged in improper or unethical conduct related to the practice of nursing. The court held that the nurse's treatment of the first patient amounted to a form of assault of both a sexual and violent nature, and his handling of the second patient, while not as violent, was not only very serious but also unethical and deemed seriously inappropriate conduct on his part. Note, the enrolled nurse who reported the abuse and director of nursing who received the notification of abuse were also themselves subject to a series of 'abusive, disrespectful, discourteous and disparaging letters, faxes and emails' from the registered nurse.[20] The regulatory authority held that the unsatisfactory professional conduct was of a sufficiently serious nature to justify removing the registered nurse's name from the roll.

More recently, in *Nursing and Midwifery Board of Australia v Millikan*,[21] a registered nurse struck a resident in the face and knocked her to the ground after she had repeatedly kicked him. The nurse failed to adequately report the incident. The Health Practitioners Tribunal of South Australia found the nurse guilty of professional misconduct because his conduct fell substantially below the standard reasonably expected of a registered health practitioner of an equivalent level of training and experience.[22]

FURTHER READING

Broomfield L, Holzer PJ. A National Approach for Child Protection: Project Report. Southbank, VIC: Australian Institute of Family Studies; 2008. www.aifs.gov.au/nch/pubs/reports/cdsmac/cdsmac.pdf. Accessed 24 June 2018.

Kaspiew R, Carson R, Rhoades H. Elder Abuse: Understanding Issues, Frameworks and Responses (Research Report No. 35). Southbank, VIC: Australian Institute of Family Studies; 2015.

Leung S, Logiudice D, Schwarz J, et al. Hospital doctors' attitudes toward older people. *Intern Med J*. 2011;41(4):308–14.

United Nations. Convention on the Rights of the Child. Geneva: Office of the High Commissioner for Human Rights; 1989.

ENDNOTES

1. World Health Organization. Fact sheet: Child maltreatment. http://apps.who.int/mediacentre/factsheets/fs150/en/index.html. Accessed 13 March 2019.
2. MacMillan HL, Wathen CN, Barlow J, et al. Interventions to prevent child maltreatment and associated impairment. *Lancet*. 2009;373:250–66; Gilbert R, Widom CS, Browne K, et al. Burden and consequences of child maltreatment in high-income countries. *Lancet*. 2009;373:68–81.
3. World Health Organization, International Society for the Prevention of Child Abuse and Neglect. Preventing child maltreatment: a guide to taking action and generating evidence. Geneva: WHO; 2006.
4. Department of Social Services. National Framework for Protecting Australia's Children 2009–2020. Canberra, ACT: Australian Government; 2009. http://www.dss.gov.au/our-responsibilities/families-and-children/publications-articles/protecting-children-is-everyones-business. Accessed 24 June 2018.
5. *Children's Protection Act 1993* (SA) s 12.
6. *Family Law Act 1975* (Cth) s 67ZA.
7. House of Representatives Standing Committee on Legal and Constitutional Affairs. Older Persons and the Law. Canberra, ACT: Australian Government; 2007. p. 159, 163, 165.
8. Ibid.
9. American Prosecutors Research Institute. *Prosecution of Elder Abuse, Neglect and Exploitation*. Alexandria, VA: APRI; 2003. p. 36, 40–2.
10. *Riverside Nursing Care Pty Ltd v Bishop* [2000] FCA 1054. (For an explanation of the rule against hearsay, see Chapter 15.)
11. *Aged Care Act 1997* (Cth) s 63-1AA.
12. Ibid. s 94A-1(1), (2).
13. Ibid. Div 95A.
14. Ibid. Div 95B.
15. For a detailed discussion of these guidelines and principles see: Kaspiew R, Carson R, Rhoades H. *Elder Abuse: Understanding Issues, Frameworks and Responses* (Research Report No. 35). Melbourne, VIC: Australian Institute of Family Studies; 2015.
16. Australian Capital Territory Government. *ACT Elder Abuse Prevention Program Policy* (2012); New South Wales Government. *Interagency Protocol for Responding to Abuse of Older People* (2007); South Australian Government. *Strategy to Safeguard the Rights of Older South Australians* (2014); Tasmanian Government. *Responding to Elder Abuse: Tasmanian Government Practice Guidelines for Government and Non-government Employees* (2012); Victorian Government. *Elder Abuse Prevention and Response Guidelines for Action* (2012); Alliance for the Prevention of Elder Abuse. *Elder Abuse Protocol: Guidelines for Action* (2013). Queensland's strategy is not publicly available, but note 'Elder abuse' website (https://www.qld.gov.au/seniors/safety-protection/discrimination-abuse/elder-abuse) and the Elder Abuse Prevention Unit (UnitingCare). See further: Chesterman J. Taking control: putting older people at the centre of elder abuse response strategies. *Aust Soc Work*. 2016;69(1):116.
17. Chesterman 2016.
18. *Gabrielsen v Nurses Board of South Australia* [2006] SA SC 199.
19. *HCCC v Gabrielsen* [2008] NSW NMT 2.
20. In light of the conduct of the registered nurse it is relevant to note that the provisions contained in section 96.8 of the Aged Care Act aims to provide protection for reporting reportable assaults.
21. *Nursing and Midwifery Board of Australia v Millikan* [2011] (SAHPT 20).
22. The disciplinary procedure was carried out under the *Health Practitioner Regulation National Law Act 2009* s 196(1)(b)(iii).

REVIEW QUESTIONS AND ACTIVITIES

1. Identify and explain the different types of (a) child abuse and (b) elder abuse.

2. Identify the voluntary and mandatory reporting obligations in your jurisdiction for reporting a child who you reasonably suspect is at risk of harm.

3. With reference to Chapters 4, 6, 7 and above, identify and discuss laws relevant to elder abuse in the context of (a) the regulation of health practitioners, (b) trespass to person, (c) negligence and (d) aged care.

Section 5   LAW AND ETHICS IN ACTION

WORKING WITH LEGAL REPRESENTATIVES

LEARNING OBJECTIVES

Upon completing this chapter you should be able to:

- describe the role of a Justice of the Peace
- identify the requirements of a statutory declaration and describe the legal effect of the document
- identify the functions of a subpoena
- discuss the requirements for evidence in a court of law and the role of professionals giving expert testimony
- describe the concepts of burden of proof and standard of proof
- describe privilege
- identify the effect of an injunction
- discuss the role of health practitioners in forensic pathology
- discuss the features of an alternative dispute resolution mechanism and distinguish this mechanism from the adversarial process.

INTRODUCTION

There are many ways in which health practitioners may become involved in litigation. They may be required to produce documents to a court, testify as a witness, provide expert opinion or appear as a party to proceedings. This chapter provides an overview of the procedural aspects of the litigation process relevant to health practitioners. It also briefly discusses alternative dispute mechanisms to litigation that occurs within an adversarial environment and is not suitable for many healthcare complaints.

LEGAL DOCUMENTS

Statutory Declarations

A statutory declaration (known colloquially as a 'stat dec') is a written statement that allows a person to declare something to be true. A statutory declaration is signed by the person who generated the document and is witnessed by a Justice of the Peace or other designated person. It must expressly state that it is a statutory declaration. Thereby it has the same legal effect as a statement made in court under oath. Proforma statutory declarations can be purchased through legal stationers or newsagencies or templates downloaded from the internet. However, provided the document is identified as a statutory declaration, is dated, signed and witnessed appropriately, there is no necessity to use a set form. A false statement made in a statutory declaration constitutes perjury and is punishable by law.

Affidavits

An affidavit is a statement in documentary form, sworn similarly to a statutory declaration, used in court proceedings. The person swearing as to the truth of the contents of the affidavit is referred to as the 'deponent'. Falsely swearing an affidavit, as with statutory declarations, is punishable by law. In some circumstances a trial may proceed with all of the evidence being given in affidavit form. It is also possible, even though the evidence is in the form of an affidavit, that the deponent is called as a witness. As an example, in a proceeding before a coroner it is possible that the inquest is conducted based on the affidavit evidence provided by the parties. A deponent, though not called to give evidence-in-chief, may be required by the court to attend the trial to be cross-examined on the contents of the affidavit. If cross-examination is not required, then the contents of the affidavit is admitted into evidence standing alone.[1]

JUSTICES OF THE PEACE

The office of Justice of the Peace is a voluntary position in each state and territory legal system. The person occupying such a role performs both judicial and administrative functions as dictated by the relevant legislation in the particular jurisdiction. Generally, the powers of a Justice of the Peace are to:[2]

- witness documents and certify them as true copies
- attest statutory declarations
- supervise the signing of affidavit documents
- certify exhibit markings for affidavits
- take dying declarations
- authorise requests to search premises
- approve applications to seize property
- issue arrest warrants and summonses, at their own discretion, in response to sworn complaints made by citizens
- approve applications for summonses by government department inspectors or by police officers
- compel the attendance of specified persons in court, as either witnesses or as defendants, through issuing a summons
- issue a warrant to remove a person to a place designated under the relevant mental health legislation
- constitute a Magistrates' Court bench (together with another Justice of the Peace), grant bail and order remands and adjournments
- act as an 'independent person' at police questioning of children and at police records of interview of adult accused persons and suspects.

DISCOVERY (DISCLOSURE) AND INSPECTION OF DOCUMENTS

It is often the case that the parties to potential litigation will not have possession of all relevant information when making decisions about whether and how to proceed with their case. The process of discovery (disclosure) of documents requires that a party produce a list of relevant documents that they have in their possession, subject to a claim of privilege.

The rules of discovery, therefore, are designed to provide each of the parties involved in the process of litigation with the opportunity of assessing the case they will be confronted with at the time of the trial. To this end, discovery permits the parties to seek information about the relevant documents in the possession of the opposing party and to submit written questions, referred to as **interrogatories** (discussed more below), to be answered upon oath. In addition, a third party, not being a party to the proceedings, may be required to provide relevant documents for the purpose of inspection.

For example, a patient injured while undergoing care within a healthcare institution may wish to initiate an action against a medical practitioner and the hospital alleging negligence. The patient therefore would require all the documents held by the hospital relating to admission and treatment within the institution. He or she may also want information from the medical practitioner and the hospital related to the specific circumstances surrounding the incident. The patient's legal counsel would seek to identify the facts in issue through the process of discovery of documents and interrogatories. The hospital and the medical practitioner may also require the medical records held by the patient's general practitioner to investigate whether the injuries existed prior to admission. They would accomplish this through serving a notice for non-party disclosure on the general practitioner.

The process of discovery is not only directed to ensuring that all parties to the litigation know the case they are to meet, it is also to ensure that 'the court will have before it all the relevant evidence required to achieve a just outcome'.[3] As stated by Lord Donaldson MR in *Davies v Eli Lilly & Co*:

> *The right [to discovery] is peculiar to the common law jurisdictions. In plain language, litigation in this country is conducted 'cards face up on the table'. Some people from other lands regard this as incomprehensible. 'Why', they ask 'should I be expected to provide my opponent with the means of*

defeating me?' The answer, of course, is that litigation is not a war or even a game. It is designed to do real justice between opposing parties and, if the court does not have all the relevant information, it cannot achieve this object.[4]

INTERROGATORIES

Interrogatories are served on the opposing party where a party does not have knowledge of the facts necessary to advance their case. Their function is to permit a party, through responses to written questions, to prove facts that they otherwise would be unable to establish. The interrogatories must relate to matters that are in issue between the parties or any facts relevant to those matters that are in issue.[5] The expectation is that whoever is required to answer the questions contained in the interrogatories will do so to the best of their knowledge and belief, demonstrating that all proper and reasonable enquiries have been made.

NOTICE OF NON-PARTY DISCLOSURE

Where a health practitioner is served with a notice of non-party disclosure, the aim is to compel all notes or documents generated in relation to the events identified to be produced. The procedural requirements for issuing such a notice will be regulated by the rules of court in the particular jurisdiction.

Such a notice is generally far-reaching in that it requires that the non-party produces all documents in their possession that are identified as relevant to the issue in question. The notice is directed to a person who is not a party to the proceedings. As an example, the legal representative for the defendant will serve notice of non-party disclosure on the plaintiff's doctor to obtain all the medical records of the plaintiff. There are grounds to object on the basis of claiming privilege; however, this objection will not apply to medical records because they have not been prepared for the purpose of the litigation.

There are, however, limitations on the circumstances in which non-party disclosure may be pursued. As an example, the process may not be used:

… when its only purpose is a fishing expedition for documents which may have been in the possession of a person not a party to the action. Documents sought must be shown to be directly relevant to an allegation in issue on the pleadings … and … probably in the possession or control of a non-party. The onus of satisfying these things lies with the party seeking discovery.[6]

SUBPOENAS

When health practitioners are involved in legal proceedings, they may be served with a document known as a subpoena. It is important that the health practitioner has an understanding of the legal effect of the document and their obligations in relation to the requested attendance and production of documentary evidence.

A subpoena is an order that compels a witness to attend court to give evidence of facts of which they have personal knowledge or to produce documents, films, tape recordings or disks. In some jurisdictions the subpoena for production is satisfied if the documents or objects are produced to the court registry before the trial date.[7]

Subpoenas to produce documents are not 'fishing expeditions' and so may be set aside if the party issuing the subpoena cannot show that it was 'on the cards' that the documents sought will assist the party's case.[8] The onus is on the party issuing the subpoena to precisely identify the particular documents required.

Within a healthcare context, where the medical files on a patient may be extensive, a subpoena to produce 'all documents' may be considered as oppressive, resulting in the subpoena being set aside.

Documents produced on subpoena are admitted into evidence in three stages. First, the documents are produced to the court. Second, the court determines whether the parties may inspect the documents before the trial and, finally, if a party attempts to tender the documents as evidence the court will determine whether they are admissible. When original hospital records are subpoenaed, the records are produced to the court registrar before the start of the trial. The records can be perused in the registry by the parties, who are able to obtain copies of all the relevant documents that they may tender in evidence. After the parties have obtained copies, the registrar will return the records to the hospital.

Subpoenas are personally delivered to witnesses or institutional representatives. The subpoena may indicate that a sum of money, referred to as 'conduct money', will be paid to cover the witness's expenses.

Where the subpoena has been served and conduct money tendered, the failure of the witness to appear will usually provide grounds for an adjournment. It is important that the witness understands the effect that failure to appear may have on the trial and the costs incurred by the parties. When subpoenaed to the Magistrates' Court, the subpoena is primarily persuasive in that a witness who fails to attend cannot be charged with contempt. However, District and Supreme Court judges do have the power to enforce appearance.

A subpoena can be served in another state at least 14 days before the date at which the attendance of the witness is required. This limitation on time may be reduced if it is determined as necessary in the interests of justice. However, the time between serving a subpoena and the appearance date must be considered in light of the personal circumstances of the particular witness. Where a witness has a long distance to travel, dependent family members or business commitments, the service of the subpoena should make allowance for these factors so that serious hardship is not experienced in the attempt to comply. Where there is a real possibility of serious hardship, an application may be made to have the subpoena set aside.

Summons

A summons is a document issued by a court declaring that legal proceedings have been begun and requiring a person to attend a court on a specified day to give evidence, respond in writing or produce documents. A person served with a summons to produce documents may object on the grounds that the content is not relevant to the legal proceedings, is classified as legal professional privilege or production would be contrary to state, territory or public interest.

RULES OF EVIDENCE AND THE STANDARDS OF PROOF

The following section is designed to provide an overview of the basic rules of evidence relevant to legal proceedings in which a health practitioner may be involved. The information is in no way to be considered as anything more than providing assistance to health practitioners in understanding the legal process and their role in that process. Where a health practitioner is involved in a legal action, they should at all times seek specific information from their legal representative or the legal representative of the party for whom they are appearing about the rules relevant to the particular jurisdiction. Many health practitioners have access to legal advice through their industrial or professional organisations. As an example, medical protection organisations, the respective unions in each of the jurisdictions and national professional colleges provide legal advice and assistance to their members.

Rules of Evidence

As a broad proposition, the rules of evidence ensure that only the proper and appropriate facts are presented to the court for consideration in the decision-making process. The rules of evidence are derived from judge-made decisions and legislation and, accordingly, each state and territory will have slightly different rules of evidence.

There are laws in relation to evidence that control the kind of facts that can be proven, the amount of evidence that is required, the manner in which such evidence is presented, the individual who must give the evidence and the mechanisms and formality by which the proceedings take place.

Admissible evidence is all the information given directly to the court or tribunal by witnesses or through documents, objects or demonstrations of which the court takes notice because it complies with the rules of evidence. It is the role of the judge to determine if the evidence is relevant and if it is admissible, with the obligation to show its relevance on the party wishing to tender the evidence.

Evidence may be relevant to the facts in issue between the parties; however, it may not be admissible on the grounds that it would unfairly disadvantage the defendant. The judge may also determine that evidence will not be admitted on the basis that its prejudicial value (the extent to which it operates against the defendant) outweighs its probative value (the extent to which admitting the evidence would assist the court in reaching the truth). Even where the evidence is admissible and relevant, the judge may exercise their discretionary power to direct the jury as to the 'weight', or persuasiveness, the testimony is to be accorded.

The Trial Process

During a trial, if there is a judge and a jury, each is responsible for making different determinations. Judges decide on questions of law, ensuring that the rules of evidence are applied and the procedural laws adhered to, and instruct the jury as to what the law is. In a criminal trial the judge determines the sentence when the defendant has been found guilty of the offence. Juries decide on questions of fact and are directed on the law by the judge.

Quite frequently trials will only have a judge hearing the case. When judges sit alone, they perform the roles of both judge and jury.

Parties to a Dispute

The parties to a dispute may be legally represented by someone who is admitted to practise law:

- **Solicitors** are legally qualified to represent and advise clients about matters of law. A solicitor deals directly with the public or corporation and is able to appear before the courts or tribunals in accordance with the relevant state or territory legislation.
- **Barristers** are also legally qualified practitioners who have undertaken additional course work and training and specialise in advocacy work. This may take the form of providing specialised legal advice or representing a client before a court or tribunal. A barrister is instructed, or 'briefed', by the solicitor who is directly in contact with the client. Barristers, in states and territories with a divided profession, are members of the Bar Association in the jurisdiction in which they practise.
- **Lawyer or legal practitioner** are general terms used to describe members of the legal profession and refer to both solicitors and barristers. In some states and territories legislation permits legal practitioners to practise as both a solicitor and a barrister; however, in other jurisdictions there is a divided profession, and a practitioner is restricted to conducting their practice as either a solicitor or a barrister.

Civil Cases

An action is commenced when one party – in a health-care context, usually the patient, client or a relative – serves initiating documents upon another party, being the health practitioner and/or the institution.

In civil cases the pleadings (claims, statements of claim, defences and replies) contain the information that effectively sets down the plaintiff's case. The pleadings contain the facts in issue – as an example, that the medical practitioner owed the patient a duty of care – and not the evidence by which the facts will be proven.

In civil actions, interlocutory steps (proceedings taken during the course of the action) provide the means by which the issues in dispute between the parties are narrowed and focused. This may include requests that the other party provides particulars, the delivery of requested documents, the inspection of documents and the interrogatories and notices to admit facts.

The Standard of Proof and Discharging the Evidential Burden

The standard of proof is the degree to which a court is required to be convinced, by the evidence, of one version of events as opposed to another. In civil actions, the standard of proof is *on the balance of probabilities.* This has been interpreted as meaning 'more probable' than not. In the criminal jurisdiction, the prosecution bears the onus of proving the guilt of the accused *beyond reasonable doubt.* The plaintiff will need to prove their case to satisfy the relevant standard of proof; it is not for the defendant to prove their innocence (although the defendant will raise defences).

SEQUENCE OF THE TRIAL

A health practitioner required to give evidence at a trial will appear in one of the following capacities: as a party to the dispute, as a non-party witness or as an expert witness.

It will assist the health practitioner if, prior to the proceedings, they are familiar with the layout of the court. Having a clear understanding of how to address the court or tribunal, where to sit, where to stand and when to face the court will serve not only to reduce the stress and anxiety of the witness but also will assist the ease with which the evidence may be elicited.

The witness should understand that their response to questions is evidence upon which a court will make a decision and therefore it must be given in a cogent and clear manner. Where the witness does not understand the question, or has not clearly heard what has been asked, it is quite appropriate to have the question repeated or to say that they have not understood.

As a general rule, witnesses remain outside the court until they are called to give their evidence. This frequently results in a proportion of the time being spent outside the court waiting to be called. For many health practitioners, the time away from their employing institution or practice is problematic and arrangements may be made to be called on short notice or to provide evidence over the telephone.

Courts have facilities for telephone evidence to be taken so that the health practitioner doesn't need to leave their place of work. There are detailed procedures in the practice directions in all jurisdictions for telephone evidence, and early arrangements will save much inconvenience. The health practitioner will take an oath or affirm over the phone and then give an examination-in-chief, be cross-examined and re-examined. There are some concerns, based on the fact that the witness is not physically observable in the court, that cross-examination is made more difficult by this mode.

The plaintiff's legal counsel opens the case for the plaintiff with an address, which sets out, in broad terms, what they will attempt to establish through the evidence of the witnesses they will call and documents they will produce.

Before giving evidence to the court or tribunal, witnesses are required to swear an oath on the Bible or to make an affirmation. An affirmation promising to tell the truth is given where the witness is not prepared to swear on a Bible. The purpose of the oath or affirmation is to compel the witness to state that they understand that the evidence must be given honestly or they will be subject to a charge of perjury if the truth is not told.

Examination-In-Chief

The examination-in-chief is conducted by the party who has called the witness. If the health practitioner is appearing for the hospital, the legal counsel representing the hospital will call that person and conduct an examination-in-chief. It is the opportunity to prove the necessary elements of the case and sometimes to disprove the elements of the other side's case. Examination-in-chief may take the form of oral evidence – that is, the testimony given on oath by the witness; written evidence in the form of affidavits and hand-up statements; or exhibits, being audiotapes or videotapes, documents, photographs, physical objects and plans.

At the beginning of the examination-in-chief the witness will be asked to identify themselves and to provide their address and their occupation to the court. If the witness is an expert witness they will be asked to identify and describe their qualifications. If the witness has provided evidence by way of affidavit they will be asked to identify the affidavit as their evidence before giving oral testimony.

During the examination-in-chief witnesses generally cannot be asked leading questions. A leading question is a question that effectively contains the answer and requires only a 'yes' or 'no' answer from the witness. An example of such a question is: 'And you went into the patient's room and adjusted the intravenous line, didn't you?' However, leading questions may be asked of *expert* witnesses during the examination-in-chief, or in relation to facts admitted and not in dispute between the parties (as an example in the foregoing discussion it is not in issue that the health practitioner went into the patient's room). The witness in an examination-in-chief must otherwise be questioned in a manner that allows them to tell their own version of the events; for example, 'Please tell the court what it was you did on entering the patient's room'.

Cross-Examination

The cross-examination of the witness is confined to the evidence elicited in the examination-in-chief or that undermines the credibility of the witness. The aim of cross-examination is to put the case of the examiner to the witness so they have an opportunity to respond to the allegations. In addition, the cross-examiner will attempt to cast doubt on the evidence given in examination-in-chief or contained in the witness's affidavit or statement materials. This is accomplished through testing the accuracy and validity of the testimony, by challenging any inconsistencies and probing for detail.

Re-Examination

The re-examination seeks to clarify and correct any damaging evidence that arose in cross-examination.

The re-examination is therefore restricted to the issues raised in the cross-examination. Leading questions are not permitted during the re-examination.

When the plaintiff's counsel has called all the witnesses they intend to rely on, and tendered all documents into evidence, the plaintiff's counsel closes their case. The defence counsel then opens the defence case. The sequence of obtaining evidence from the witnesses is the same as for the plaintiff. After a witness is called, they will give their examination-in-chief, undergo cross-examination and then be re-examined. The defendant closes the case with the plaintiff having a right of reply.

Where there is a jury trial, the judge will sum up for the jury. The jury at a later point in time will return a verdict to the court.

In a civil trial, if the plaintiff is successful, the judge will make a decision regarding liability as to the amount (quantum) of damages. In a criminal trial it is the role of the judge to determine the sentence once the jury returns a 'guilty' finding.

CATEGORIES OF EVIDENCE

Direct Evidence

Direct evidence is evidence of a fact in issue. The facts in issue are all the facts that a plaintiff in a civil action or the prosecutor in criminal proceedings must prove in order to win the case or, alternatively, those facts that must be proven to establish a defence. In giving direct evidence a witness is testifying that they have perceived with their own senses an occurrence or event of which they have first-hand knowledge. It is distinct from circumstantial and hearsay evidence. A witness stating that they saw the doctor strike the patient is an example of direct evidence.

Circumstantial Evidence

This involves a witness giving evidence of facts that are not in issue but from which a fact in issue may be inferred. The judge or jury must first assume the witness is telling the truth and then infer the connection between the witness statement and the fact in issue. Consider an example where a patient has been found dead in her hospital bed and the postmortem

reveals the cause of death as being an overdose of an intravenous narcotic. Where the witness testifies that he saw the nurse leaving the room with the empty syringe at the time of the death, the court is asked to infer that this fact is connected to the death of the patient.

Best Evidence and Secondary Evidence

The distinction between best evidence (the original document) and secondary evidence (the copy) is not as significant today as it has historically been. The 'best evidence' rule requires that the original document is tendered in preference to the copy.

Perjury

All witnesses must answer the questions asked by legal counsel as truthfully as possible. The failure of the witness to tell the truth will result in a charge of perjury.

Original and Hearsay Evidence

Original evidence is the evidence a witness is able to give about an incident they observed or experienced first-hand.

Hearsay evidence is evidence that is based on second-hand knowledge and is generally inadmissible. The reason underpinning the exclusion of hearsay evidence is that opposing legal counsel cannot conduct a cross-examination on information that has been relayed and interpreted from one person to another. The veracity of the evidence cannot be tested by the court where the witness is simply repeating a story told to them by another. Where a witness is attempting to recount an incident 'second-hand', it is not possible to obtain information about the surrounding circumstances. It is generally, therefore, considered as unreliable and unsuitable to be placed before the court. However, there are exceptions to this rule. One exception is where specific legislative provisions, such as section 92 of the *Evidence Act 1977* (Qld), permit the admission of documentary hearsay evidence in civil proceedings. Such an exception is relevant to health practitioners who, for example, document care in the medical records of patients and later may be unavailable (e.g. due to death, illness, being out of state, unknown whereabouts) to be called as a witness in civil proceedings where medical negligence is alleged.

WITNESSES – PROFESSIONAL EXPERTISE

Expert opinion must be confined to those areas in which the witness has expertise. If the witness attempts to give evidence on matters outside their area of expertise this would be considered as opinion evidence and thereby inadmissible.

Expert Evidence

Expert evidence is received by the court where there is a need for the assistance of a person who possesses a special knowledge, skill or experience in the particular area under consideration. The expert evidence, however, is not admissible as the ultimate determinant of the matter before the court. The underlying proposition is that the subject matter of the opinion provided by the expert witness forms part of a body of knowledge or experience that is outside the range of knowledge and experiences of the court[9] and is sufficiently recognised and organised to be accepted as reliable.[10] Once it is established that the issue is one for which the court would require an expert opinion, the qualification of the expert witness is a matter for the trial judge to determine.[11]

Expert witnesses therefore provide the court with an opinion on an issue that, if presented by a lay witness, would be held in most circumstances to be inadmissible. The role of an expert is to interpret factual information and form an opinion relevant to the issues in the action. As described by Lord President Cooper in *Davie v Edinburgh Magistrates*:

> … *their duty is to furnish the judge or jury with the necessary scientific criteria for testing the accuracy of their conclusions, so as to enable the judge or jury to form their own independent judgment by the application of these criteria to the facts proved in the evidence.*[12]

The obligations of the expert witness to the court are included in the practice directions in some jurisdictions. An expert 'has an overriding duty to assist the court in matters relevant to the expert's area of expertise; is not an advocate for a party; and has a paramount duty to the court and not to the party who retains the expert'.[13]

When an expert opinion is sought, the legal representative will brief the expert with the documents and materials necessary to prepare the opinion. In a medical negligence action, this may include the treatment notes, extracts from the medical records, treating medical reports and all relevant test reports and results. The expert should have a clear understanding of the facts of the case about which the opinion is sought and be provided with a list of assumptions and specific questions relevant to assisting the court to determine the issues in dispute.

In all Australian jurisdictions the parties are required to exchange proofs of expert evidence as a condition of admitting the expert testimony at trial. Legal professional privilege does not prevent the exchange, which is required by the rules of court.[14] However, the rules will determine the extent of the disclosure. From the point of view of the expert witness, it is to be assumed that the report they have written will be available to the other side before the pre-trial conference. This exchange and disclosure is fundamental to the efficiency of the case flow management scheme and highlights the very important issue that the expert has an overriding obligation to the court to be independent.

In a number of jurisdictions court rules and directions permit expert witnesses to consult with one another and produce individual or joint reports identifying the issues upon which they agree, the issues upon which they disagree and the basis for their respective opinions. Section 65 of the *Civil Law (Wrongs) Act 2002* (ACT) provides that in a personal injuries claim for damages the parties may, if they agree, appoint one expert to give evidence; however, if they cannot reach an agreement, the court has the power on its own initiative to appoint an expert. In the case of *Halverson & Ors v Dobler Halverson (by his tutor) v Dobler*[15] the New South Wales Supreme Court took the plaintiff's expert evidence concurrently with the defendant's expert evidence. Through this process the court was not only able to directly question the experts but also to observe and listen to the exchange between the expert witnesses as they considered the relevant issues.

Appearing as a Witness

The following may assist those preparing to appear as a witness:

1. Familiarise yourself with the court environment.
2. Review any relevant documents.
3. Clarify with the legal representative the reason you are appearing to give evidence.
4. Conduct yourself in a calm and organised manner.
5. Speak clearly.
6. Know the facts.
7. If you do not hear or understand a question, seek clarification.
8. Do not estimate unless you are specifically asked to do so.
9. Tell the truth.
10. Expect to be vigorously cross-examined.
11. Be reasonable when answering questions and be seen to be reasonable.
12. Make concessions to your original view only if new facts or more information make it appropriate to do so.
13. Do not use abbreviations.
14. If you are representing the institution and bringing documents or records as a result of a summons the following will apply:
    - You will not need to be sworn in or take an oath.
    - You will be asked your full name and the institution you represent.
    - You will identify your role in the institution and your relationship to the documents.
    - The documents will then be tendered (given to the court).

Privilege

The communication between certain identified parties, or the communication that occurs in specific circumstances, may be referred to as 'privileged'. Examples of where the term 'absolute privilege' attaches may vary between jurisdictions but include:

- communications between solicitors and clients *in the course of litigation* (note: the communication must have taken place with reference to litigation that is *actually taking place* or is *in the contemplation of the client*; attempts to claim this form of privilege over medical records have proven unsuccessful because the documents have not been generated, nor did they come into existence, as part of the litigation process)

- official communication between ministers of the state and the Crown
- communication that takes place in parliament as part of parliamentary proceedings
- statements made during judicial and quasi-judicial proceedings
- communication occurring between parties that is classified as privileged through the relevant legislation. As an example of this type of privilege, see section 20(14) of the *Health Services (Conciliation and Review) Act 1987* (Vic), which states:

Evidence of anything said or admitted during the conciliation process–
(a) is not admissible in proceedings before a court or tribunal; and
(b) cannot be used by the Commissioner as a ground for a exercising power of investigation or inquiry.

In the context of health care, the qualified privilege will protect the communication between employers and employees, including assessments of work performance, written references and reports required as part of the employment. However, the protection is constrained by the requirement that the maker of the statement honestly and on reasonable grounds believed that what they wrote or said was true and necessary for the purpose of their vindication, though in fact it was not so.

Other examples of such privilege in the healthcare context include that it may be used as a defence to an action in defamation – for example, where the health practitioner claims qualified privilege in relation to the disclosure of patient information or in response to requests for information contained in a professional assessment of a colleague.

Privilege may also be used as a justification for refusing, in legal proceedings, to disclose information communicated by the patient to the health practitioner during the patient's period of hospitalisation or treatment.

Other forms of evidentiary privilege include the following:

- *Privilege against self-incrimination*. In all jurisdictions other than South Australia there are legislative provisions that protect the individual from having to disclose information that will incriminate them.

■ *Statements made 'without prejudice'.* The effect of 'without prejudice' correspondence or negotiations is to shield the content from admission in relation to an issue in dispute between the parties in the future. In this way, both sides are able to attempt negotiations in a manner that maximises the possibility of reaching a settlement. In most Australian jurisdictions, 'without prejudice' meetings are a regular part of the disciplinary process. After the notification of a complaint, and before a charge is laid, either the health practitioner or the regulatory authority may initiate a 'without prejudice' meeting that will be attended by the registrant, their union, professional indemnity or legal representative and the representative of the regulatory authority.

■ *Health practitioner and client privilege.* Health practitioners are often in a unique position in relation to the level of trust they engender from patients. This often results in patients and clients disclosing personal information to the health practitioner in the belief that they will not divulge that information at any future time. The dilemma for the health practitioner arises when they are compelled as a witness at trial to answer a question put to them by the legal counsel that will necessitate breaking the confidence. There are obviously personal, professional and ethical issues raised by this situation. Privilege attaches to the communication between health practitioners and their patients in the Australian Capital Territory,[16] New South Wales,[17] Northern Territory,[18] Tasmania[19] and Victoria.[20] Health practitioners not working in these states or territories can be compelled to disclose the content of conversations they have had with their patients.

In Tasmania the *Evidence Act 2001* protects any person who has the possession, custody or control of any record of communication made between a doctor and their patient from being compelled to disclose the content. This legislation is very broad and would appear to include such people as practice managers, secretaries and other health practitioners who may gain access to the information through their employment.

In addition to the foregoing, in New South Wales and Victoria there is limited privilege for sexual assault communications between a person who is working as a health practitioner and the victim of a sexual assault.[21]

Injunctions

An injunction is a legal order to hold or preserve property or the status of a situation until the matter is resolved by a court. Where the order is for a person to refrain from carrying on an activity, it is referred to as a **restrictive injunction**. Alternatively, where the order requires an individual to carry out an action, it is called a **mandatory injunction**. The usual course in an emergency is to apply for an **interim injunction** until the court determines if an order for an **interlocutory injunction** should be made, pending the dispute going to trial. A **perpetual injunction** determines the permanent rights of the parties.

In a healthcare context, an application for an injunction may be sought in response to many circumstances. For example, a patient with anorexia may seek an injunction to compel a health practitioner to stop a particular treatment in the form of forced feeding; relatives of a patient on life support may seek an injunction to halt ventilatory intervention where the medical treatment is thought to be futile; or an injunction may be sought to prevent the disposal of chemical substances allegedly linked to a patient's injury.

Injunctive relief is granted at the discretion of the court. Therefore, the burden lies on the applicant to make a case to exercise the discretion, and this will depend on the type of injunction sought. Where an interim injunction is sought in an emergency, the court will consider the probability of the rights of the applicant being destroyed unless the relief is granted. The mere threat of damage will not, in itself, be sufficient for the court to grant an injunction. The court must be satisfied that the applicant is eligible to apply and that the defendant intends to 'unjustly' harm the applicant if the injunction is not granted.

Forensic Science

The meaning of the term 'forensic' is commonly misinterpreted by many health practitioners. The traditional notion of 'forensic' is associated with death, including homicide. However, the Latin term *forensis* means 'forum', and the word 'forensic' tends to pertain to public debate in courts of law. Hence, any discipline of science that practises within a legal arena is arguably practising forensic science.

'Forensic pathology' is mainly concerned with the scientific investigation of death, as opposed to 'clinical forensic practice', which is concerned with survivors of violent crimes and liability-related trauma.[22] Clinical forensic practice is developing as a recognised component of health care in the United States, Canada and Australia and has been recognised as a respected discipline in public health in the United Kingdom, East Asia and Russia for some decades. Forensic specialists work as clinicians who evaluate survivors of crimes such as rape, domestic violence (including abuse of children, spouses and the elderly), suicide attempts, motor vehicle injuries, occupation-related injuries, medical malpractice and injuries sustained while in institutional care. The process involves the awareness and recognition of unidentified or unrecognised trauma and the collection of evidence from living patients. The role of a forensic clinician includes determining the circumstances associated with the trauma (including the actual causes of the injury), identifying human rights violations and pinpointing unsafe conditions and products. Thus a patient who visits a health practitioner or is admitted to hospital for care with injuries that may be liability-related is considered to be a clinical forensic patient.

There are a number of health-related disciplines that are developing specialty skills and education related to forensic science. For example, in the United States nurses with some education in forensic science have been working in emergency departments and detention centres where, during the course of their nursing, they will identify and care for victims of crime. Knowledge of specific injuries enables precise observation, collection of evidence and documentation. Other health practitioners with specific expertise in this area include pathologists, psychologists, psychiatrists and social workers.

Many health practitioners, despite lack of specialised forensic education, will at some time care for a clinical forensic patient. It is important that they understand their role in the preservation, handling, proper storage and protection of physical evidence. Hospitals and healthcare facilities may have specific policies and procedures as to the correct manner of removing and dealing with evidence. The obligation is on the health practitioner and the institution to be mindful of the importance of the evidence and to preserve it in the most viable form until the appropriate legal authorities assume control.

ALTERNATIVE DISPUTE MECHANISMS IN HEALTH

When a patient or client sustains damage or suffers an adverse event while under the care of a healthcare institution or provider, they may wish to have the issues addressed without resorting to the legal system. A high proportion of negligent conduct never becomes the subject of a claim and, of those that reach the courts, the costs – financial, professional and emotional – are often high for all the parties involved. In response to the increasing numbers of complaints lodged in relation to the care received by healthcare consumers in both the public and private sectors, the national Medicare funding arrangements prescribed the establishment of independent health complaints bodies in every Australian state and territory.

In all jurisdictions, alternative dispute mechanisms have been created as a means by which consumers can have their complaints answered and resolved. And, with the exception of New South Wales, conciliation is the predominant mode of complaints resolution in all states and territories.

FURTHER READING

Cairns BC. *Australian Civil Procedure*. 9th ed. Sydney, NSW: Thomson Reuters; 2011.

Faunce T. Carney v Newton: expert evidence about the standard of clinical notes. *J Law Med*. 2007;15:360.

Freckelton I, Selby H. *Expert Evidence: Law, Practice, Procedure and Advocacy*. 4th ed. Sydney, NSW: Lawbook Co; 2009.

Ligertwood ALC, Edmond G. *Australian Evidence: A Principled Approach to the Common Law and Uniform Acts*. Sydney, NSW: LexisNexis Butterworths; 2010.

ENDNOTES

1. ACT: O 40 r 15; FCR: O 14 r 19; NSW: Pt 38 r 9: NT: r 40.04; Qld: r 439; SA: r 83.12; Tas: r 463; Vic: r 40.04; WA: O 36 r 2.
2. Note, the specific duties of a Justice of the Peace may vary between the states and territories.
3. Vickery P. Managing the paper: taming the Leviathan. *J Judic Admin*. 2012;22:51–61.
4. *Davies v Eli Lilly & Co* (1987) 1 WLR 428; 1 ALL ER 801 at 804.
5. *Davis v BO's Plant Hire Pty Ltd (in liq)* (1997) 1 Qd R 481.
6. *Uthmann v Ipswich City Council* (1998) 1 Qd R 435.

7. *Service and Execution of Process Act 1992* (Cth) s 34; Practice Direction No 3 of 1980 (Qld).

8. See, for example, *Attorney-General (NSW) v Stuart* (1994) 34 NSWLR 667.

9. *Clark v Ryan* (1960) 103 CLR 486.

10. *Fisher v Brown* (1968) SASR 65; Freckelton I, Selby H. *Expert Evidence*. Sydney, NSW: Law Book Co; 1998. para 1–132.

11. *R v Parenzee* [2007] SASC; *Milirrpum v Nabalco Pty Ltd* (1971) 17 FLR 141 at 160 (NT Sup Ct) per Blackburn J.

12. *Davie v Edinburgh Magistrates* (1953) SC 34 at 40.

13. Cairns BC. *Australian Civil Procedure*. 4th ed. Sydney, NSW: LBC Information Services; 1996.

14. *Trebilcock v Nominal Defendant* (1991) 58 SASR 213.

15. *Halverson & Ors v Dobler Halverson (by his tutor) v Dobler* [2006] NSWSC 1307.

16. *Evidence Act 2011* (ACT) Div 3.10.1A.

17. *Evidence Act 1995* (NSW) Pt 3.10 Div 1A.

18. *Evidence Act* (NT) s 12.

19. *Evidence Act 2001* (Tas) s 127A.

20. *Evidence Act 2008* (Vic) Pt 3.10 Div 1A.

21. *Criminal Procedure Act 1986* (NSW) Ch 6, Pt 5 Div 2; *Evidence Act 1995* (NSW) s 126H; *Evidence (Miscellaneous Provisions) Act 1958* (Vic) Pt II Div 2A.

22. Hammer RM, Moynihan B, Pagliaro EM. *Forensic Nursing: A Handbook for Practice*. 2nd ed. Burlington, MA: Jones and Bartlett Learning; 2013, p. 6.

REVIEW QUESTIONS AND ACTIVITIES

1. What are the types of subpoenas and what may a health practitioner be compelled to do in response to being served with a subpoena?

2. What is a statutory declaration?

3. Describe the difference between giving evidence in examination-in-chief and being cross-examined.

4. What is 'hearsay evidence' and why is it excluded from adversarial proceedings?

5. As a health practitioner what is your role as an expert witness?

6. You are required to participate in a 'without prejudice conference'. What is the purpose of such a meeting between the parties to a legal action? What is the status of information disclosed during such a meeting?

18

CASE STUDIES: GUIDED APPLICATION OF LEGAL AND ETHICAL PRINCIPLES

LEARNING OBJECTIVES

Upon completion of this chapter you should be able to:

- discuss a variety of case scenarios that may raise ethical and/or legal issues
- reflect upon the application of ethical or legal principles to such case scenarios
- demonstrate and apply a reasoned approach to resolving ethical and legal dilemmas.

INTRODUCTION

In this chapter readers will find case studies and guided answers written by experts from the following disciplines: medicine, midwifery, nursing, paramedicine, pharmacy, physiotherapy, podiatry and speech pathology. Some cases focus on ethical issues, others on legal issues, and others on both ethical and legal issues. The case studies are intended to link back to the discussion in the previous chapters of this book and to provide practice area examples of issues that may be faced in a variety of healthcare settings.

Readers are encouraged to read, reflect upon and discuss the ethical and/or legal issues raised by the case studies and how one may approach the respective issue(s) before reading the guided answer provided. In doing so, it may be helpful to refer to the ethical decision-making process outlined in Chapter 3 as a broad framework to approaching the respective case studies. This may include the following:

- Identify what the ethical/legal issue is (or issues are).

- Identify the personal reaction to the case.
- Gather any relevant facts regarding the situation.
- Identify the values at stake in the scenario.
- Identify the options available in the case.
- Consider what should be done and relevant justifications for doing so (i.e. why).
- Consider if the problem could have been prevented.

Readers are also encouraged to: (1) refer back to discussion in relevant chapters of this book to consider the relevant law as it may be applied to the respective cases; (2) discuss further the applicability of specific ethical guidelines or codes of practice relevant to the area of practice being discussed; and (3) use the case studies as a 'springboard' to further discussion that moves beyond the text and the ethical and legal concepts herein.

When constructing a response to the case study, readers may want to contemplate what they would do, reflecting and incorporating their own experiences to inform the exercise, noting *there is no one right answer*.

Readers may wish to consider all the case studies, focus on a specific practice area, or consider a variety of cases from different practice areas. Note, while cases are presented in the context of specific practice areas, the issues raised in one area (e.g. good record keeping, elder abuse, child abuse, mandatory reporting) are likely to be relevant to other practice areas also. The reader may therefore also wish to consider case studies from other practice contexts.

In addition to the above, readers may find benefit in having guided answers written by the contributors that reflect upon considerations relevant to the case studies and their particular practice areas. Guided answers following the scenarios therefore offer the knowledge, experience and insight of the respective contributors regarding the ethical and legal issues raised and relevant considerations to the practice area being discussed (e.g. in relation to the law and/or specific elements of a relevant code, ethical guidelines or other relevant policy). They follow the ethical decision-making process outlined in Chapter 3 and noted above; however, they also demonstrate that the process should not be applied mechanically. Therefore, differences in focus and approach may be seen throughout. The guided answers nevertheless move from identifying relevant issues to discussing initial 'gut' reactions, to engaging with a reasoned consideration of challenging ethical, legal and professional issues, linking back to material throughout the book to enable readers to further reflect on how one might approach such scenarios.

CASE STUDIES

Medicine

(Contributor: Dominique Martin)

CASE 1: MENTAL HEALTH AND INVOLUNTARY TREATMENT

Trent is a 27-year-old man who is brought to the emergency department of a rural hospital late one night by the police. The police explain that they were called to Trent's house after neighbours overheard him shouting that he was going to kill himself. Trent appears unhappy and withdrawn. Initially, he refuses to speak to the medical and nursing staff about his health. He announces that he was intoxicated and upset about a relationship breakup but is now feeling calmer and would like to go home. He is breathalysed and found to have a blood alcohol concentration of 0.06% – just over the upper limit acceptable for driving. The doctor speaks with him and determines that Trent is depressed but not mentally disordered. Although Trent insists he 'didn't mean' what he said earlier about killing himself, the doctor fears that he may be concealing suicidal ideation. Trent promises he will go home and go to bed, explaining that he has to be at work the following morning. But the doctor asks him to stay the night in the emergency department for observation and a further review by the psychiatrist in the morning. Trent refuses and announces that he will go home.

What Are the Legal Issues That Arise From This Case?

There may be legal issues regarding keeping a person against their will or whether this would be acceptable pursuant to an 'involuntary' admission to prevent Trent from harming himself or others (see Chapter 15).

What Are the Ethical Issues That Arise From This Case?

- Efforts to prevent harm by keeping Trent in hospital until healthcare staff are confident he will be safe may conflict with duties to respect Trent's autonomy.
- If Trent is forced to remain at the hospital this may conversely cause harm to him.

What Could Be the Personal Reaction to This Case?

As a healthcare worker, making risk evaluations such as the one that the doctor faces in this case can provoke a lot of anxiety. People may be fearful of allowing Trent to go home in case he harms himself. However, keeping him at the hospital against his will is a violation of his right to make decisions for himself, if he is competent to do so. Although the probability of harm occurring may be low, if the severity of the potential risk is significant – in this case, life-threatening – people may wish to 'err on the side of caution', even if doing so entails restricting someone's freedom.

What Facts May Be Relevant Regarding This Situation?

Factors that may influence the assessment of Trent's risk of self-harm include his past medical and psychosocial history (e.g. whether he has a history of self-harm) and whether he has access to things that might be used to cause serious harm to himself such as a gun or medication.

Aspects of his current medical and psychological assessment are also relevant because they might influence the doctor's confidence in their assessment of Trent's current state of mind and ability to predict his likely behaviour, and whether a more expert assessment can be arranged earlier than the morning.

Having an alternative management plan that would protect against the risk of harm while respecting Trent's wish to leave hospital is also relevant – for example, whether there is a relative or friend who can provide support for Trent at their home or at his overnight.

What Values May Be at Stake?

- Autonomy, liberty/freedom, respect, dignity
- Care, beneficence
- Honesty, trust

What Are the Options in This Case?

- Trent may be held at the hospital involuntarily overnight pending further assessment.
- Consult further with Trent to determine if he will agree to stay voluntarily for further assessment in the morning.
- Discharge him home alone.
- Discharge him with an accompanying relative or friend if available.
- Conduct further assessment in hospital overnight.

What Should Have Occurred in This Case?

Determine the option that will best provide care for Trent. In some jurisdictions this may involve a temporary period of involuntary care to protect Trent from the threat of self-harm pending further assessment of his mental wellbeing.

Could the Problem Have Been Prevented?

It is often difficult to prevent the dilemma inherent in situations such as this in which a person poses a risk to themselves and refuses treatment. Respectful treatment of people in such cases, including providing explanations of the reasons for asking Trent to stay overnight, may lead to greater acceptance of care and avoid conflict or involuntary admission.

CASE 2: MANDATORY REPORTING

Candice is a junior surgical registrar in New South Wales at the beginning of her training to become a surgeon. After three weeks on the colorectal surgical ward she notices that one of the consultants, Dr Mitchell, regularly smells of alcohol during evening ward rounds. Candice asks one of the more senior registrars about this and is told that Dr Mitchell often has a 'nip of whiskey' in his office at the end of the day to celebrate the successful completion of difficult operations. Candice observes no evidence that Dr Mitchell is impaired when performing evening ward rounds, nor does his performance seem impaired when a late evening surgery is unexpectedly required.

What Are the Legal/Ethical Issues That Arise From This Case?

This case raises concerns about Dr Mitchell's professional conduct and the appropriate response to these by the junior doctor, Candice. At law the question is whether Candice has a legal obligation to report Dr Mitchell in accordance with the mandatory reporting duties outlined in the *Health Practitioner Regulation National Law Act* (see Chapter 4).

Ethically, Candice may have concerns about reporting Dr Mitchell – for example, if she is uncertain whether he is in fact intoxicated at work or whether intoxication at work necessarily meets the standard for 'notifiable conduct'. Reporting him if his behaviour is not inappropriate could cause harm to him, to patients and other staff – for example, if he is distressed or suspended temporarily from work. However, failure to report Dr Mitchell may result in harm to patients if he is not performing his work safely and competently.

Candice may also be concerned about the potential impact on her career or position if it is known that she reported him.

What Could Be the Personal Reaction to This Case?

The possibility that a surgeon may be practising while intoxicated by alcohol might cause disgust or horror. You might wonder how it is possible that no one has reported Dr Mitchell before if his behaviour is well known. You may be familiar with real-world examples like this and the factors that sometimes influence decisions about reporting in such cases.

What Values May Be at Stake?

- Prevention of harm ('nonmaleficence')
- Care, beneficence
- Respect for patients
- Trust, integrity, professionalism

What Are the Options in This Case?

- Approach Dr Mitchell to discuss her concerns.
- Approach another senior colleague for advice or to clarify the situation.
- Say nothing.
- Report concerns to hospital management and/or the Australian Health Practitioner Regulation Agency (AHPRA).

What Should Have Occurred in This Case?

As a medical practitioner, Candice has a legal obligation to report Dr Mitchell if she has 'formed a reasonable belief' that he has practised 'while intoxicated by alcohol'. Reporting Dr Mitchell is ethically appropriate given Candice's duty to prevent harm.

Could the Problem Have Been Prevented?

Continual training and education of health practitioners regarding appropriate behaviour at work is required. So too are counselling and support services for practitioners who have drug or alcohol problems. However, this does not guarantee that such ethical issues will not arise. It is therefore important to also have mandatory reporting requirements and procedures in place to deal with such issues when they do arise.

CASE 3: DEATH AND ORGAN DONATION

Jonathan is a single, 23-year-old man who lives with his parents and younger sister in Melbourne, Victoria. He suffers a devastating brain injury as a result of a motorcycle accident. Jonathan is admitted to hospital for neurosurgical intervention and is intubated and mechanically ventilated because he cannot breathe for himself. After three days of treatment in the intensive care unit his condition deteriorates and he is declared dead according to neurological criteria. His heart continues to beat, and a ventilator maintains oxygenation of his organs and tissues. Jonathan is registered on the Australian organ and tissue donor registry, and the donation coordinator at the hospital approaches his family to discuss the possibility of Jonathan becoming an organ and tissue donor. Jonathan's father and sister are happy for donation to proceed and agree that this is what he would have wanted. However, his mother declares, 'I just want the machines to be unhooked so I can hold him while he dies and let him go in peace. We want to take his body home and bury him. I don't want anyone to cut him up – he's suffered enough.' Although Jonathan's father and sister are unhappy, they accept his mother's decision to refuse donation.

What Are the Legal Issues That Arise From This Case?

It is important to understand: the law regarding the circumstances under which organs may be removed and donated; the importance of consent in removing human tissue and organs; and the role of family/next of kin in decision making (see Chapter 13).

What Are the Ethical Issues That Arise From This Case?

Respecting Jonathan's decision to become an organ donor after death in this case will conflict with respecting his mother's decision (supported by the family) to refuse.

Overriding Jonathan's decision to donate in favour of his mother's wish may cause harm to his family in the longer term if his father and sister – or even mother – have regrets about not respecting his wish. His family will also miss the benefits that many families experience when their loved one becomes a donor, including a sense of comfort knowing that despite their loss, other lives have been saved and improved through the benefits of organ transplantation. However, overriding his mother's decision may also cause harm to his family through acute distress and anxiety and also to the community if publicity about the case and his mother's reaction fosters distrust or negative attitudes towards organ donation in others.

The case also raises issues relating to the rights of people to make binding decisions about the treatment of their body after their death, including decisions about removing organs for transplantation.

What Could Be the Personal Reaction to This Case?

Many people may feel that it is unfair or disrespectful of Jonathan's mother to override his decision and may be concerned that allowing his mother to do so may prevent people from receiving lifesaving organ transplants.

On the other hand, others may appreciate the difficulty of the situation for Jonathan's family. The tragic loss of his life and the distress that his family may have experienced in witnessing the often highly invasive treatments he has undergone in the preceding few days may make further decision making at this time an additional emotional burden.

What Facts May Be Relevant Regarding This Situation?

It will be important to check that his mother understands the process for organ donation if this were to proceed, as well as the potential risks and benefits of donation for the family and community, to ensure she makes a decision that is well informed and likely to be sustained, so as to avoid later regret.

It will also be important to check that the family has had adequate time to reflect on the information about donation and Jonathan's status as a 'registered donor'.

What Values May Be at Stake?

- Compassion, care, beneficence
- Prevention of harm
- Respect, dignity, autonomy
- Trust
- The public good

What Are the Options in This Case?

The health practitioners may allow more time for decision making and to provide additional supports to the family. The health practitioners may otherwise respect the family's decision not to proceed with organ donation.

What Should Have Occurred in This Case?

In Australia, Jonathan's status on the donor registry does not have legal authority. Removing his organs against the wishes of his next of kin may have legal repercussions and could exacerbate grief and distress within his family. After supporting his family to make a decision, this should be respected. Ensure that his family has access to appropriate care such as grief counselling.

Could the Problem Have Been Prevented?

In most cases in Australia families respect the wish of their loved one to be a donor when they know this is what they would have wanted. It is possible that if Jonathan had spoken more with his mother about his wish to be a donor she may have been more comfortable respecting his decision at the time of his death.

Midwifery
(Contributor: Sally-Ann de-Vitry Smith)

CASE 1: TESTIMONIALS AND CONFIDENTIALITY

Alicia, a homebirth midwife, used her mobile phone to take a photo of a mother she cared for named Jackie and her baby immediately after the birth. Alicia requested verbal permission to take the photo and later posted it on her midwifery Facebook page. Jackie did not provide written consent for the photo to be used. Jackie was extremely happy with her homebirth and posted a testimonial on Alicia's Facebook page saying Alicia's care was 'beyond amazing' and that she was a fantastic midwife. In her post Jackie included a link to an anti-vaccination article and indicated Alicia had supported her choice not to vaccinate her baby.

What Are the Legal/Ethical Issues That Arise From This Case?

The case raises a number of issues that can be identified as both legal and ethical:

- breach of privacy
- patient confidentiality
- permission to take and use photos of a client
- use of client testimonials
- promotion of anti-vaccination materials.

What Could Be the Personal Reaction to This Case?

A 'gut reaction' regarding Alicia's request and verbal permission to take a photo may initially question what the issues raised are, and whether they are serious. That is, in today's world, posting on social media is common, and the practice has blurred the boundary between public and private spheres. Does it seem reasonable to use a photo you have been given verbal permission to take? Does a midwifery client have the right to hold anti-vaccination beliefs and share them publicly? If a client finds a midwife's care is exceptional, should she be able to let other women know?

What Facts May Be Relevant Regarding This Situation?

A personal photo of a client was taken by the midwife with verbal permission. However, the midwife posted the photo on her Facebook page without consent from the client. The client posted a testimonial on the midwife's Facebook page and included a link to anti-vaccination materials.

What Values May Be at Stake?

- Respect for confidentiality and privacy
- The ethical use of personal images
- Preventing the promotion of misleading or deceptive materials
- Using client testimonials for self-promotion

What Are the Options in This Case?

- Laws pertaining to confidentiality and privacy should be considered. When there has been a breach of privacy or confidentiality a remedy may be available to the patient that requires rectifying the breach and/or may lead to compensation (see Chapter 5).

- Photos must be used in accordance with the consent provided, and unauthorised images of clients must not be posted in any medium without consent because this is considered a breach of the client's privacy and confidentiality. The images of the client (Jackie) and her newborn must be removed from the Facebook page.

- Midwives providing or distributing anti-vaccination information on social media may be in breach of professional obligations. The Nursing and Midwifery Board of Australia (NMBA) may impose conditions or restrictions on their registration. 'Any published anti-vaccination material and/or advice which is false, misleading or deceptive which is being distributed by a Midwife (including via social media) may also constitute a summary offence under the National Law and could result in prosecution by AHPRA'.[1] The midwife must immediately remove the anti-vaccination link from her Facebook page.

- AHPRA governs the use of testimonials in the *Guidelines for Advertising Regulated Health Services*. Section 133 of the National Law states: 'A person must not advertise a regulated health service, or a business that provides a regulated health service, in a way that uses testimonials or purported testimonials about the service or business'. The ban on testimonial use means testimonials cannot be used on personal Facebook pages, in print or on radio, television, websites or personal or work-related social media accounts including Facebook, LinkedIn and Twitter. The ban includes clients posting comments about a midwife on their business website. Of note:

  - Midwives are accountable for social media content and comments on their accounts, even if they did not post the information.
  - Midwives should remove any testimonials posted on their social media.

  - Testimonials used to advertise a midwife's service through social media may contravene the National Law (see Chapter 4).
  - Midwives are not responsible for removing unsolicited testimonials published on a website or in social media they have no control over.[2]
  - Midwives should not encourage patients to leave testimonials on their social media.

Could the Problem Have Been Prevented?

The midwife should understand the expectations of midwives regarding vaccination advice. Midwives are expected to use the best available evidence when providing health information to the public. The *Australian National Immunisation Handbook* provides evidence-based guidelines supporting the safe and effective use of vaccines. According to the NMBA, any anti-vaccination material distributed by a midwife – including on social media – may constitute a summary offence and could result in prosecution.[3]

To prevent the problems occurring, the midwife could have discussed her professional obligations regarding social media with the client, ensuring the client understood it was not appropriate to post testimonials or information on the midwife's social media platform. It is in the best interest of midwives to:

- comply with the National Law, *Midwifery Code of Ethics*, *Midwifery Code of Conduct* and the *Guidelines for Advertising Regulated Health Services*
- comply with ethical and legal obligations concerning patient confidentiality and privacy
- consider online information as 'permanent and searchable'[4]
- show professionalism online
- stay informed about the policies and guidelines for social media and review the AHPRA *Registered Health Practitioners: Social Media Policy*.[5]

CASE 2: CARE OUTSIDE THE GUIDELINES

Molika is 39 years old, pregnant with her second baby and has chronic hypertension. Her previous pregnancy resulted in an emergency caesarean for obstructed labour. Molika's baby boy, Rhys, weighed 4,140 grams and is now 18 months old. Molika's previous birth experience was very traumatic and she is terrified of having another operative hospital birth. She has requested a homebirth with a publicly funded homebirth service. Katarina is the midwife taking Molika's history and has told Molika her risk factors may preclude a homebirth. On hearing this news Molika becomes distressed and teary and says she refuses to consider a hospital birth.

What Are the Ethical/Legal Issues That Arise From This Case?

Molika has a legal right to make decisions regarding her care following a discussion about the risks and benefits of any aspects of care. (See Chapter 7 discussion regarding consent.) However, the midwife has a duty of care towards Molika and must meet reasonable standards of practice (see Chapter 6). Molika has risk factors that would normally preclude a homebirth. According to the *National Midwifery Guidelines for Consultation and Referral*,[6] she should be referred to a medical practitioner.

What Could Be the Personal Reaction to This Case?

Midwives follow informed choice principles and respect the woman's right to make decisions regarding her care. Molika is upset and this is difficult for the midwife, who wishes to respect her choices but must also follow the policies of the service she is employed by and national guidelines.

What Facts May Be Relevant Regarding This Situation?

Molika has a history of caesarean section and has chronic hypertension. Midwifery care during pregnancy and labour is governed by the *National Midwifery Guidelines for Consultation and Referral*,[7] the *Code of Conduct for Midwives*,[8] the *Midwife Standards for Practice*[9] and the *Code of Ethics for Midwives*.[10] According to the *National Midwifery Guidelines for Consultation and Referral* this scenario falls under level B for caesarean section history and level C for chronic hypertension. Level C requires referral to a medical practitioner for secondary or tertiary care.

What Values May Be at Stake?

Midwives are guardians of normal birth. They consider birth a normal physiological process and wish to work with women to provide the care they desire and respect their right to autonomy. Midwives must also consider what is the safest option for women and their babies.

What Are the Options in This Case?

Molika may choose to follow the recommendation to accept a referral or she may reject the care pathway recommended in the guidelines and choose care the midwife considers outside their scope of practice and ability to manage safely.

If Molika chooses care outside the recommendations provided in the guidelines, the midwife must attempt to discuss the risks and benefits of her decision and explore available options and possible resolutions that meet Molika's needs, expected standards of care at law and the midwifery professional standards.

Molika's concerns, the advice and information provided and her decision should be fully and carefully documented (see Chapters 5 and 7). After this discussion, the midwife would outline the course of action in compliance with the law and midwifery standards of practice.

If Molika chooses not to follow recommended advice, then Katarina, as the midwife, should follow the *National Midwifery Guidelines for Consultation and Referral*:

1. **Advise** Molika of the recommended guideline including the underpinning reasoning and evidence without understating or overstating the risk.
2. **Support** Molika to access relevant, high-quality, unbiased evidence-based information.
3. **Consult** by seeking advice from a midwife and/or medical practitioner.

Molika has the right to accept or reject the midwife's advice.

During consultation with another midwife or a medical practitioner, Katarina will identify the next steps and the safest and most ethical actions. Katarina may also recommend Molika consults with other professionals to gain information to assist her decision-making process. The remaining steps Katarina should follow are:

4. **Share** the advice from the consultation with Molika and ask her to share the advice she was given.

5. **Document** the advice, process and outcomes of this decision and record relevant details. The Australian College of Midwives recommends using the *record of understanding* provided in Appendix B.

6. **Provide** a reasonable period of time for Molika to review the information and advice she was given. Then discuss and document Molika's decision.

After completing steps 1–6, Molika may decide to select actions outside the guidelines and midwifery standards. In this circumstance Katarina may decide if she will continue or discontinue Molika's care.

In making this decision, Katarina must be informed by her ethical judgement, scope of practice, ability to justify her decision making to a reasonable body of peers and her midwifery support network.[11]

The midwife's wellbeing and the impact on the woman need to be considered. Continuing midwifery care in any form does not mean the midwife endorses the woman's decision to follow a course of action that increases the risk of harm to her or her baby; this should be clearly outlined. If Katerina decides to continue care, she must:

- continue to inform the woman about changes in indications, health and wellbeing for her and/or her baby
- continue to make recommendations for safe care consistent with the guidelines and any relevant broader evidence base
- engage other caregivers who may have become involved in providing advice or care (e.g. obstetricians, general practitioners, hospital-based midwives and/or other midwives)
- plan for an emergency, including those that may be outside the midwife's scope of practice or competence
- document all discussions and decisions.[12]

If Katerina decides to discontinue care, she must:

(a) as soon as possible, clearly communicate her inability to continue to provide care and the reasons why

(b) provide written advice confirming that midwifery care is being discontinued. A specific date should be given for the cessation of care. The date should give the woman a reasonable length of time to

find another caregiver. If the woman is unable to arrange alternative care, the midwife should make a reasonable attempt to find a registered maternity care provider who is willing to see the woman and provide care

(c) send a written referral to the registered maternity care provider identified in (b) above, confirming the date on which the midwife will discontinue midwifery care of the woman. In the event that no registered maternity care provider has been identified, seek the woman's consent to send a written referral to the nearest appropriate public maternity service

(d) retain a copy of the correspondence stipulated in (b) and (c) above.[13]

If appropriate, the midwife's insurer should be notified of changes in circumstances related to the woman's care.

Could the Problem Have Been Prevented?

It may not be possible to prevent this ethical challenge. It is the midwife's responsibility prior to commencing care of clients to explain her scope of practice, the boundaries of midwifery care and the function of the *National Midwifery Guidelines for Consultation and Referral*. It would be beneficial for Katarina to read and become familiar with the Australian College of Midwives' position statement about caring for women who make choices outside professional advice.[14]

CASE 3: REFUSAL OF TREATMENT

Connie was diagnosed with bipolar disorder as a teenager. She had a severe episode of disturbed mood after discontinuing her medication when her pregnancy was diagnosed and has been prescribed pharmacological treatment for her bipolar disorder by her treating psychiatrist. At her antenatal appointment with her midwife, Connie indicates she is not taking the medication prescribed to treat her bipolar disorder because she is concerned about how it will affect her baby. Connie's psychiatrist believes she is taking the medication.

What Are the Legal/Ethical Issues That Arise From This Case?

Connie is not taking medication prescribed to control her bipolar disorder because she is concerned about the effect on the fetus. From an ethical perspective she has a right to personal autonomy. However, her psychiatrist does not know that Connie is not taking her medication, and there may be risk to Connie and her fetus. Does the midwife have an ethical or legal obligation to let the psychiatrist know that Connie is not taking her medication? What is the midwife's duty of care? Is patient privacy and confidentiality relevant? Is Connie competent to refuse treatment? (See Chapters 5, 6 and 7.)

What Could Be the Personal Reaction to This Case?

Midwives are trained to respect a woman's right to make decisions regarding her care. However, they may be challenged if the mother's choices are not perceived as in the best interests of their fetus or if the best option is not easy to determine.

What Facts May Be Relevant Regarding This Situation?

Connie has been prescribed a medication to treat bipolar disorder but is not taking the medication. Connie's psychiatrist is not aware of this decision. Connie tells her midwife she is not taking the medication.

As a person with mental illness, Connie has the right to personal integrity, autonomy and the right to choose or refuse treatment. Medication administration is restricted to therapeutic purposes and requires informed consent.

Connie's capacity and competence to make decisions regarding her care need to be determined. If Connie's cognitive function is normal, her wishes should be respected. The rights of Connie's unborn fetus are not present in law until the infant is born.

What Values May Be at Stake?

- Advocacy: midwives act as advocates for women and support ethical principles including informed consent where a woman has a comprehensive understanding of the implications of treatment, both positive and negative, and can make her own decision based on accurate information.[15]
- Autonomy: midwives respect women's right to make decisions about their care including to choose or refuse treatment and to accept responsibility for the outcome of their choice.

- Beneficence: midwives act in the best interests of the women under their care.
- Non-maleficence: midwives act to avoid harm to the women under their care.
- Respect: midwives understand women have the right to be treated with dignity, truthfulness and honesty.

What Are the Options in This Case?

The midwife can discuss options with Connie including the importance of notifying her psychiatrist that she is not taking the medication prescribed to control her bipolar disorder. With Connie's consent, a consultation could be organised with her psychiatrist. At this consultation Connie would be able to obtain information on the risks and benefits of taking her medication.

If Connie has the capacity and competence to make an informed decision regarding her treatment, then her decision should be respected. Connie needs to be informed about how to take preventative action such as avoiding sleep deprivation. Connie and her partner need to understand how to monitor her condition and the actions to take if her condition deteriorates.

It is important that Connie understands the risk of relapse is higher postpartum, particularly in the first month. If an acute relapse occurs postpartum and places mother and baby at serious risk, involuntary admission may be necessary.[16]

Could the Problem Have Been Prevented?

Ideally, management of Connie's bipolar disorder would have been discussed preconception and covered preventing relapses through monitoring moods, identifying triggers, being aware of early warning signs, psychoeducation, psychological therapy and medication adherence.[17]

Early management of Connie's bipolar disorder would ensure she was aware of the increased risk of relapse with abrupt discontinuation of some pharmacological treatments as well as the risks and benefits of pharmacological treatments. Although the fetal effects of medications for bipolar disorder are not easy to quantify, Connie should have been given up-to-date evidence-based information so she could make informed decisions.

Close liaison between Connie's maternity care providers and specialist psychiatric care is required for optimum care.[18]

Midwifery care is provided through professional relationships and respectful partnerships with women.[19] Midwives must objectively resolve ethical dilemmas, putting the interests of women and their families first, with respect for their decision autonomy and rights to self-determination. Many situations are complex and challenging, yet midwives must continue to provide objective and compassionate care regardless of their own viewpoint and opinion.

CASE 4: CONSENT TO TREATMENT OF A MINOR

Lillian is 15 years old and 18 weeks' pregnant. Lillian has presented to a midwifery-led antenatal clinic for pregnancy care. The midwife has provided information about the 20-week fetal ultrasound. Lillian says she wants to have the ultrasound and wishes to know the gender of her infant. Lillian's mother indicates she refuses to consent for Lillian to have the ultrasound because she is concerned it may be dangerous for the fetus.

What Are the Legal/Ethical Issues That Arise From This Case?

Lillian is a minor and wishes to have a mid-trimester ultrasound; however, her mother is her legal guardian and refuses to provide consent. It must be determined whether the wishes of Lillian (minor) or her legal guardian (mother) should be followed. (See Chapter 7 regarding consent.)

What Could Be the Personal Reaction to This Case?

Although Lillian is a minor, she also has a right to personal autonomy and for her wishes to be respected if they do not place her at risk of harm.

What Facts May Be Relevant Regarding This Situation?

In Australia a person is deemed to become an adult at 18 years of age and they can provide consent for their own medical treatment. When a person is under the age of 18 years, consent is generally provided by parents or legal guardians. However, in some circumstances minors can provide consent to their own medical treatment. The ability of an adolescent female under 16 years of age to provide consent to maternity care is recognised by common law. This law is based on what

is known as Gillick competence (see Chapter 7). The Gillick principles were endorsed in Australian common law following a decision by the High Court of Australia concerning a child's capacity to make decisions, known as Marion's case (1992).

A parent's ability to consent to treatment of their child can only be exercised in the best interests of the child's physical, psychological and emotional wellbeing. In Australia the Supreme Court in each state and territory has the power to override the decision of a parent or legal guardian if their decision is not considered in the best interests of their child. This is known as a court's *parens patriae* jurisdiction.

The use of obstetric ultrasound has resulted in significant improvements in the care of pregnant women and their fetus(es). The mid-trimester ultrasound is undertaken to identify fetal abnormalities and provide information about the aetiology and implications of the diagnosis. Routine medical ultrasound is not contraindicated during pregnancy and has a high level of safety. No detrimental biological effects have been proven, although there is the potential for subtle, unrecognised effects.[20]

Verbal informed consent is generally considered sufficient for low-risk obstetric ultrasound; however, some institutions may require written consent.

What Values May Be at Stake?

Autonomy: the ability of a minor to make decisions regarding their medical care versus the autonomy of a parent to make the decision on their behalf.

What Are the Options in This Case?

Ideally, a mutual decision could be reached and Lillian's mother would agree to support her wishes. The midwife may provide information about the safety, risks and benefits of the 20-week fetal ultrasound to Lillian and her mother. If, following this discussion, a consensus is not reached, an obstetrician and/or sonographer may be requested to discuss the ultrasound with Lillian and her mother. The Royal Australian and New Zealand College of Obstetricians and Gynaecologists (RANZCOG) recommends all consenting patients be offered ultrasound assessment for fetal abnormalities, number of fetuses, gestational age, cervical length and location of the placenta between 18 and 22 weeks. Therefore, it is reasonable for Lillian to be booked for the routine mid-trimester fetal ultrasound. The discussion and outcome must be documented comprehensively.

Could the Problem Have Been Prevented?

If Lillian had received earlier antenatal visits, there would have been more time to receive information regarding the purpose of the fetal anatomy ultrasound, understand the implications, ask questions and make an informed choice.[21]

CASE 5: PROFESSIONAL BOUNDARIES

Anna works in a midwifery group practice serving a rural community. Anna is passionate about midwifery and works hard to provide excellent care for women and their families. Anna has developed a strong relationship with Julia, one of the mothers she has cared for during pregnancy, birth and the postnatal period. Julia is from a similar background to Anna and they are the same age. They have a friendly midwife–client relationship.

Julia has invited Anna, her midwife, to the christening of her baby and said she would like to stay in touch and continue to meet each other as friends now that her midwifery care is about to come to an end.

What Are the Legal/Ethical Issues That Arise From This Case?

This scenario gives rise to an ethical and professional dilemma regarding how to determine the appropriate professional relationship and boundaries between a midwife and her client.

What Could Be the Personal Reaction to This Case?

The midwife and her client have developed a friendly relationship and it may feel difficult for the midwife to decline an invitation from the client and her requests for an ongoing relationship.

What Facts May Be Relevant Regarding This Situation?

The *Code of Conduct for Midwives* outlines the legal requirements, professional behaviour and conduct expectations for midwives. Principle four requires midwives to maintain professional boundaries around the professional relationship between midwives and

women. Having this boundary is an integral component of the professional relationship.[22] Maintaining professional boundaries promotes woman-centred practice and protects the midwife and her client. According to the NMBA, maintaining professional boundaries requires midwives to:

- recognise the inherent power imbalance that exists between midwives, women in their care and significant others, and establish and maintain professional boundaries
- actively manage the woman's expectations, be clear about professional boundaries that must exist in professional relationships for objectivity in care and prepare the woman for when the episode of care ends
- recognise when over-involvement has occurred, and disclose this concern to an appropriate person, whether this is the person involved or a colleague
- reflect on the circumstances surrounding any occurrence of over-involvement, document and report it and engage with management to rectify or manage the situation.

Over-involvement with the client occurs when a midwife confuses their personal needs with those of the client and breaches the professional relationship boundary. Over-involvement may include favouritism, gifts or inappropriate relationships.[23]

What Values May Be at Stake?

Professional behaviour: midwives act 'with integrity, honesty, respect and compassion'.

What Are the Options in This Case?

Anna (the midwife) explains the nature of professional boundaries and a professional relationship as identified in the *Code of Conduct for Midwives*.[24] Following this discussion, Anna respectfully and kindly indicates her responsibility to avoid an ongoing personal relationship.

Could the Problem Have Been Prevented?

This problem could have been prevented if the midwife (Anna) had informed Julia (the client) of her obligations under the *Code of Conduct for Midwives* at the beginning of their professional relationship.

Nursing

(Contributor: Jackie Dempsey)

CASE 1: STEALING AND SELF-ADMINISTRATION OF SCHEDULE 8 DRUGS

Jenny is a 30-year-old registered nurse. She has worked in intensive care at a large public hospital in Sydney for eight years. She is often in charge of the busy unit and as such she carries the Schedule 8 drug cupboard keys. She often checks out patient medications with the other registered nurses. Staff have raised concerns that the Schedule 8 drug count is often inaccurate, with one or two drug ampoules missing. It has also been noted that Jenny takes a lot of breaks from the unit and on her return appears to be under the influence of drugs. None of the staff have approached Jenny with their concerns because she is the senior registered nurse and they say they are too busy to do so.

What Are the Legal Issues That Arise From This Case?

Issue 1: A registered nurse appears to be taking Schedule 8 drugs and self-administering them while at work. Stealing Schedule 8 drugs is illegal. Self-administering a Schedule 8 drug is illegal.

Each state and territory has a Poisons Act and Poisons Regulations (see Chapter 12). There may also be relevant policy that must be followed (e.g. see *Medication Handling in NSW Public Health Facilities*[25]). Policies may include such things as expected best practice principles for medication handling, dispensing, supplying, administration and recording of various schedule drugs including Schedule 8 drugs. Mandatory requirements include accurate record keeping of drugs dispensed and the procedures to be followed if the drug count is incorrect.

In addition, the NMBA has its *Code of Conduct for Nurses* and the International Council of Nurses (ICN) has its *Code of Ethics for Nurses* to which all registered nurses must comply pursuant to the National Law (see Chapter 4). The code of conduct sets out domains that includes that nurses must practise legally. Section 1.2 of the code requires that nurses must practise 'honestly and ethically and should not engage in unlawful behaviour as it may affect their practice and/or damage the reputation of the profession'. It also specifically states that nurses 'must comply with relevant poisons legislation, authorisation, local policy and own scope of practice including to safely use, administer, possess, prescribe, sell, supply and store medications and other therapeutic products'. Further, 'nurses must not participate in unlawful behaviour and understand that unlawful behaviour may be viewed as unprofessional conduct or professional misconduct that may have implications for their registration'. (Readers may also wish to refer to Chapter 10 to reflect upon the general elements of a crime and whether the criminal law may also be applicable here.)

Issue 2: The other staff have failed to notify AHPRA contrary to legislative mandatory notification requirements (see Chapter 4).

Issue 3: Patients are being put at risk of harm and possible injury arguably through the negligence or omission to act by the other registered nurses/staff. (See Chapter 6 regarding the principles of negligence.)

What Are the Ethical Issues That Arise From This Case?

Registered nurses are under an ethical duty to act professionally in accordance with the ICN *Code of Ethics for Nurses*. Jenny is failing to do so. In addition, the registered nurses have not raised their concerns with their manager about Jenny's behaviour – putting their patients at risk and breaching the code of ethics.

What Could Be the Personal Reaction to This Case?

Jenny is stealing and using Schedule 8 drugs from the medicine cabinet. The staff who suspect this may feel strongly that this is wrong and be concerned that this is illegal. However, staff may also feel conflicted about reporting her – she is a senior nurse, they may doubt whether they are correct, and they may fear there will be ramifications from reporting.

What Values May Be at Stake?

- Stealing and self-administration of a Schedule 8 drug as a registered nurse will affect the nurse's ability to practise safely and will put patients at risk.
- Family members of patients would not want their loved ones cared for by a health practitioner who is intoxicated.

- Other healthcare workers' responsibilities are compromised by colleagues engaging in unsafe and/or illegal behaviours.
- Management has a duty to protect patients.
- Society at large does not accept that health practitioners may place the public at risk due to personal behaviours.

What Should Have Occurred in This Case?

The Health Practitioner Regulation National Law has the overall objective to *protect the public* and ensure that all health practitioners are properly trained and accredited (see Chapter 4). Registered nurses should, at first instance, notify their unit/hospital manager of their reasonable belief about a colleague's behaviour and missing Schedule 8 drugs in accordance with state and hospital policy. Pursuant to both the National Law and the code of conduct, registered nurses have a duty to act including a mandatory or voluntary notification to AHPRA if a nurse knows or reasonably suspects that a colleague is intoxicated while practising or has a health condition that could affect their ability to practise safely or could put people at risk.

The staff may also be falling below the reasonable standard of care expected of their profession if they are negligent in overlooking Jenny's behaviour or the missing drug ampoules, and/or in their omission to report. They should ensure they are always acting to a reasonable standard of care when practising their profession (see Chapter 6).

Could the Problem Have Been Prevented?

One way to prevent such problems would be to have a policy that two different keys are required to open medicine cabinets, with no one person having both required keys. Doubling up when removing Schedule 8 drugs, recording when they are dispensed and tracking use may add some protections. Nurses (and other health practitioners) should be educated about the risks to their own and patient health and safety related to drug use.

CASE 2: STEALING A PATIENT'S MONEY

Taylor is a 50-year-old registered nurse. She has been working at an aged care facility for five years as a nurse administrator. It is a work requirement that Taylor is a registered nurse. Carmel, a 70-year-old resident, sustained brain damage following a motor vehicle accident several years ago. Consequently, she has no comprehension of financial matters. She can feed herself but requires help with all other activities of daily living. Carmel does not have any family to help her with financial matters. Taylor decides to become Carmel's financial advisor and has Carmel sign a power of financial attorney to enable access to Carmel's bank accounts on the pretext of helping Carmel. Taylor goes to Carmel's bank and withdraws $20,000 and uses the money to pay Taylor's outstanding bills and for a holiday.

What Are the Legal Issues That Arise From This Case?

- Does Carmel have the capacity to enter into a power of financial attorney with Taylor given Carmel's brain damage? (Consider the discussion of capacity in Chapter 7.)
- Can Taylor, as a registered nurse, have Carmel's power of financial attorney? (Is it appropriate for Taylor to access or use Carmel's money?)
- Stealing Carmel's money is a crime (see Chapter 8).

What Are the Ethical Issues That Arise From This Case?

What ethical duties does Taylor have to the patient with a disability? Is this a case of boundary crossing?

What Could Be the Personal Reaction to This Case?

Taylor appears to be acting opportunistically. There does not appear to be good will or care for the patient. A person observing this may immediately perceive this as 'wrong'.

What Values May Be at Stake?

- Patient safety
- Upholding the rights of people with a disability
- Honesty, integrity of care
- Protecting vulnerable patients

What Should Have Occurred in This Case?

Carmel does not have the legal capacity to enter into any legal agreement given her brain damage. To enter into any agreement, a person must have the competence to do so. That means they must have the ability to understand what they are entering into. Given Carmel's inability to understand what she is doing, the financial attorney agreement is not legally binding. Therefore, Taylor does not have a lawful authority to deal with Carmel's money and should not be doing so.

The NMBA requires all registered nurses to comply with its codes and guidelines. In the *Code of Conduct for Nurses* at section 1.2, a nurse's behaviour must be lawful. Specifically, nurses must respect their relationship with their patients 'by not taking possessions and/or property that belong to the person and/or their family'. In the same code at section 4.1, nurses are required to maintain professional boundaries by 'recognising the inherent imbalance that exists between nurses, people in their care and significant others and establish and maintain professional boundaries'. Further, at section 4.4, nurses must not become financially involved with a person in their care – for example, by signing powers of attorney. In the ICN *Code of Ethics for Nurses* there are four fundamental responsibilities. One of the main responsibilities is that nurses demonstrate professional values such as respectfulness, responsiveness, compassion, trustworthiness and integrity.

Note also, if Taylor is caught stealing Carmel's money and is convicted of a crime, the National Law requires that a health practitioner must, within seven days, give the National Board written notice of the event. In addition, the *Code of Conduct for Nurses* (section 1.1e) requires nurses to 'inform AHPRA of charges, pleas and convictions relating to criminal offences'. See the NMBA Registration Standard: 'Criminal history'.

CASE 3: SEXUAL RELATIONSHIP WITH A PATIENT

Morgan is a 40-year-old nurse who has been registered for 10 years. Morgan has been looking after Nancy, a 30-year-old patient who had surgery a few days ago and is recovering from her surgery. Morgan has looked after Nancy on every shift and finds her very attractive. Nancy likes talking to Morgan, who seems genuinely interested in her. Over the course of several nights Morgan has confided in Nancy about relationship troubles and leaving Morgan's partner. Nancy agrees that it's the best option and gives Morgan her telephone number so they can meet up when she is discharged from hospital. On her last night in hospital Morgan kisses Nancy several times. Following Nancy's release, they meet up and begin a sexual relationship that goes on for several months. Eventually Nancy wants to end the relationship, but Morgan refuses to do so and keeps on contacting her. Nancy decides her only option is to make a formal complaint to the NMBA and to lodge an official complaint about Morgan's unprofessional behaviour by having a sexual relationship with her as a former patient.

What Are the Legal/Ethical Issues in This Case?

Morgan is in breach of the NMBA *Code of Conduct for Nurses* and the ICN *Code of Ethics for Nurses*. This may result in disciplinary proceedings pursuant to the National Law, which could result in Morgan's registration being cancelled (see Chapter 4).

What Could Be the Personal Reaction to This Case?

Nancy returned Morgan's advances, agreed Morgan should leave a current relationship, and suggested they meet up when Nancy was released. Did she 'encourage' Morgan? She only reported Morgan when she wanted to end the relationship and Morgan did not agree. Was Nancy really taken advantage of, or is this a matter of revenge?

Morgan shouldn't have been telling Nancy about relationship problems in the first place; Morgan developed a liking for Nancy and was flirting with her, which constitutes overstepping boundaries as a health practitioner.

What Values May Be at Stake?

The relationship between health practitioner and patient is inherently unequal. The patient is often vulnerable and may depend emotionally on their caregiver. To receive health care, patients are required to reveal information that they may not reveal to anyone else. A breach of sexual boundaries between a health practitioner and their patient exploits the inherent power imbalance. Public confidence may also be at stake. Members of the community should never be deterred from seeking health care, permitting required intimate examinations or sharing deeply personal information because they fear potential abuse.

What Should Have Occurred in This Case?

Section 4 of the *Code of Conduct for Nurses* specifically refers to professional boundaries for nurses. Section

4.1d states that nurses must 'Avoid sexual relationships with persons to whom they have currently or previously entered into a professional relationship. These relationships are inappropriate in most circumstances and could be considered unprofessional conduct or professional misconduct.'

Section 4.1e requires a registered nurse to 'recognise that over-involvement has occurred and disclose this concern to an appropriate person whether that be the person involved or a colleague'. Section 4.1f requires the nurse to 'reflect on the circumstances surrounding any occurrence of over-involvement that has occurred, document and report it, and engage in management to rectify or manage the situation'.

Morgan should not have discussed private life details with a patient. Morgan should not have accepted the patient's telephone number. Morgan should not have kissed the patient and, regardless of Nancy's responses, should have declined to become involved with her in or out of the hospital environment or engaged in any sexual activity with her, noting that sexual relationships between nurses and people with whom they have previously entered into a professional relationship are generally inappropriate. Such relationships automatically raise questions of integrity regarding exploiting the vulnerability of people who are or who have been in their care. Consent has not been considered an acceptable defence in the case of sexual or intimate behaviour within such relationships.

CASE 4: HOW YOUR PRIVATE LIFE CAN AFFECT YOUR PROFESSIONAL LIFE

Jane is a 60-year-old registered nurse. She has been working at the local general hospital for 30 years. She is divorced with few friends. She is lonely and looking for some spice in her life so joins an online dating service. She has been on several dates with Trevor and really enjoys his company. However, Trevor has a very chequered work history and finds it difficult to hold onto a job. Lately he has taken to stealing money whenever possible. One night, Trevor drives into a service station, goes into the shop armed with a gun and steals the contents of the till. Trevor is later charged with armed robbery, found guilty and jailed.

While Jane did not take part in the robbery she did nothing to stop Trevor either before the robbery or after it. She is charged as an accessory after the fact, receives a conviction and is placed on probation for two years. The local paper runs the story of the case detailing the convictions and clearly identifying Jane as a registered nurse. The NMBA is notified of Jane's conviction and, after an investigation, forms the view that she is 'not a fit and proper person to be a registered nurse' in accordance with the National Law.

Her registration is cancelled.

What Are the Legal Issues That Arise From This Case?

While Jane did not actively take part in the robbery, her suitability to hold registration is subject to the conditions of the Health Practitioner Regulation National Law (see Chapter 4). Specifically, regard may be had to an individual's criminal history to the extent that 'it is relevant to the individual's practice of the profession' and whether the person is 'an appropriate person to practise the profession or it is not in the public interest for the individual to practise the profession'.

What Are the Ethical Issues That Arise From This Case?

The ICN *Code of Ethics for Nurses* has four principal elements that outline the standards of ethical conduct including that the nurse demonstrates professional values such as respectfulness, responsiveness, compassion, *trustworthiness* and *integrity*. The code is a guide based on social values.

What Could Be the Personal Reaction to This Case?

One may look at Jane and feel sorry for her. She was 60 and lonely. She wasn't looking for a criminal to date; she was looking to 'spice up' her life. One might see her as somewhat 'innocent' other than by association. However, instinctively one may also consider that as soon as there was an indication of criminal activity on Trevor's part, Jane had a professional obligation not to be involved and to report what she knew.

What Values Are at Stake?

Nurses who involve themselves in illegal and unethical behaviour bring the profession and themselves into disrepute by engaging in unethical behaviour.

What Should Have Occurred in This Case?

Nurses must abide by the law in the state or territory where they are employed. Jane should have notified the police as soon as possible of Trevor's conduct and advised her employer of what had occurred. Being honest about what has occurred evidences insight into the behaviour, even if there has previously been a lack of judgment. Following her conviction, she should have notified AHPRA and/or the NMBA, especially if the conviction could result in imprisonment for 12 months or more.

Could This Situation Have Been Prevented?

Only to the extent as stated above that as soon as Jane realised Trevor was engaging in criminal behaviour she should have acted. It is not possible to govern people's personal lives to the extent of determining their relationships.

Paramedicine

(Contributor: Ruth Townsend)

CASE 1: MENTAL HEALTH

Jane is a 48-year-old female with a history of anxiety and depression. She is a single mother to two young boys aged 10 and 12. One of the boys rings for an ambulance today because Jane has locked herself in the bathroom and is threatening self-harm. On arrival, the paramedics ask Jane to unlock the bathroom door. She complies. When the paramedics ask Jane if she would like to go to hospital she says no because she has to look after her children. The paramedics observe a large amount of various types of pills both in and out of the packaging on the bathroom floor. Jane denies taking any medication and there is no clinical evidence that she has done so. Jane tells the paramedics that she has been managing her depression and anxiety for years and she will be okay. She doesn't want to go to hospital. One of the paramedics thinks she should be transported. The other does not.

What Are the Legal Issues That Arise From This Case?

The main legal issues relate to assessing the patient as being acutely mentally unwell under the respective Mental Health Act of the jurisdiction the paramedics are operating in. There are some broad elements that apply to all Acts in Australia and they are that the patient is demonstrating the acute symptoms as set out in the legislation as per the table in Chapter 15. Additionally,

the task of the paramedics is to assess Jane's capacity to make decisions. An adult is presumed to have capacity to make decisions regarding their own body, so for the paramedics to involuntary treat and transport Jane, they would need to assess that Jane is lacking the capacity to make decisions for herself (capacity is discussed in Chapter 7).

What Are the Ethical Issues That Arise From This Case?

Jane may be perceived to be exercising her autonomy in making a decision that best suits her. However, one of the paramedics wants to override her autonomy because they believe that Jane is not able to make decisions in her own best interests. It may be that the paramedic is aware that sometimes suicidal patients may not wish to go to hospital because they know this will affect their ability to commit suicide. The paramedic may be concerned that Jane says she feels okay and doesn't intend to commit suicide, so she is left on her own. How do the paramedics determine what Jane's plans are?

There is also an ethical issue regarding the care, health and safety of the children. Although the children are not patients of the paramedics, the paramedics do have a professional responsibility to ensure they are safe. There is a lot of medication lying around, so it would be prudent of the paramedics to remove it. The paramedics may also be able to contact a relative or friend to help with the children and/or social services. There may be issues of privacy to consider regarding the sharing of Jane's personal information with a relative or friend, so it is important to consider what information will be shared and what actions may be taken to mitigate any breach of Jane's confidence (e.g. get her consent to share information).

Noting from Chapter 3 that here one may frame the dilemma as a normative question(s) (i.e. what 'should' or 'ought' one do in the context), the paramedics must act to protect Jane's interest – that is, they have a legal duty of care to Jane. This is a legal requirement established under civil liability law. Further, as registered health practitioners, they have a professional duty under the Health Practitioner Regulation National Law (Part 1, s 5) to meet a professional level of performance, which is to practise with 'the knowledge, skill or judgment possessed, or care exercised by, the practitioner in the practice of the health profession in which the practitioner is registered' that meets the standard 'reasonably expected of a health practitioner of an equivalent level of training or experience'.

They also have an ethical obligation to act in Jane's primary interest. This is set out in the code of conduct for paramedics.[26] A breach of this ethical requirement could result in the paramedics being required to explain their decision making to a panel of their peers (professional standards panel).

What Could Be the Personal Reaction to This Case?

The paramedics' first reaction to this case may be to think that Jane does not have capacity and therefore must be transported. Under criminal law the paramedics can act to stop Jane from harming herself even if she objects, but paramedics are also bound by other laws that require them to uphold the rights of individuals who have capacity to make decisions for themselves even if it results in their death. Therefore, the paramedics must be thorough in their assessment of her capacity and make an informed and justifiable decision to transport her.

What Facts May Be Relevant Regarding This Situation?

Making an informed decision will require the paramedics to gather all the relevant facts of the situation including Jane's mental health history as far as they are able to. There are limits to the amount of information that may be available to the paramedics because of the nature of the environment in which they work. They need to have made all reasonable attempts to gather all relevant information to inform their decision making.

What Values May Be at Stake?

- Autonomy/liberty/respect/dignity of Jane to make decisions for herself
- Non-maleficence – for the paramedics to do Jane no harm by either transporting her against her will when she is competent to refuse, or leaving her at home when she should be getting access to treatment
- Beneficence – to act to benefit the patient by either respecting her wishes or transporting her for further care and treatment to prevent her from harming herself

What Are the Options in This Case?

The possible actions and alternatives in this scenario are that the paramedics leave Jane at home as she has asked, thus upholding her autonomy to make decisions for herself, but with support for both Jane and the children by asking for a friend or relative or social services to attend. The alternative is to transport Jane to hospital as an involuntary patient. The ethical motivation behind this decision should be one of the paramedics acting in the patient's best interests, not in their own interests (i.e. they do not want to get in trouble for not transporting Jane). If they do transport Jane, they will still have to arrange care for Jane's children.

CASE 2: PRIVACY

Paramedics are called to a major road crash with multiple occupants reportedly injured. On arrival at the scene they find a car with all the windows shattered. In the front is a driver trapped but alive. The cause of death of the passenger is obvious even a fair distance from the vehicle. There are two children in the back. The paramedics are unable to tell at first glance if the children are alive or dead. There are bystanders at the scene. Some are taking photos. One of the paramedics notices that their colleague has their phone in their hand and appears to be taking photos of the incident as well.

What Are the Legal Issues That Arise From This Case?

The main legal issues pertain to the privacy of the patients and how to protect such privacy.

While the paramedics are needed to treat the casualties, they do routinely ask the public to move away from the site; the police will generally keep the public well back from the scene. There may be the necessity to ask the police to erect privacy screening to prevent the public from being able to photograph the accident.

Regarding the paramedic who has the phone in their hand, it should first be confirmed whether the paramedic is calling the communication centre to ask for backup or whether photographs are being taken (one cannot assume). If photographs are being taken, the purposes of this should be established, noting the paramedic is not allowed to take any identifying images to share publicly without the permission of the patients (see Chapter 5).

What Are the Ethical Issues That Arise From This Case?

If photographs are being taken for the wrong purposes, this gives rise to the ethical issue that one of the paramedics appears to be prepared to breach the privacy and confidence of their patient. Paramedics are privy to a great deal of personal information from vulnerable people, often in serious and time-critical situations. Upholding a patient's privacy and confidence is essential to maintaining a professional relationship and for the public to have confidence that paramedics will act to protect their patients' interests first and not exploit the circumstances of their patients (who are often having their worst day) for the paramedics' own interests.

What May Be the Personal Reaction to the Case?

It would be expected that the paramedic not holding the phone in this case would be upset if their partner was behaving in an unethical manner or contrary to the law. Apart from the obvious potential breaches of privacy for the patients, the paramedics are at a major trauma scene, with multiple potential patients. Time is critical. Managing a health practitioner who is acting poorly is not something that should even have to be thought about, and the time spent considering it is a poor use of already limited resources. This amplifies the unethical nature of the action.

What Values May Be at Stake?

- Trust – the privacy and confidentiality of patients
- Confidence – the public's confidence in the profession not to breach a patient's privacy and confidentiality
- Care, beneficence, non-maleficence – to put the patients' interests first
- Justice – there is an issue of resourcing here. Time spent being concerned about the potentially unlawful and unethical actions of the paramedic is time not spent in attending to patients.

What Should Have Occurred in This Case?

The paramedic without the phone should establish what their partner is doing. If the partner is in fact taking inappropriate photographs then the response must be firm: 'I do not think you should. It is a breach of privacy and we don't have time for that. We have patients to treat and a duty to protect them.'

Could the Problem Have Been Prevented?

Clear protocols, laws and codes of conduct exist in relation to privacy and confidentiality of patients at the scene of an emergency (as they do for health care generally). Ensuring paramedics are aware of their legal and ethical obligations is essential to upholding such obligations. It is also important to ensure that clear communication is had so that emergency situations are handled effectively and with trust.

CASE 3: END OF LIFE AND FAMILY CONFLICT

Emily is a 48-year-old married mother of two who has end-stage breast cancer. In these end stages of her life, Emily is being cared for in her home by her husband, Andy, with regular support from the community palliative care team. Emily has appointed Andy as her guardian/surrogate decision-maker in a formal instrument executed as per the legislative requirements. Her end-of-life wishes include no further active treatment and to die at home. However, Emily's mother, Clare, who is only intermittently involved with Emily, has arrived to visit Emily today and, noting Emily's very poor condition, has called an ambulance without discussing it with Emily or Andy. The crew arrive at Emily's house to find Emily unconscious with shallow breathing. Clare is demanding that the paramedics aggressively treat Emily and transport her to hospital because she believes Emily is in pain. Clare threatens to sue the paramedics if they do not do as she demands.

What Are the Legal Issues That Arise From This Case?

The main legal issue is that Emily has legally stipulated her wishes regarding her refusal of consent for further treatment. She made this decision when she was competent to do so and was aware of the implications of her actions (i.e. that it could result in death) (see Chapters 7, 8 and 12). Clare is seeking to override Emily's wishes. Clare has no legal standing in this matter because Emily has executed the documents required for healthcare staff (including the paramedics) to act according to her wishes with no prospect of any further legal action being able to be taken. That is, the paramedics cannot be litigated for failing to provide active care to Emily because she has legally refused that care (see Chapter 12). Additionally, the paramedics cannot be sanctioned by their professional body for refusing to actively treat Emily because in upholding her wishes they are upholding the law and therefore there is no sanction that could apply.

Legally the paramedics would be able to administer further pain relief (e.g. an opioid) that may have the incidental effect of hastening Emily's death, but the paramedics would not be in breach of the law if this were the case and could not be considered to have 'caused' Emily's death if they were to do so. The cause of Emily's death would be the advanced breast cancer.

What Are the Ethical Issues That Arise From This Case?

The ethical issue is that Emily has exercised her autonomy, as is her legal and ethical right, to refuse medical treatment, even if doing so will result in her death. Clare is seeking to override Emily's wishes. Ethically, it may appear that Clare is trying to act in Emily's best interests (with beneficence), but the beneficent action here is to uphold Emily's wishes. The paramedics should work to advocate for Emily and act in her best interests which, in this case, would be in accordance with her wishes. Clare is suggesting that Emily is in pain and needs care that can only be provided in hospital. The paramedics are able to provide comfort to Emily while also respecting her wish to die at home.

What Should Have Occurred in This Case?

The paramedics have an ethical obligation to act in the primary interest of Emily. In terms of dealing with Clare, the code of conduct for paramedics[27] provides guidance on the expected standard of professional behaviour in dealing with relatives at section 3.9:

> 3.9 Relatives, carers and partners
> Good practice involves:
> (a) Being considerate to relative, carers, partners and others close to the patient or client and respectful of their role in the care of the patient or client

But at section 3.12 it also refers to end-of-life care:

> 3.12 End-of-life care
> Practitioners have a vital role in assisting the community to deal with the reality of death and its

> consequences. In caring for patients or clients towards the end of their life, good practice involves:
> • taking steps to manage a person's symptoms and concerns in a manner consistent with their values and wishes
> • when relevant, providing or arranging appropriate palliative care
> • understanding the limits of services in prolonging life and recognising when efforts to prolong life may not benefit the person
> • for those practitioners involved in care that may prolong life, understanding that practitioners do not have a duty to try to prolong life at all cost but do have a duty to know when not to initiate and when to cease attempts at prolonging life, while ensuring that patients or clients receive appropriate relief from distress
> • accepting that patients or clients have the right to refuse treatment or to request the withdrawal of treatment already started
> • striving to communicate effectively with patients or clients and their families so they are able to understand the outcomes that can and cannot be achieved
> • when relevant, facilitating advance care planning
> • taking reasonable steps to ensure that support is provided to patients or clients and their families, even when it is not possible to deliver the outcome they desire
> • communicating with patients or clients and their families about bad news or unexpected outcomes in the most appropriate way and providing support for them while they deal with this information, and
> • when a patient or client dies, being willing to explain, to the best of the practitioner's knowledge, the circumstances of the death to appropriate members of their family and carers, unless it is known the patient or client would have objected.

What Could Be the Personal Reaction to This Case?

The paramedics' first reaction to this case may be to consider the option of transporting Emily to hospital. However, a response that considers all the facts of the situation informed by the paramedics' knowledge of their legal and ethical responsibilities should help them to arrive at the decision to support Emily and help her to die comfortably at home.

What Facts May Be Relevant Regarding This Situation?

The type of facts that are relevant to making an informed decision include:

- Reading Emily's advance care plan – note that even if the paramedics do not read it but form a reasonable belief that it exists, and that Emily's wish is to die at home, they will be unlikely to be exposed to any legal sanction for not transporting Emily. Further, Emily's husband is her surrogate decision-maker under a formal instrument, so if Emily is unable to refuse consent for treatment because she is unconscious, Andy will, in some jurisdictions, be able to act to refuse transport on Emily's behalf.
- Understanding the legality of respecting Emily's wishes to remain at home and the option to transport her to hospital.
- Understanding the ethical dilemmas involved in this case.

What Values May Be at Stake?

- Autonomy – that Emily has made an informed decision to refuse further treatment. This decision should be respected and thus upheld.
- Beneficence – to act in Emily's best interests here is to uphold her wishes.
- Non-maleficence – to do no harm in this scenario is to uphold Emily's wishes and to provide comfort and support to her mother, who is clearly distressed by the situation.
- Justice – that upholding Emily's wishes is an appropriate use of public resources. Transporting her and treating her in hospital is utilising public resources that may be able to be used on another person who wishes to have that treatment.

What Are the Options in This Case?

The paramedics may leave Emily at home and provide her with pain relief to ensure she is comfortable. The alternative is to transport Emily, but this would be both unlawful and unethical and is therefore not a viable alternative.

Compare the answer below to that above in the 'Medicine' case study regarding a junior doctor (case 2). The law and ethical issues are the same in both scenarios.

CASE 4: IMPAIRMENT OF A FELLOW WORKER

Raj has been working with the same paramedic partner, Jim, for a number of shifts. Raj notices that Jim appears to be impaired from time to time at the beginning of this shift regardless of whether it is a day or night shift. Raj believes that Jim is using drugs and is working while under the influence. Raj is concerned that Jim may place patients, himself and Raj at risk of harm.

Consider the reasoned approach and think about how different considerations may lead to the same/different outcomes.

What Are the Legal Issues That Arise From This Case?

The main legal issue arising from this case is that there is an obligation on registered health practitioners under the Health Practitioner Regulation National Law to mandatorily report practitioners who practise while they are intoxicated by alcohol or drugs (s 140 (a)). This is known as notifiable conduct (see Chapter 4). The reason why this behaviour is considered notifiable conduct is because it is likely to place the public at risk of harm. One of the key objectives of the National Law is to protect the public from risk of harm from incompetent or unprofessional practitioners.

What Are the Ethical Issues That Arise From This Case?

Raj is faced with having to report his partner at work without being sure that drugs or alcohol are the cause of his partner's appearance and behaviour. However, under the National Law there is a protection for staff who make a report if they have formed a reasonable belief that the practitioner is at risk of harm to self or others. This belief does not need to be beyond doubt but neither should it be a mere 'feeling'.[28] The reason this protection exists is to ensure that staff report and allow the matter to be investigated. If there is no case, there is no harm. But if there is a case, then a harm to the practitioner and/or the public may have been prevented from occurring.

Here one may frame the dilemma as a normative question(s) (i.e. what 'should' or 'ought' one do in the context). Raj has an obligation to report not only at law but also ethically. This is because Jim has the potential, by way of the privilege of his position, of putting the health of others at risk. By acting to notify AHPRA of his concerns, Raj is not only protecting the public but is also potentially protecting Jim. The code of conduct for paramedics (s 9.3) makes reference to 'other practitioners' health':

Health practitioners have a responsibility to assist their colleagues to maintain good health.
Good practice involves:
(a) providing practitioners who are patients or clients with the same quality of care provided to other patients or clients
(b) notifying the Boards if treating another registered practitioner who has patients or clients at risk of substantial harm when practising their profession because they have an impairment (refer to the Boards' guidelines on mandatory reporting); this is a professional as well as a statutory responsibility under the National Law
(c) notifying the Boards and encouraging a colleague (who is not a patient or client) who you work with to seek appropriate help if it is reasonably believed the colleague may be ill and impaired; and if this impairment has placed patients or clients at risk of substantial harm, refer to the notification provisions of the National Law and the Boards' guidelines on mandatory notifications.

Where there is a statutory obligation to report in the public interest, even if it means disclosing private information about a professional partner, the dilemma becomes one of ethical theories. A utilitarian would value the sharing of the information to do the most good and create the most happiness. The deontologist would argue that the trust and confidence relationship between the practitioner and patient (as it could potentially become between Raj and Jim) is a sacred one and should not be breached.

What Could Be the Personal Reaction to This Case?

The first response by a practitioner to a case like this is to stop and consider the potential consequences of making a mandatory report on their colleague. The mandatory reporting requirement for impairment of a health practitioner is a controversial topic. This is because the mandatory reporting requirements raise

the potential for professional conflicts to arise between competing duties for practitioners. For example, practitioners have an obligation to maintain patient confidentiality (their partner's private health information) but also a duty to report practitioners they believe may place patients at risk because of their own impairment. This potentially creates a tension between treating practitioners' duty to their patient and their duty to the safety of the public.

However, the overriding objective of the legal and ethical position in these matters is to ensure the protection of the public and patients – including practitioner patients who should, as noted in the code of conduct, be entitled to receive the same care for any health issues they have as any other patient. There is some concern among practitioners that notifying the regulator of their condition may mean they are unable to practise their profession, but there are many ways in which the regulator will deal with an impaired practitioner that allows for the practitioner to get the care and treatment they need while protecting the public.

What Facts May Be Relevant Regarding This Situation?

Raj should assess whether he has enough 'evidence' of Jim's behaviour to form a 'reasonable belief' that Jim is practising while intoxicated and that his impairment affects or is likely to detrimentally affect his capacity to practise the profession (see Chapter 4). The qualification of the 'likelihood' of the impairment causing a harm is another measure that the practitioner can weigh up before making a report.

What Values May Be at Stake?

The values that are at stake in this scenario are trust between two professional practitioners, and issues of confidence and privacy. Should Raj share his belief with the regulator or should he act as Jim's practitioner and not only recommend that he seek treatment but also enact the privacy and confidentiality provisions that are afforded to all practitioner–patient relationships?

What Are the Options in This Case?

The options in this case are for either Raj to report Jim or not. The matter will rest with Raj, but the duty to report is a mandatory one. This means that if the Paramedicine Board becomes aware that Raj knew about

Jim's impairment and did not report it, then they could potentially ask Raj to explain his decision making in front of a panel of peers at a professional standards review. Arguably the greater risk in not reporting is to the public. If Raj knows Jim poses a potential risk and does nothing and that risk eventuates, then is Raj as culpable as Jim?

CASE 5: NEGLIGENCE

Jack and Bridget were called to a patient who 'appears intoxicated'. Upon arrival Jack attempts to approach the patient. When asked, the patient says his name is Rod, but his speech is noticeably slurred. As Jack gets closer he thinks Rod smells like alcohol. Rod is not able to stand and is rambling and pointing to his head. Jack thinks that maybe Rod has fallen and hit his head and upon examination notices an egg-like lump. Jack tells Rod that he should go to hospital and get it checked out because 'there could be something serious going on inside your skull that I can't see'. Rod pushes Jack away from him and says that he's just had too much to drink and that he will be alright when he sobers up. Jack calls the police for assistance. Rod refuses to get in the ambulance, so the police take Rod to the cells for the night 'for his own safety'. During the few hours that Rod is in the cell, he develops an intracerebral haemorrhage that results in him losing the use of the left side of his body. Unfortunately, it was not until Rod became unconscious in the police cells that the paramedics were called back and were then able to treat and transport Rod. By then significant time had passed and significant damage was done. Rod sues Jack (the ambulance service) and the police for negligently failing to take him to hospital.

What Are the Legal Issues That Arise From This Case?

What are the limits of Jack and Bridget's duty of care to Rod? Were they negligent in the exercise of that duty? That is, did they fall below the standard of care expected of them and, if so, did such failure (breach) cause Rod's harm? (See Chapter 6.)

Rod may argue that he was not competent to refuse transport on the night of his accident and that Jack should have known this. Jack believes that Rod understood the implications of refusing transport to hospital and that Jack therefore did not breach his duty by not taking Rod to hospital. Jack argues that if he had transported Rod he would have been committing a battery. Rod argues that he wasn't competent to refuse

consent because he had obviously sustained a head injury. He also argued that the risk of harm to himself in not going to hospital was foreseeable and not insignificant. Jack argues that both of those things may be true but if Rod was competent to refuse transport then he was effectively stating that he was prepared to accept those risks. Jack adds that it was not his actions that caused Rod to develop a brain injury; rather it was the intoxication and subsequent fall that led to the damage. Rod argues that he lost a chance at sustaining less damage by not being taken to hospital sooner.

What Are the Ethical Issues That Arise From This Case?

The ethical issues with this matter relate to Rod's autonomy and the weighing of harm versus benefit. Jack argued that he was upholding Rod's autonomy by not insisting that he be transported to hospital. Questions arise regarding the extent to which paramedics have the power to compel a patient to go to hospital. In this case, the paramedics did not believe they had the legal power to compel Rod, and so Jack relied on Rod's refusal of treatment and transport as a justification for him not treating and transporting Rod. But should Jack have done it anyway because Jack should have known, as any reasonable paramedic in the same situation would have known, that Rod's decision-making capacity was most likely very low?

Should the police have transported Rod to hospital even though Rod was refusing? They instead thought that Rod was simply drunk and that he would sober up safely in the cells. But because police are not trained health practitioners, should Jack have made it clearer that he had concerns for Rod because of the observable head injury?

What Could Be the Personal Reaction to This Case?

The paramedics' first reaction to this case may be to think that Rod did not have capacity to refuse treatment and transport because he was clearly intoxicated. When they realised that Rod was quite feisty (which could have been another sign of his head injury) they made the decision not to transport him ostensibly as a nod to Rod's autonomous right to refuse. However, it may have been that Jack and Bridget did not want to 'force' Rod into the ambulance because they were concerned about him becoming physically aggressive. To what extent is it okay for the paramedics to protect themselves from potential harm while also working to protect the interests of the patient?

What Facts May Be Relevant Regarding This Situation?

The type of information that should be gathered in this scenario is largely clinical. To make a safe clinical decision the practitioners should ensure they have undertaken a comprehensive physical assessment of the patient and followed their clinical practice guidelines for managing a patient like Rod.

What Values May Be at Stake?

The values at stake in this scenario include respecting Rod's autonomy to make decisions for himself and the obligation of Jack and Bridget to act in Rod's best interests and in a way that did not expose Rod to additional harm.

What Are the Options in This Case?

The possible actions and alternatives in this case were to either transport Rod or not transport him. With hindsight we now know that not transporting Rod to definitive care in the first instance resulted in a harm to him that was greater than it arguably would have been if he had received treatment sooner. However, the paramedics treating Rod at the time did not have the benefit of hindsight to help them in their decision making. They did not leave Rod to fend for himself as they could have done. Instead they arranged for police to come and take Rod to a place that they thought would be safe. This was, under these circumstances, likely the best result for Rod. If he had been left alone, or had gone home alone, he likely would never have received further treatment and could potentially have died because of his, arguably, self-inflicted (i.e. not created by the poor care of the paramedics) injury.

Pharmacy

(Contributor: Maree Donna Simpson)

CASE 1: PHARMACISTS AND COMPLEMENTARY MEDICINES

Australian pharmacists are registered health practitioners who are required to complete four years of university education and a fifth year of intern training and practice. The focus of their education is on: evidence-based practice; health and disease states; management of disease states, both medicinal and non-pharmacological; the features of various dose forms such as tablets, creams, transdermal patches; and the benefits of each for a particular patient and a specific disease or condition. Medicines in Australia are regulated on the basis of risk, safety and permitted access into several different schedules (see Chapter 12), while complementary medicines such as herbal products and vitamins may be either 'listed' (Aust L) or a smaller proportion may be 'registered' (Aust R), which differ in the needs for evidence of efficacy. Complementary medicines are widely available in health food stores, supermarkets and online, though some consumers may wish to purchase them from pharmacies to ask for additional advice regarding interactions with existing prescribed or over-the-counter medicines, or suitability with life stages such as pregnancy or lactation.

As practitioners trained to practise in an evidence-based manner, some pharmacists may struggle with whether to stock and/or recommend complementary medicines. The different regulation of medicines and complementary medicines may pose ethical, professional and legal issues for pharmacists.

What Are the Legal Issues That Arise From This Case?

Medicines are intended to be supplied for a therapeutic purpose, so if complementary medicines have little evidence, could or should the law protect Australian consumers from these substances? Further questions that arise include:

- Should the law be changed? (See Chapter 14.)
- Should only registered complementary medicines be available?
- Some complementary medicines are used in lower amounts as culinary items (e.g. cinnamon). How might the law address this?
- What might be the penalty, if any, for a person possessing a complementary medicine?
- Should complementary medicines for which good evidence exists be available on the Pharmaceutical Benefits Scheme (PBS)? (See Chapter 2.)

What Are the Ethical Issues That Arise From This Case?

The *Code of Ethics for Australian Pharmacists* (2017)[29] aligns with values of care, integrity and competency, which expect pharmacists to demonstrate beneficence (act in the best interests of the patient), to do no harm (non-maleficence) and to respect patient autonomy (see Chapter 3). Several ethical questions arise:

- Is it ethical to stock complementary medicines for which there may be limited evidence?
- Is it ethical if the current evidence is mixed – some good, some bad? Does it vary by disease state?
- Could it be ethical if the disease state was self-limiting such as a tension headache? What if it were for a life-limiting disease state for which all allopathic remedies had been tried without success? Might it be ethical if the patient had a strong preference for and belief in complementary medicines?
- What role does the ethical principle of beneficence play in decision making when most medicines (allopathic or complementary) have some adverse effects?

Pharmacists are expected to operate and make decisions within an evidence-based framework; however, there is some evidence in the areas of placebo and nocebo responses that an inactive substance (a placebo), even when identified to the patient as such, will have a positive response in a proportion of patients. Questions that arise concerning professional issues include:

- Is it professionally appropriate to refuse to stock and recommend complementary medicines that may offer a positive patient outcome to some consumers?
- Could it be professionally negligent (see Chapter 6) to not consider and identify a relevant complementary medicine to a consumer? When/how might this occur?

What Should Occur in This Case?

Complementary Medicines in Pharmacies. Although we may not usually think about it, the patient's response to a medication is not just an interaction of medicine and disease state. Rather, it also reflects the patient–health practitioner relationship in which trust is usually identified as pivotal. Many pharmacists may choose to stock complementary medicines and allow pharmacy assistants to address patient needs, while a subset will also choose to recommend relevant complementary medicines while alerting the patient to the evidence currently available.

The availability of complementary medicines reflects considerations of safety, all things considered. This need not imply that there are no interactions with other medicines or disease states – for example, St John's Wort with psychotropic medicines such as some anti-depressant medicines.

Should Complementary Medicines Be Listed on the PBS? On the basis of available evidence, the majority of complementary medicines could not meet the requirements to be listed on the PBS.

What Role Could the Law Play? The law could resolve the issue by prohibiting medicines that do not have an evidence base for assisting health issues but is unlikely to do so for many reasons. This includes a long history of traditional use and the likely backlash from consumers. This is well illustrated for non-prescribed medicines that contained combinations of paracetamol, aspirin or ibuprofen with low doses of codeine. On 1 February 2018 these products were up-scheduled to Schedule 4 or prescription-only medicines but with significant consumer angst and some professional concern.

CASE 2: PHARMACISTS' PERSONAL VERSUS PROFESSIONAL VIEWS AND PRACTICES

Pharmacists in Australia supply medicines on prescription (Schedules 4 and 8) and also those that are non-prescribed (unscheduled, Schedules 2 and 3) (see Chapter 14). Prescription-only medicines may be available on the PBS or as private prescriptions where consumers meet the cost themselves (see Chapter 2). The PBS places certain expectations and conditions on approved pharmacies that supply PBS items to consumers. Some pharmacists are conflicted when their own moral views differ from professional views and struggle for legal and ethical solutions, and a small number communicate quite firmly with consumers seeking these products. Unfortunately, many of the issues that engage a pharmacist's moral views affect women; for example, pharmacists may choose not to stock or supply the oral contraceptive pill unless it is being used for non-contraceptive purposes, or not stock/supply emergency hormonal contraception (two types). This is arguably discriminatory because they often do stock medicines for erectile dysfunction such as sildenafil (Viagra) to assist males.

What Are the Legal Issues That Arise From This Case?

An approved pharmacy, holding approval to supply pharmaceutical benefits, must carry a sufficient stock and range to serve the needs of the community as identified in the *National Health Act* (1953) and the *National Health (Pharmaceutical Benefits) (Conditions of approval for approved pharmacists) Determination 2017* (PB 70 of 2017) (see Chapter 2). Many oral contraceptives are available on the PBS whether as combined tablets (oestrogen and progestogen) or as progestogen-only products. An approved pharmacy that does not stock oral contraceptive products may be in breach of these requirements.

It may be more complicated where a pharmacy stocks oral contraceptive products but interrogates patients about their intended use and refuses to dispense where the sole use is as a contraceptive. In this regard, providing privacy is also an important issue and it is expected that the pharmacist would discuss issues of supply with patients in a counselling room or an area of the pharmacy where conversation is not readily overheard.

Non-prescribed emergency hormonal contraception is available in Australia as a Schedule 3 medicine. There are two categories, levonorgestrol and ulipristal, supplied under an S3 protocol developed collaboratively with pharmacy peak professional bodies.

What Are the Ethical Issues That Arise From This Case?

Pharmacists may believe that the ethical principle of non-maleficence (do no harm) allows them to refuse supply of oral contraceptives and emergency hormonal contraception. Pharmacists are, however, expected to respect a patient's dignity and right to autonomy.

If a pharmacist is going to refuse to supply contraception they could refuse supply courteously without rejecting the patient's views and beliefs.

The Pharmaceutical Society of Australia's *Code of Ethics for Pharmacists* reminds pharmacists of their duty to their patients. Pharmacists are expected to inform the patient 'when exercising the right to decline provision of certain forms of health care based on the individual pharmacist's conscientious objection, and in such circumstances, appropriately [facilitate] continuity of care for the patient'.[30] Continuity of care would be expected to apply to the ongoing use of an oral contraceptive product prescribed by the patient's general practitioner.

What Could Be the Personal Reaction to This Case?

In 2011 a survey of Australian pharmacists identified that 22% perceived that it was reasonable for a pharmacist's religious faith to affect emergency hormonal contraception supply. However, emergency hormonal contraception is time-sensitive and is most effective if taken within 72 hours of unprotected sex (levonorgestrol) or within 120 hours (ulipristal). The over-the-counter availability of emergency hormonal contraception provides women with access in a timely manner, which can be critical for women in rural and remote communities where timely access to medical care can be difficult.

It is anticipated that a pharmacist would not just refuse to supply an oral contraceptive or emergency hormonal contraceptive request or prescription but would have identified strategies for patients to obtain those products in cases of need, especially if the pharmacy is the only one in a geographically sizeable area. Note, the *Australian Charter of Healthcare Rights* could play a role in the pharmacist's decision making since the charter applies to all health settings anywhere in Australia, including public hospitals, private hospitals, general practice and other community environments (see Chapter 2).

What Are the Options in This Case?

Australia has a high rate of unplanned pregnancies, with almost half the women of childbearing age disclosing an unplanned pregnancy.[31] Timely access to emergency hormonal contraception can reduce the high rate of unplanned pregnancies among women in Australia. Levonorgestrel has been available as an S3 pharmacist-only medicine since 2004; however, ulipristal acetate has only been available as an S3 medicine since February 2017 (see Chapter 14). Access to reliable contraceptive options can also reduce the high rate of unplanned pregnancies.

Pharmacists have an obligation under the PBS to carry an appropriate range and volume of medicines, including oral contraceptives and their continued supply. However, it is recognised that some pharmacists may be conscientious objectors to the use of exogenous hormone products in women for contraceptive reasons.

One or more of the following may be potential solutions to 'conscientious objection' among pharmacists:

- pharmacists stocking medicines consistent with the needs of their community
- multiple pharmacists working concurrently, with supply being undertaken by the non-objecting pharmacist(s)
- a formalised strategy to courteously direct to another predetermined point or points of supply
- every pharmacist respecting a patient's right to autonomy, respect, confidentiality and privacy, whether supplying or not.

CASE 3: PATIENTS WITH DEMENTIA

A patient who the pharmacist has known for more than 10 years approaches the counter looking distressed. He advises the pharmacist that he has a diagnosis of Alzheimer's disease at age 63 years. He also presents a prescription for a cholinesterase inhibitor and asks whether it will help and whether other medications or supplements may assist.

What Are the Ethical Issues That Arise From This Case?

There are several ethical challenges for pharmacists and all are likely to need to be considered during the course of this condition. First is the capacity of the patient to give informed consent (see Chapter 3); second is to understand the offer of, for example, a generic brand to lessen the cost of the medicine by avoiding the brand price premium.

A further concern is: When should the pharmacist interact with the carer/guardian and not the patient for decisions about medicines?

There is also the issue of when professional services such as dose administration aids are no longer useful for managing a patient's medicines and for contributing to patient adherence to the medication regimen since the patient may no longer remember why or how to use them.

Is it fair and just, however, to stop these services if a carer (professional or family) has learnt to use them and depend on them?

What Are the Professional Issues That Arise From This Case?

Just as there are ethical dilemmas, there are also professional challenges that need to be navigated by pharmacists. The Professional Practice Standards[32] offer guidance for pharmacists in providing therapeutic goods (medicines and devices), health information and professional services.

But how much advice should a pharmacist offer and to whom might he/she offer that advice when the professional focus requires that the patient be the primary concern? This presents a professional challenge.

Physical assault by individuals with Alzheimer's is a common experience during care-giving. The most commonly presented behaviours include hitting, grabbing, pinching, scratching and throwing items, and carers or family are often quite affected by the change in their patient or loved one.

Professional services are provided *to* an individual patient but can they be provided *for* an individual patient so the carer can continue to receive dose administration aids for example?

What Are the Legal Issues That Arise From This Case?

As memory and capacity are increasingly affected, ideally appointing an enduring power of attorney and drawing up an advance care directive as early in the condition as possible would be helpful, though ideally every individual would do so as a prudent member of society as a normal life practice (see Chapter 12).

Then there are issues of personal rights and freedoms versus societal protection: issues of voting, driving and continuing to work. Pharmacists may be placed in difficult circumstances when a condition and/or medications may affect an individual's judgment and capacity to drive safely at any time but possibly more so in a condition such as Alzheimer's when the affected individual's insight may be impaired.

Another issue that is sometimes raised with pharmacists is how to remove the individual with Alzheimer's from the electoral roll. Carers/guardians might find the following link useful: https://www.aec.gov.au/FAQs/Electoral_Roll.htm.

Does the patient's right to confidentiality override other responsibilities such as to carers or to the public?

What Are the Options in This Case?

Unfortunately, this is not a 'one size fits all' situation because a diagnosis of Alzheimer's disease does not result in the same experience or disease 'milestones' for every individual affected. While the layperson's usual expectation is that people living with Alzheimer's lose their memories, and they do, behavioural challenges are often more problematic and pose more legal concerns, ethical dilemmas and professional quandaries for the health practitioners who interact with them.

Is the New Prescription Medicine Going to Help?

This is a good question, but we need to remember that just as 'drugs don't have doses, people do', these medicines do not assist every patient. They may delay apparent progression but do not cure nor manage long term, and ethically this is a challenging situation. Pharmacists need to abide by their code of ethics, considering and balancing beneficence and non-maleficence.

Further, many patients will be started on antipsychotics such as risperidone for behavioural issues. But prescriptions are often longer term than the 12-week course covered by the PBS, and these patients are often older and may be supported by a government-funded pension (see Chapter 2).

There are supplements that may assist. One such product is Souvenaid, which is a nutritional drink that contains omega-3 fatty acids, B group vitamins and other nutrients thought to support brain functions affected in early Alzheimer's disease.

How Can Lack of Capacity to Give Informed Consent Be Addressed?

The Pharmacy Board of Australia advises in its code of conduct that 'when working with a patient or client whose capacity to give consent is or may be impaired or limited, obtaining the consent of people with legal authority to act on behalf of the patient or client and attempting to obtain the consent of the patient or client as far as practically possible'[33] is expected (see Chapter 3).

How Might Professional Issues Be Addressed Such as Caregiver Assault?

There are strategies to reduce the risk of assault such as a relaxed and kindly approach, alerting the individual with Alzheimer's of the intended action and avoiding confrontational tone and language. Beyond these simple actions, referring the carer/family member back to the person's neurologist or general practitioner for an assessment may assist. Symptoms such as agitation, restlessness or aggression in Alzheimer's can be a major source of distress for caregivers and increase the likelihood of an institutional placement. Other questions that may be asked include: 'How might a carer know how much effort they can use to keep the patient safe and keep themselves from physical harm also?' and 'Are there limits to self-defence?'.

CASE 4: AN IMPAIRED PHARMACY STUDENT

You are a pharmacy owner and consistently take pharmacy students from several universities for placement. You have been approached by a specific student three times in the past in a phone call but today she approaches you in person. She tells you she is a final-year student and that she must dispense medicines and counsel patients on prescription medicines as part of her placement. You are puzzled because the university placement coordinator clearly identified her as a second-year student who should be observing your interactions and role-playing similar cases with you or your staff to put counselling theory into practice. In talking with her you are concerned that she may be affected by a mental health issue. During your conversation with her she does not, however, disclose any health issues, even though you asked if there are any health issues you needed to consider. The longer you talk with her, the more concerned that you become. Her manner is vague and unfocused and her responses do not necessarily answer the questions you have asked, nor are they close to being related to the topic. You decide to make a voluntary AHPRA notification of the student as an impaired student because you are quite concerned for the safety of the student and the public.

What Are the Legal Issues That Arise From This Case?

Pharmacists are registered health practitioners with AHPRA and have mandatory and voluntary reporting of impaired practitioners (see Chapter 4). However, any person may make a voluntary notification to AHPRA about a student when they believe that the student meets one of three conditions. In this case the condition would be that she 'has or may have an impairment that they believe may harm the public'.

Titles of registered health practitioners are protected, and it is an offence to impersonate a health practitioner in a manner likely to deceive a member of the public. The student claiming she has more experience than she has is of concern. In denying a health condition that may affect practice, the student has possibly demonstrated a lack of awareness and insight.

The National Pharmacy Board's role focuses on registering students and managing notifications about students in certain circumstances:

- students whose health is impaired to such a degree that there may be substantial risk of harm to the public
- students who have been found guilty of an offence punishable by 12 months' imprisonment or more
- students who have a conviction of, or are the subject of, a finding of guilt for an offence punishable by imprisonment
- students who have contravened an existing condition or undertaking.

This is a challenging situation and one where a resolution might seem to be discriminatory, but it is essential to remember that registered health practitioner students are registered as students while they undertake their course studies, and regulatory authorities are concerned with protecting the public.

What Are the Ethical Issues That Arise From This Case?

Privacy and confidentiality – the student need not disclose a health condition, and some students do express concerns about discrimination based on health (see, for example, the discrimination case that highlighted the difficulty of balancing the rights of medical students with a disability with the rights of the community to safe health care at https://theconversation.com/a-fine-balance-disability-discrimination-and-public-safety-25653) (see also Chapter 3).

What Are the Professional Issues That Arise From This Case?

Public safety is a professional concern because pharmacists and students are expected to practise only to their capabilities. The capabilities of a second-year student would be anticipated to be quite different from a fourth-year student, so a second-year student may place the public at risk from lack of knowledge, skills and judgment.

What Are the Options in This Case?

In this case the student probably had an untreated mental health issue as evidenced by her behaviour, but what may have been the position had the student merely misrepresented their capabilities? The National Law protects the public by ensuring that only registered health practitioners who are suitably trained and qualified can use protected titles such as pharmacist, nurse or doctor (see, for example, *Health Practitioner Regulation National Law Act* (NSW) s 113) (see also Chapter 4).

Could the student sue the pharmacist for reporting her to the National Board? Note the following from the National Law (s 237):

> *The National Law provides protection from civil, criminal and administrative liability for people who make a complaint or raise a concern about a registered health practitioner or student if the complaint or concern raised is made 'in good faith'. A complaint or concern raised about a practitioner 'in good faith' is one that is made honestly, sincerely and fairly.*

CASE 5: PHARMACISTS AND FAMILY

You are an early career pharmacist working in a busy rural private hospital pharmacy as a staff pharmacist (see Chapter 2). You have been assigned by the pharmacist-in-charge to the maternity ward and orthopaedic ward for patient education, medication supply (for an individual patient) and imprest (a method under which medicines are supplied and maintained in a ward or clinic by staff from the central pharmacy). You are looking through the pathology reports for your patients when you notice your uncle's name – he is an inpatient in the surgical ward. Out of curiosity you go past the surgical ward on your way to the orthopaedic ward, where you find your uncle. You look up his diagnosis and see that it is advanced colorectal cancer. You go home and tell your mother because it is her brother after all. She goes to see her brother, who is most upset that his sister is aware of his health condition.

Sometimes family members may not be perceived to be in the same role as another patient. However, this is no excuse for breaching patient privacy, and the relationship with the person offers no protection.

What Are the Ethical Issues That Arise From This Case?

In this situation, is it fair and just for a health practitioner to respect privacy and confidentiality of other patients but not their family member's? Has patient autonomy been considered and respected? Has the pharmacist acted in a beneficent manner? How can the practitioner maintain integrity and tell 'the truth' when patients are individuals and medications may give different outcomes with different people and conditions? (See Chapter 3.)

This action breaches the Pharmacy Board of Australia's code of conduct.

What Are the Legal Issues That Arise From This Case?

If personal information about an individual is collected for one purpose such as to facilitate medical treatment in a hospital, it should not be disclosed for another purpose (such as a discussion with a family member) unless the individual has consented to this, and clearly in this case the uncle had not done so (see Chapter 5).

Under the National Law, a breach of privacy laws by a pharmacist may amount to unprofessional conduct or professional misconduct. There is legal guidance in this situation – for example, the Australian Privacy Principles in the *Privacy Act 1988*. The Australian Privacy Principles, which are contained in Schedule 1 of the Act, outline how organisations and health service providers must manage an individual's personal information (see Chapter 5).

What Are the Options in This Case?

This situation may have both personal and professional outcomes and may well not have occurred if the practitioner had followed the guidance in various pharmacy profession codes and by various pharmacy bodies. Such action by a recently registered pharmacist may quite likely have had significant consequences including some or all of the following:

- a complaint against the practitioner made to the National Pharmacy Board, which may result in outcomes ranging from no further action to cancellation of registration (see Chapter 4)
- action by a healthcare body such as a health complaints commission

- appearance in court (see Chapter 1)
- a formal warning by the hospital
- reputational risk and challenges of further future employment.

Physiotherapy

(Contributors: Clare Delany, Brett Vaughan)

CASE 1: FAMILY INSISTING ON ACTIVE PHYSIOTHERAPY WHEN NOT CLINICALLY INDICATED

Madonna is 85 years old. She was admitted to the general medicine ward one week ago with end-stage emphysema. Each day at least two members of her large extended family (three brothers and four adult children) have been by her bedside. She is on low-flow oxygen. However, she has started to show signs of increased congestion and possible pneumonia. Her family have requested antibiotics, suctioning and physiotherapy twice daily. Madonna is very short of breath and can only talk briefly before becoming short of breath – she understands English but tends to talk only in Italian now when she does speak. Suctioning is highly distressing for Madonna and she is exhausted and visibly traumatised by the experience. She does not have the energy for breathing exercises or other active physiotherapy treatment. The physiotherapist thinks that Madonna's treatment is futile and causing Madonna pain and discomfort; and Madonna clearly doesn't want it. But the family is insisting that Madonna has been like this before and she needs this active treatment so she can get well enough to spend one more Christmas at home.

What Are the Legal Issues That Arise From This Case?

The two main legal issues raised by this case are:

- capacity to give informed consent
- whether and in what circumstances family members can insist on a particular treatment in the absence of advance care directives – that is, act as substitute decision-makers.

Chapter 6 discusses the importance of informed consent and the significance of a person possessing sufficient capacity to understand information and provide voluntary consent to accept or refuse treatment. Chapter 7 reminds us that discussions about treatment with family is a legitimate part of their decision-making process but that as a competent adult Madonna should be consulted first as to her wishes and preferences. In this case, a translator may be required to assist in this process of finding out what Madonna understands and what her preferences are. Chapter 7 outlines some strategies that could be employed here including the use of a translator and/or diagrams.

The second legal issue concerns whether, in this situation, the family can insist on specific treatments on behalf of Madonna. Chapter 7 provides examples of different types of guardians and the legislation underpinning their legal standing. Guardian(s) may be appointed when the patient lacks the requisite capacity to decide in part or in whole for themselves.[34]

What Are the Ethical Issues That Arise From This Case?

The normative questions that arise from this case are:

- Should the physiotherapist continue giving active treatment to Madonna when she does not believe it is in Madonna's best interests and when she believes it is burdensome for her?
- Who should decide Madonna's treatment?
  - What capacity does Madonna have to contribute?
  - Can families insist on active physiotherapy for their mother?

What Could Be the Personal Reaction to This Case?

A fundamental ethical principle of health care and, in this case, physiotherapy treatment, is to provide a benefit for the patient rather than cause harm. Health practitioners are not obliged to provide treatments that they believe are burdensome or harmful for a patient and that the burdens of the treatment outweigh the benefits. However, considerations of burdens and benefits may be contested. In this case, the therapist and Madonna's family may hold different views about what counts as a burden or a benefit. For example, the physiotherapist in this case may view the suction and other active treatments as unnecessary or futile because they will not delay the inevitable progress of her lung disease and are clearly distressing for Madonna. The therapist may believe that an appropriate goal of care is to take a more palliative approach that enables Madonna to be more comfortable and have greater quality of life.

Madonna's family may value length of life over quality. They are obviously distressed about their mother's deteriorating health and are expressing a wish for treatment to provide every possible chance for recovery and to prolong her life. They are also influenced in their reaction, perhaps by previous times when she did recover from an exacerbation of her condition.

In this case description Madonna's concerns and wishes for treatment are not obvious, other than clear distress from the active respiratory interventions.

Identifying these emotional responses is an important step in ethical analysis of this case because it may help to explain the source of apparently divergent views and assumptions about what matters for Madonna. For example, a physiotherapist's view on what is important for a patient with end-stage lung disease is grounded in knowledge of physiology, pathology and illness trajectory. Madonna's family is likely to be motivated by wanting to prolong her life. They may see their role as a loving family to keep trying everything possible to give her a chance to be home with them.

What Facts May Be Relevant Regarding This Situation?

In this case there is not one clear ethically appropriate response. The physiotherapist and Madonna's family are both responding in a way that they believe is best for Madonna. Before the next step of weighing up these differing values to decide on a response, it is important to gather other information and facts about the situation. Fact gathering helps to unpack and illuminate the source of underlying values and can help all people involved to be more aware of the reasoning behind stated positions and to know what the effects will be of either continuing to treat or ceasing active physiotherapy treatment.

Relevant fact questions in this case are:

- What is known about what Madonna understands, her wishes and what she is hoping for?
- Does Madonna have an advance care directive or has she previously expressed any wishes about the scope and intensity of end-of-life care?
- How advanced is Madonna's lung disease?
- What is the likely trajectory of the condition?

- What does the physiotherapy treatment comprise? How will it affect Madonna's quality of breathing and comfort?
- Has Madonna been in this situation before and recovered enough to go home?
- Who has spoken to the family to find out what they understand and are hoping for?
- What has the family been told about the lung disease?
- Have they been given consistent information or have some members of the treating team given different prognoses?

What Values May Be at Stake?

A common feature of ethical dilemmas is that people hold differing values and perspectives about the 'right' thing to do. Identifying those values helps to understand the drivers of conflicting or competing views and may help to illuminate where there is agreement between people's perspective. This can lead to an outcome that does not simply override one for another. As outlined above, the physiotherapist believes that active treatment is both futile and burdensome for Madonna. Her perspective about futility is possibly grounded in the fact that it will not prevent Madonna's disease process. In contrast the family may view the physiotherapy treatment as the only mode of treatment that can help Madonna and that if they were to cease that treatment, then Madonna would most certainly die. The value they are holding on to is to give Madonna every possible chance, or perhaps to do their duty as a family to try everything possible for Madonna.

What Are the Options in This Case?

Possible options for responding in this case are (1) the physiotherapist explains that continuing with suction and active breathing exercises is not appropriate for Madonna because it will not prevent the inevitable decline and it is too burdensome for her; (2) the physiotherapist continues to provide active treatment according to the family's wishes; or (3) the physiotherapist speaks with the family about their understanding about physiotherapy treatment and liaises with social work, palliative care and the medical team to find out who has been involved and whether there is a need to provide more supports for Madonna and her family so they can understand Madonna's current situation.

What Should Occur in This Case?

Options 1 and 2 require the therapist to choose one value over another. If she chose to cease active physiotherapy against the family's wishes, the outcome would be that Madonna is relieved of treatment she finds distressing. However, the family may be distressed, and this distress may extend beyond the immediate time and be a source of regret about how they did or did not help their relative at the end of her life. If the physiotherapist continued treatment against her own better judgment, this may lead to moral distress, frustration and resentment.

The third option involves finding out more about the situation by seeking Madonna's current or previously stated views, seeking to understand the family's perspective and values and seeking input from the wider health team. This information gathering will most likely identify a modified position that can accommodate different perspectives. This is likely to be a treatment plan with agreed criteria for when treatment should cease or how it can be slowly limited so as to provide some benefit with less burden.

CASE 2: A SPORTS THERAPIST'S OBLIGATIONS TO REPORT A PLAYER WHO IS UNFIT TO PLAY

Sandra has joined as a physiotherapist for the Australian netball team. She has travelled with the team to a training camp in northern Queensland. Spending time with the team for three weeks has helped her build relationships with the athletes and the wider health practitioner and training team. Sandra is worried about one of the players. Hayley is 23 years old and has been with the team for five months. Hayley had surgery six months ago for a right anterior cruciate ligament (ACL) tear. The surgery was performed by the surgeon who has been involved with the Australian team for the past 20 years. He is due to retire next year. Hayley reported that her rehabilitation was going well and that she'd been doing her own exercises and following a program given to her by another physiotherapist from the Australian team when she had had a previous ACL repair on the same knee three years earlier. Hayley played her first full game two days ago.

When Sandra examined Hayley following the game she noticed some effusion in her right knee and, more alarmingly, considerable movement within the knee suggesting ligament laxity. But Hayley insisted it felt fine and that she was ready to play in the first team selection game the next day. She told Sandra that because she hadn't been involved in the original rehabilitation program she didn't have the right to interfere with her chance of playing. She was highly anxious and insisted that Sandra declare her fit for playing. Sandra was certain that Hayley shouldn't be playing. She was also concerned that the surgical repair had not been successful and that there was ongoing instability. There had been some disquiet about the surgeon lately within the team, but no one was prepared to say anything because he was soon to retire.

What Are the Legal Issues That Arise From This Case?

This case raises legal questions about the scope and limits of confidentiality and privacy. These questions concern the scope of the duty for health practitioners to prevent injury on the sports field and contractual-based reporting obligations within sports teams.

Sandra has a legal obligation to undertake a clinically appropriate and thorough examination. As part of this legal standard of care (Chapter 6), Sandra is required to document her examination findings with respect to the ligamentous laxity and the advice she provides to Hayley about fitness to play. In Chapter 5 it was explained that the duty to maintain confidentiality requires that information should not be disclosed to others without the client's permission. This reinforces the ethical considerations of respecting Hayley's preferences while also ensuring Hayley is not harmed, especially if that harm can be prevented.

To assist in resolving these conflicting obligations, it will be important to know about the contractual obligations Sandra has as the team physiotherapist. Chapter 6 describes the legal tests applied to determining the engagement. This will subsequently influence liability.

What Are the Ethical Issues That Arise From This Case?

The key ethical issues arising from this case concern confidentiality and privacy.

- Should Sandra report her findings about Hayley's knee including that she considers her unfit to play, and that the surgery has been unsuccessful?
- Can Hayley insist that Sandra not pass on the clinical assessment of her knee to others within the team?

What Could Be the Personal Reaction to This Case?

From a physiotherapy discipline perspective, Sandra may be concerned about minimising the risk of re-injury for her patient, and she may feel an obligation to ensure the surgeon is aware of her assessment. However, Hayley is no doubt motivated to stay in the team and to be included.

What Facts May Be Relevant Regarding This Situation?

Gathering relevant facts is an important task when weighing up competing values. In this case, it is important to have a good understanding of Sandra's contractual arrangement with her employer including requirements to share information about fitness to play. Within specific contractual arrangements, Sandra has professional autonomy to assess and manage players' health and fitness within her scope of practice. This case highlights the need to be clear about the balance between keeping players' information that is shared within a clinical encounter as confidential and sharing that information with health staff, coaches and others.

What Values May Be at Stake?

The values at stake include, on the one hand, respect for Hayley's privacy and respect for her choice to play, even if it means taking a risk of re-injuring her knee. On the other hand is the therapist's professional goals and values to minimise harm and ensure players are physically ready to play.

What Are the Options in This Case?

After weighing up these competing values the options will most likely involve Sandra documenting her concerns and informing Hayley of any obligations to pass on information. It is also important to uphold Hayley's wish for confidentiality. One harmful outcome if this value is ignored is to diminish trust between Sandra and Hayley.

What Should Occur in This Case?

A final action will be a process of managing the risk of re-injury against the harms of breaching confidentiality without Hayley's informed consent.

CASE 3: WHEN PATIENT-CENTRED CARE CONFLICTS WITH EVIDENCE-BASED CARE

Christian is a 53-year-old businessperson who has attended an inner-city physiotherapy centre four times over the past two years with recurring low back pain. Each time Christian has requested massage and mobilisation, and his physiotherapist has always complied with this request. But today he is seeing a different physiotherapist who is doing a locum for two weeks at the practice. Isabella graduated two years ago and is currently doing a Master of Physiotherapy focusing on the evidence for exercise for low back pain. She is not prepared to give Christian massage only. She believes it is a waste of time and that given Christian has had back pain over such a long time, he should be doing exercises. Christian says he is not interested in doing exercises. He travels too much for his work and finds them inconvenient. Christian insists on his regular treatment of massage and threatens to go elsewhere.

What Are the Legal Issues That Arise From This Case?

From a legal perspective, Chapter 7 outlines the requirements for valid consent for care. In this case, Christian appears to be *competent* to make treatment decisions and has expressed his preference for a particular type of treatment. Drawing on Chapter 7, as part of obtaining consent Isabella would be required to explain alternative treatment approaches that may assist Christian. However, if Christian makes his preferences clear, then Isabella would need to decide and justify her final decision, drawing on the ethical considerations discussed above.

What Are the Ethical Issues That Arise From This Case?

The ethical issues raised by this case concern a conflict between a therapist's values of providing evidence-based care that has shown to be effective and respecting the wishes of a patient who requests a suboptimal treatment. The ethical question could be expressed as:

- Should the therapist insist on providing evidence-based care according to the known evidence and studies or should she do what the patient requests?

What Values May Be at Stake?

There are several competing ethical values that are relevant to this case. Isabella is strongly committed to providing treatment that is known to be evidence-based. She is uncomfortable in providing what, she regards, is suboptimal treatment. Christian is a competent adult who has a right to make decisions about his health including what he considers to be helpful treatment.

Health practitioners are not ethically obliged to provide treatment they do not agree with or that they think will be harmful.

What Facts May Be Relevant Regarding This Situation?

Relevant factual questions in this case include asking:

- How harmful would it be for Christian to receive massage rather than exercises?
- How strong is the evidence for exercise as being the preferable treatment?
- Does the evidence apply to Christian's situation?
- Are there any harmful effects of refusing this request?
- Do the harms of refusing treatment outweigh providing the massage requested (including diminishing the therapist–patient relationship; Christian moving to another practice)?

What Are the Options in This Case?

Weighing the above values and factual considerations is important in negotiating a pathway for respecting both the health practitioner's and the patient's values and preferences. In this case, the harms of insisting on evidence-based treatment over the patient's preferences may outweigh the benefits. Losing Christian's trust, ignoring his choices and causing him to seek alternative treatment are all harms that should be considered.

CASE 4: WHO DECIDES? WHEN PARENTS AND THERAPISTS DISAGREE ABOUT TREATMENT FOR A CHILD

Casey is a seven-year-old girl with cerebral palsy. Casey is able to walk for short distances but it is an effort and she is slow. Casey's parents are concerned she is not keeping up with her friends at school and that she is missing out on games and play in the school yard. They have located a light and easily manoeuvrable (and expensive) wheelchair they can import from America and they think this will make all the difference for Casey. They are willing to pay and are excited about their internet searching – they enthusiastically present the idea to Jo, who has been Casey's physiotherapist for years.

Jo is very concerned about this. She thinks that Casey has been making great progress with her walking and needs to keep going to build up her strength, stamina and balance. She thinks that once Casey starts regularly using a wheelchair she won't want to keep up with the walking and she will lose all of the rehabilitation gains of the past three years. She is especially concerned about the wheelchair Casey's parents have chosen. She thinks it is a bit gimmicky, way too expensive and will make things 'too easy' for Casey. She thinks occasional time in a wheelchair for rest but not for mobility is the best way to go for Casey at the moment.

What Are the Legal Issues That Arise From This Case?

From a legal perspective, consent is an issue in this case. According to Chapter 7, Casey may be regarded as Gillick competent and able to provide valid consent. This suggests that Jo should at least enquire as to Casey's wishes and capacity to understand choices available to her.

Although Casey's parents have a legal authority to make decisions about health care on behalf of their daughter, this legal power or discretion to decide is not without limits. Chapter 16 discusses what would constitute neglect with respect to children and the voluntary or mandatory reporting of potential or actual child abuse. There may be situations where the care decisions made by parents will cause harm to a child. Consideration of whether Casey's parents' requests constitute harm or neglect will need to be made.

Chapter 5 highlights the need to document discussions about the benefits and risks of both the wheelchair approach and the walk-based rehabilitation approaches, and that the care decision was made by Casey's parents.

What Are the Ethical Issues That Arise From This Case?

This case involves disagreement about what constitutes the most benefit for a young child. The therapist believes continued active treatment with small periods of time in a wheelchair is the best treatment for Casey because it will allow Casey to keep up her capacity to walk. Casey's parents are placing their hopes on a particular form of equipment – a new wheelchair – to give Casey more mobility and capacity to participate more at school and with her friends.

What Could Be the Personal Reaction to This Case?

The drive to maximise a child's potential and to keep as many options available for healthy functioning is a strong principle of physiotherapy care. When gains have been made over a period of rehabilitation, the physiotherapist's initial reaction may be to resist losing those gains and to keep striving for physical strength and functional progression. The therapist may also be concerned that the wheelchair will hasten irreversible and more generalised muscle weakness. Casey's parents may be influenced by other values of quality of life for Casey. They value seeing Casey joining in with her friends as much as possible. They find it distressing to see Casey having to work hard to achieve walking and they wish to decrease the burden of walking and to provide a less taxing way for her to participate.

What Facts May Be Relevant Regarding This Situation?

The two competing positions about what will ultimately improve Casey's life appear to be grounded in different values being placed on participation with others and the value of maintaining functional strength to avoid more severe future functional loss. The relevant questions to probe these two value positions are:

- What does Casey want and what does she value?
- What is known about loss of function that will occur should Casey spend more time in a wheelchair?
- What will Casey's life be like if she spends more time in a wheelchair? How will that affect what she can and can't do?
- What have Casey's parents been told and what do they understand about Casey's condition and the impact of continuing with walking training versus using the wheelchair?
- What is Casey's home and sibling situation? How will continued walking versus wheelchair dependency affect that situation?

What Values May Be at Stake?

Casey's parents are prioritising her capacity to participate with friends and at school over strength gains or avoidance of developing muscle weakness. The value expressed by the physiotherapist is that it is more important to focus on maintaining muscle strength and mobility to avoid premature weakness and ultimate loss of function. Casey will also have formed values about what is important for her and, at seven years old, she could be consulted separately from her parents. Involving children in decisions that affect their own welfare offers positive benefits to those children. Among other things, it allows children to obtain needed practice and skills in making responsible decisions, contributes to their perception that they have some control and influence over their lives, and results in a greater sense of self-esteem and competence while reducing anxiety and fear of the unknown.

An overriding consideration in this case concerns Casey's parents' discretion to decide what is best for their child. Parents do have moral authority to make decisions for their children based on what they think is best for them. However, moral authority or decision-making discretion is not absolute. Parents can make choices for their children that are suboptimal, as long as the choices are not harmful. Thinking about parental requests or choices in this way helps to focus on the bottom line of whether parents are wanting something that is going to cause harm to their child or whether their request is perhaps suboptimal but nevertheless within their discretion to choose. It is ethically justifiable to override their decisions if they cause significant harm to the child.

What Are the Options in This Case?

The options in this case are to (1) support Casey's parents in their choice to buy a wheelchair and to adjust the rehabilitation program from a focus on walking to managing the wheelchair and (2) to insist on continued walking-based rehabilitation.

What Should Occur in This Case?

In this case, the parents are choosing what the therapist regards as a suboptimal treatment. However, depending on the responses to the fact-based questions, it appears unlikely that the parents' choice of a wheelchair could be considered a 'significant harm' leading to a clear

need to refuse their request. It would in fact be impossible to prevent Casey's parents from buying the wheelchair. A middle position that provides a balance between competing values is to inform Casey's parents of the concerns about functional decline from relying on a wheelchair and to work with them to enhance Casey's capacity to participate at school and to continue to build her strength. Building the trust and maintaining a good relationship between the therapist and the family is another value that must be balanced between competing ethical values about the best treatment for Casey.

CASE 5: STANDARDS OF CARE AND PHYSIOTHERAPY TREATMENT

Dan is a 40-year-old self-employed builder. He presented to a physiotherapist in his home town in rural New South Wales with severe acute right-sided low back pain extending into his right buttock. Dan was having trouble sitting or bending over so he was unable to work. The physiotherapist provided Dan with some information about massage and manual treatment and otherwise did not warn Dan of a risk of exacerbating the injury. She did not check for nerve involvement and did not refer Dan for a scan or seek a second opinion. Dan had two treatments on two consecutive days with the physiotherapist and, within that time, the pain worsened. He returned to the physiotherapist following a week's bed rest with less pain but increased neurological deficits. The physiotherapist had not followed up with Dan by calling between visits. Two weeks later Dan attended the emergency department of a public hospital in severe pain. After a magnetic resonance imaging (MRI) investigation, he underwent surgery for a prolapsed L4–5 disc. Dan was left with residual neurological injuries, including a foot drop. The physiotherapist worried that she might be blamed for exacerbating the patient's problem and whether she should have insisted on an MRI scan before any manual treatment. Dan is seeking advice as to whether to sue the physiotherapist on the basis that the initial treatment was negligent.

What Are the Legal Issues That Arise From This Case?

Case 5 raises a number of clear legal issues concerning whether the physiotherapist has been negligent.

Duty of Care. There is no doubt in law that a health practitioner owes a duty of care to their patient. There is no factual basis to believe that the facts of this case fall outside of the duty of care, and the physiotherapist owed a clear duty of care to Dan.

Standard of Care. As health practitioners the standard of care expected of physiotherapists is that they are expected to treat patients in a manner that could reasonably be expected of a person professing to be an ordinary, skilled physiotherapist (Chapters 4 and 6). Legal requirements set out in Chapter 6 describe overall standards of care as being met if they represent those of an ordinary skilled person exercising and professing to have the special skill. These standards are based on:

- the standards of care set by the profession (physiotherapy guidelines, position statements and expert opinion about the particular area of clinical practice)
- the best available evidence about what constitutes appropriate physiotherapy assessment, diagnosis and management of lumbar spine pain
- the documentation made by the physiotherapist as to the assessment, tests used, test results, treatment, advice, warnings and information given.

Wrongful Acts or Omissions? (Breach of Duty of Care). To determine liability, it is necessary to evaluate whether the acts or omissions of the physiotherapist fell below the standard of care of a reasonable physiotherapist. Identifying the exact breaches is crucial to determining this question. Dan's lawyer has suggested that, in this case, negligence may comprise:

- an omission to appropriately test for nerve involvement (neurological testing)
- failure to diagnose appropriately
- failure to refer to a medical colleague for a second opinion or for a scan
- failure to provide sufficient information about the nature of the problem and the options for treatment and further assessment.

It is reasonably foreseeable that such breaches may lead to harm and that the risk was not insignificant.

A court would therefore ask what a reasonable physiotherapist would have done in the circumstances. In relation to the failures to test, diagnose or refer for a second opinion/scan, whether the acts or omissions fell below the reasonable standard of care of a physiotherapist will

be determined by reference to evidence of what the profession would consider to be acceptable practice. Such practice does not need to be universal but needs to be widely supported. (See Chapter 6.)

In relation to the failure to give adequate advice or warnings, the court will determine whether the actions of the physiotherapist were reasonable. Chapter 5 outlines the requirements for giving information and obtaining informed consent. This includes the need to warn the patient about the potential risks of treatment and alternatives to the proposed care. The scope of advice and information a physiotherapist is expected to give is detailed in that chapter. It includes:

- information about the nature of physiotherapy treatment and other care options
- warnings as to possible adverse outcomes of treatment or no treatment
- estimation as to the degree of uncertainty or outcome associated with treatments
- time and cost involved and any aspect of the procedure that is especially costly or protracted.

Chapter 5 also reminds us that the information provided to the patient needs to be in language that the patient may understand.

Applying this all to the facts of the case, the practitioner would be reasonably expected to inform the patient of the risk of exacerbating their complaint and/or progression to a disc herniation. Failure to provide this information may mean that valid consent has not been obtained.

It is likely that the physiotherapist's acts and omissions will be found to have fallen below the expected standard of care of a reasonable physiotherapist.

Did the Breach Cause Harm/Injury?

In negligence it is important to determine not only whether the acts or omissions fell below the standard of care but also whether such breaches *caused* the harm/injury/loss suffered by Dan. Two main questions arise in the circumstances:

1. Did the failures in relation to diagnosis, testing and treatment exacerbate Dan's injuries? The answer to this question will be determined by reference to medical evidence. If yes, then the physiotherapist will be liable to compensate Dan.

2. Given adequate information and/or warnings, would Dan have proceeded with treatment? The answer will be determined by looking at evidence (if any) of what Dan would have done. If Dan would not have had treatment, would have delayed treatment and sought a second opinion, or would have asked for alternate treatment, it is likely that the physiotherapist will be held liable to compensate Dan for his harm/losses.

Note, Dan only needs to succeed in any one of the arguments that a particular breach caused his injury/harm/loss in order to receive compensation.

Podiatry

(Contributor: Nikolaus Nikolopolous)

CASE 1: INCOMPLETE PATIENT NOTES

This is John's first job as a podiatrist. He is working at a well-known clinic with some of the most experienced practitioners in the area. Being new, he does not have his own case load and is being referred clients by his colleagues in the practice. Upon reviewing the medical and treatment history of one such client, he notices that the history and note taking is incomplete and that the notes have not been signed. On most notes there is simply a line stating 'to be completed later'. He notices that this stretches to almost 12 months ago, with repeated incomplete, unclear entries. John instantly becomes anxious. He is uncertain as to the client's history and previous treatment, does not want to seem foolish asking the client about previous treatments and does not want to make his colleague look bad by indicating that the notes are below standard. He is also concerned because he does not want to cause any trouble – this is his first job, he is grateful to be working where he is and does not want to jeopardise his employment and future.

What Are the Ethical Issues That Arise From This Case?

- Does John need to inform the client that their medical and treatment history is incomplete?
- Does John have a responsibility to ensure that the medical and treatment history is such that he is able to perform his duties at a reasonable standard based on the information contained within?

- Does John have a responsibility to make his colleague or anyone else, such as a regulatory body, aware of his findings?

What Could Be the Personal Reaction to This Case?

It is understandable that John may feel anxious. He is balancing the needs of his client with the fact that he is a new practitioner, in a new role, working with colleagues who are more experienced than he. He knows that there is somewhat of a power imbalance.

John wants to be liked and to forge a successful career as a podiatrist and is worried about the possible repercussions of raising this as an issue.

He is feeling very uncomfortable about the fact that the client may be put at risk by way of an incomplete medical and treatment history. This could also lead to errors in treatment and decision making and he knows that his colleague is falling short of the expected standards.

What Facts May Be Relevant Regarding This Situation?

The information in the client's file is incomplete. John will rely on this information to treat the client. The notes indicate that there are areas to be completed at a later date, but this is yet to occur. The practitioner in question is very experienced and may have a leading role in determining John's progression and future as a podiatrist. John's colleague may have just had a few bad months and is planning on completing and finalising all notes as required.

What Values May Be at Stake?

The stakeholders are the client, John, the clinic management and staff.

From the client's perspective, it is their right for information to be correct, contemporaneous, accurate and be able to be relied upon (see Chapters 3 and 5).

John may consider that he has been put in a difficult position. It is his responsibility to ensure that information is able to be used for the purposes for which it has been provided.

Based on workplace arrangements and employment law contracts, other staff may be liable for the behaviour of those who work on the premises.

What Are the Options in This Case?

- John may choose to undertake his treatment, complete his notes and do nothing else.
- John could discuss the matter with his colleague and not bring it to the attention of anyone else.
- John may bring the matter to the attention of clinic management.
- John could report his colleague to AHPRA – the Podiatry Board of Australia.

What Should Occur in This Case?

Medical records are expected to be accurate, up-to-date and contemporaneous. They serve as a form of communication between practitioners, a record of what has occurred during treatment, the history of the patient, relevant treatment and socio-demographic details. There are clearly defined standards that need to be met across jurisdictions regarding the keeping of medical records and note taking. The key factors are that such information should be clear, concise, accurate and relevant (see Chapter 5 and the Podiatry Board of Australia's *Podiatry Guidelines on Clinical Records*). In a practical sense, this means that information must be objective in nature, must be included at the time and must be able to be evaluated by independent parties – that is, by someone other than the person who made the notes.

In this situation John has a responsibility both to the client and to the clinic. He has a professional obligation to ensure that information within the record at the time of his accessing the record is accurate, on point, relevant and able to be used to further the best interests of the client.

John may consider undertaking one or all of the following:

- informing the client that there are elements within the medical history that need to be reviewed and to do so
- identifying the areas for review and completing these accurately while not informing the client
- notifying clinic management of the issues and doing nothing else
- reporting his colleague to AHPRA, which John has an obligation to do.

Ultimately, the responsibility at this point in time rests with John, as he is aware of the matter and is treating the patient. He is required to complete areas requiring review, ensure that information is relevant, inform the client of gaps in the medical record in so far as these gaps and omissions affect the client, notify clinic management and report his colleague to AHPRA.

Could the Problem Have Been Prevented?

This ethical problem could be prevented by ensuring that all practitioners are aware of the relevant guidelines for note taking, by ensuring there are regular audits of medical files, that staff attend professional development sessions regarding these matters and that there is an environment where practitioners feel comfortable bringing these issues to the attention of fellow colleagues and also clinic management.

CASE 2: ISSUES OF CONSENT

Jemima's toe hurts, so she makes an appointment to see you. She thinks it may be infected and wants to have the problem sorted because she is a keen runner, and this has stopped her in her tracks. During the consultation, you tell Jemima that she has an ingrown toenail. Given that she is a runner, you suggest that she might benefit from a musculoskeletal and biomechanical assessment. You undertake the assessment and determine that she requires foot orthoses. Prior to treating her toenail, you check that Jemima has completed all of the necessary paperwork and you discuss issues of consent, even though she has already signed the practice's informed consent form. You request that Jemima returns in a week so you can check the state of her foot. She does so and during this consultation you present her with a pair of foot orthoses. Jemima looks at you quizzically, saying that she doesn't recall requesting a pair of orthoses. You respond by indicating to her that she signed the consent form, that you discussed the nature of treatment regarding orthotics and that you undertook assessments leading to orthotic prescription. You give Jemima an invoice for the orthoses.

Jemima is very upset, telling you that she consented to treatment for her toenail, not for a pair of foot orthoses. You tell her that 'consent is consent' and that she signed the informed consent form.

What Are the Legal/Ethical Issues That Arise From This Case?

This case gives rise to both ethical and legal issues concerning consent.

The nature of consent and, in particular, informed consent refers to a client having all the material information in order to make an informed decision and consent to treatment or refuse treatment (see Chapters 3, 5 and 6). This means that information provided has to be relevant to the course of treatment, the course of care and include factors that may influence a person's decision making regarding a particular course of care.

The major issue in this case is whether informed consent provided for treatment relates to the treatment of the toenail and the prescription of the foot orthoses or for the former alone.

What Could Be the Personal Reaction to This Case?

It may well be that the practitioner in this situation has not sought to take advantage of the client and clearly believes that based on the information provided to Jemima and her agreement to sign the consent form that she does in fact understand and has in fact provided informed consent regarding all treatment.

Jemima's personal reaction may be that she provided informed consent in relation to treating her toenail and at no time did she provide consent for orthoses to be made. To her mind, it was a discussion and assessment regarding musculoskeletal and biomechanical factors.

What Facts May Be Relevant Regarding This Situation?

Jemima has attended the practice for treatment for a particular problem and she is aware that she is to be treated for her ingrown toenail.

Any additional treatment is information to be taken on notice and is subject to additional consent.

What Values May Be at Stake?

From the client's perspective, values at stake include autonomy with respect to the decision-making and informed consent processes.

From the practitioner's perspective this would relate to ensuring there is respect for autonomy and that all matters relevant to consent have been considered. The practitioner may indeed feel aggrieved by the fact that the client may be suggesting that the practitioner acted improperly.

What Are the Options in This Case?

One option would be for the client to pay for the orthoses upon establishing that this is a course of care that she will benefit from.

Another option may be for the practitioner to provide all the information at this stage, receive informed consent regarding this form of treatment, prescribe the devices, issue the orthoses and deal with the necessary financial arrangements.

The practitioner may choose to absorb the costs of treatment and not pursue the matter further.

Jemima may choose to refer the practitioner to AHPRA and the Podiatry Board of Australia for breach of the code of conduct.

What Should Have Occurred in This Case?

The practitioner should have a clear and unambiguous understanding of the granting of informed consent. In the absence of specific informed consent regarding this course of care, the client may assert that she did not provide consent for the foot orthoses.

Informed consent was provided for the specific complaint during initial attendance, with risks, treatment procedure and information provided on that front. This informed consent is not overarching and does not include forms of treatment that significantly depart from the reason for which the original consent was granted. The extensive financial imposition on the client may also aggravate the situation.

In this case, the practitioner should discuss the fact that additional informed consent should have been sought and provide options to Jemima to provide or refuse such consent. Insisting that Jemima provided informed consent for orthotic treatment would be inappropriate.

Could the Problem Have Been Prevented?

The clinic and practitioners may consider having various documents that provide information about a variety of courses of care and specific consent forms related to such care. Consent forms that are completed by clients may indicate their consent to treatment related to the reason for their presentation and whether they consent to alternate courses of care. Where additional treatment is to be provided or additional costs incurred, additional informed and financial consent needs to be sought.

CASE 3: SOCIAL MEDIA

Stephanie is very excited because she has just opened her new clinic and is well on the way to establishing a great reputation, a great service and a great future. She was also very keen to take advantage of her special skills in promotion and marketing, particularly those related to social media. As luck would have it, one of her first clients is a well-known sportsperson. Stephanie is thrilled and is keen to not only provide the best service to the client but also feels this may be a perfect opportunity to promote her clinic. Towards the end of the consultation, she asks if it would be okay to take a photograph with her famous client – after all, the client is pleased with the service and has just told Stephanie that she would come back when required. Stephanie takes the picture and her client leaves. Later that same day, Stephanie decides to upload the photograph to the clinic's social media account. Underneath the photograph she writes 'Leading the way, treating Australia's finest'. The picture is clear, so there is no doubt as to who the client is. She posts the photo and goes on her merry way. Stephanie has now received a letter from her client's representatives stating that she has used the photograph for purposes other than that for which it was taken, that the client did not provide consent for the photograph to be used in such a manner and that she will be referred to AHPRA regarding her conduct. Stephanie is very stressed about the situation and is unclear as to what to do next.

What Are the Legal/Ethical Issues That Arise From This Case?

Stephanie has taken an image and used this image to promote her clinic. This raises legal and ethical issues with respect to client confidentiality, autonomy, consent and breach of advertising standards (see Chapters 3, 4 and 5).

What Could Be the Personal Reaction to This Case?

Stephanie may feel that upon receiving consent to take the photograph she would be able to use that photograph in any way she felt necessary, given that the client was comfortable with the photograph being taken.

From the client's perspective, it is reasonable to assume that consent was provided for the taking of the photograph but not for its distribution. The client did not waive their right to confidentiality and at no stage was it made clear that the photograph would be used for marketing and mass distribution.

What Facts May Be Relevant Regarding This Situation?

Matters to be considered include Stephanie's request to take the photograph. It could be argued that in her position as a care provider she should maintain a level of professionalism that relates to the treatment alone. Further, she is a position of power and influence over her client, who may feel compelled to agree to having the photo taken.

The photograph was taken for a specific purpose, for her personal collection, and as such its use should be limited to this. Alternatively, no consent was provided for the photograph to be used in the manner it has.

The client's image has been used for marketing purposes and may be indicating that there is a commercial agreement between the parties.

What Values May Be at Stake?

From the client's perspective, the image has been used in a manner for which consent has not been granted. Confidentiality has been breached, and issues regarding autonomy arise.

In Stephanie's case, she has potentially breached her obligations regarding maintaining client confidentiality and the code of conduct and advertising standards as set out by the Podiatry Board of Australia.

The management company may indicate that the image is being used to suggest a commercial relationship between the parties and therefore suggest that this is actionable.

What Are the Options in This Case?

The client could consider personal action against Stephanie and refer her to AHPRA. As such, Stephanie may be sanctioned for breach of code of conduct and social media guidelines by AHPRA.

The management company could take legal action against Stephanie. To minimise risk, Stephanie could delete the post and provide a formal apology to her client and representatives. Alternatively, she may enter into a commercial arrangement with her client – subject to lawful execution.

What Should Occur in This Case?

Issues regarding matters of confidentiality and breach of standards should be considered and it would be wise for Stephanie to remove all posts. This would be in keeping with the request of the client and respecting autonomy in the decision-making process.

Stephanie should apologise to all parties concerned regarding her actions. Even if inadvertent, she has breached her profession's regulatory standards.

Stephanie needs to be counselled about the guidelines regarding the use of social media, matters of practitioner–client confidentiality, interaction with clients and the relevant codes of conduct.

Could the Problem Have Been Prevented?

The need for health practitioners to be comprehensively aware of issues of confidentiality and avenues for the breach is imperative. Stephanie must have a working knowledge of, and is subject to, guidelines regarding advertising, the code of conduct and use of social media.

The situation would have been prevented if Stephanie had not engaged in behaviour that is contrary to the reason for which the client attended.

CASE 4: ACCEPTING GIFTS

According to George, the best thing about being a podiatrist is being able to help people. George loves how appreciative his clients are; it simply makes him feel great. He has a fantastic relationship with his clients – they know all about his family and he knows of theirs. During a consultation, one of George's clients, Sophie, decides to give him a gift. She knows that George loves to play the guitar and as a 'thank you' she presents George with a brand-new acoustic guitar. George tells Sophie that he is grateful for the gift but that he cannot accept it. Sophie tells George that she is so pleased with him that it is the 'least she could do' and that if he does not accept the gift she will be offended. Unsure of what to do next, George accepts the gift. This whole episode is really playing on George's mind. He doesn't know what to do, so he approaches you for advice.

What Are the Legal/Ethical Issues That Arise From This Case?

- Does accepting the gift put George in a position where he may be seen to have an actual or perceived conflict of interest?
- Will the client expect preferential treatment on a professional or personal level after giving the gift?
- Does the acceptance or otherwise of the gift depend on its monetary or other value?

What Could Be the Personal Reaction to This Case?

George may feel very proud of the fact that his client validates his efforts by giving him the guitar. It is also understandable that George may feel uncomfortable with the size of the gift or with the idea of receiving a gift regardless of its size or value. George may question how his acceptance of such a gift would influence the client–practitioner relationship. George may also feel rather embarrassed about the whole situation.

Sophie is clearly so pleased with the level of service that she may consider this a mere token of her appreciation. Sophie may consider that the non-acceptance of such a gift would mean that George is not validating her actions and feelings. Sophie may feel that she deserves preferential treatment as a result of the gift.

What Facts May Be Relevant Regarding This Situation?

George regularly shares information about his life with his clients. It helps build the relationship with his clients and at no stage has he ever been inappropriate.

Sophie is clearly doing everything she can to indicate to George that she is appreciative of his help. Sophie has provided the guitar to George and George has accepted this.

What Values May Be at Stake?

The stakeholders are the client, George, the clinic management and staff.

Sophie may feel it is her right to provide a gift and that refusal of such a gift would be offensive.

George feels that even though he has accepted the gift, he has a responsibility to ensure that neither Sophie nor any other client feels obliged to provide such gifts. George is being remunerated for his work as part of his employment and he must manage this matter so that he is not put in a position of conflict.

Based on workplace arrangements and employment law contracts there may be guidelines regarding giving and accepting gifts.

What Are the Options in This Case?

George may choose to receive the gift, as he has done, and enjoy playing the guitar or he may choose to return the gift to the client. George may also check as to whether his workplace has a gift registry whereby all gifts of a value and/or type need to be registered. George may also pass on the gift in such a manner so that it is not of direct benefit to him – for example, by donating it to charity. He may turn to the code of conduct as set out by the Podiatry Board of Australia for guidance.

What Should Occur in This Case?

Practitioners should not act in any manner that may place them in a perceived or actual conflict of interest (refer to the code of conduct as set out by the Podiatry Board of Australia). This may include accepting gifts and the perception that clients may need to provide gifts to receive standard or preferential treatment.

In this situation George should contact the client and make it clear that, while he is appreciative of her actions and the intent behind the giving of the gift, he cannot keep the guitar. George may provide alternate options such as passing the guitar on to charity in the client's name. Otherwise, George may choose to have the gift returned to the client, indicating that gift-giving of this nature and of this magnitude is potentially contrary to his profession's code of conduct.

It is important to recognise that in this situation George has a responsibility to his profession, his client and his workplace to ensure that, among other possibilities:

- a culture of gratuitous gift-giving is not established
- the client and/or other clients do not feel obliged to provide gifts
- he does not benefit in a manner contrary to the code of conduct through his relationship with this client. (Note, it is expected that he is being paid. But even if he was a volunteer, George is still bound by his profession's code of conduct.)

Could the Problem Have Been Prevented?

This ethical problem could be prevented by ensuring George's workplace has a clear policy with respect to the giving and accepting of gifts. This may include guidelines regarding what is acceptable. Typically, a travel souvenir of modest value given to a practitioner by a client would be considered differently from giving a brand-new guitar.

George must have a working knowledge of, and is subject to, his profession's code of conduct. Even in the absence of specific workplace policies regarding such matters, George is still expected to act in accordance with relevant regulatory codes.

CASE 5: POSSIBLE ELDER ABUSE

Jack has recently moved in with his daughter and her family. In the space of a year, he has become widowed, sold the family home and left his old neighbourhood. This is Jack's third visit to your clinic and you feel like you are building a solid rapport with him. Today though, Jack seems somewhat withdrawn. You ask him if he is okay and he responds that things are a little tricky at home; he feels like he is imposing on his daughter and her family. While chatting to Jack, you notice some marks around his neck. Concerned that he may have fallen, you ask him about these marks. Jack tells you not to worry about it: 'It's nothing,' he says.

As you examine the back of his right leg you notice a series of bruises, and looking at his hands, they too appear bruised. You ask Jack how he got the bruises. While doing his best to avoid your question, he does tell you that they are not the result of a fall. Concerned that he may be in some sort of danger you feel that you should do something. You suspect that Jack may be a target of elder abuse. What should you do?

What Are the Legal/Ethical Issues That Arise From This Case?

- Should you report your suspicions to anyone? What if you are incorrect? (ethical, legal)
- Do you have a mandatory reporting obligation? (legal) (see Chapters 4 and 16)
- Are you interfering with the client's right of autonomy? (ethical)

What Could Be the Personal Reaction to This Case?

You feel uncertain about what to do. Jack has not told you anything and you cannot be sure of what is happening. You suspect he may be a victim of abuse and feel it is your responsibility to act somehow. However, is it your position to delve into Jack's private life?

Jack may feel embarrassed because of his situation. He may not want to involve the authorities or cause trouble for his family and/or social network. Jack may not trust you enough to divulge the true state of affairs.

What Facts May Be Relevant Regarding This Situation?

- Jack has attended his consultation with multiple marks on his body.
- You do not know the origin of these marks.
- Jack has indicated that 'things are tricky' at home.

- Jack has indicated that these injuries were not sustained during a fall.
- Jack has said you should not worry about the origin of his injuries.
- You suspect that the injuries sustained may be a result of elder abuse.

What Values May Be at Stake?

Your ultimate responsibility as a practitioner is for the care and wellbeing of your patient. This relates to their physical, emotional and financial wellbeing in the context of your role as a podiatrist.

As a care provider, you are called upon to make an assessment in the best interests of your patient. This assessment is based on the facts as they stand. Your commitment to your patient is an overarching obligation.

What Are the Options in This Case?

- You may choose to do nothing based on assurances from Jack that everything is fine.
- You may choose to make enquiries of Jack's family, to contact family members or next of kin to assist in determining whether Jack is at risk and to find out what happened.
- You may refer the matter directly to welfare authorities and/or the police based on your suspicions.

What Should Occur in This Case?

The identification of, protection from and reporting of elder abuse is not subject to an accepted national framework, as is the matter of child abuse (see Chapter 16). However, your obligation is to act in the best interests of your patient. If you feel that your patient is genuinely at risk, practitioner– patient confidentiality may be breached in good faith.

Incidents of elder abuse may be dealt with under the criminal law, potentially as episodes of domestic violence. As such, there would be a call for notification to be made to the police in situations where elder abuse is suspected.

Could the Problem Have Been Prevented?

Practitioners must be aware of what behaviour classifies as elder abuse, the overt signs and signals and those that may be difficult to detect.

Practitioners must be clear on when they may need to make a report based on information received during the practitioner–patient relationship and based on their observations. Establishing a referral pathway for instances where elder abuse is suspected would assist in providing some clarity and support for practitioners and appropriate outcomes for patients.

Practitioners must also have a clear understanding of principles underpinning and regulating the exchange of information between practitioner and patient, such as confidentiality. In addition, practitioners must have a working knowledge of, and are subject to, their profession's code of conduct. Refer to the APHRA website (Podiatry Board of Australia), even in the absence of specific workplace policies regarding such matters.

Speech Pathology
(Contributors: Trish Johnson and Suze Leitao)

CASE 1: INADEQUATE FUNDING AND SERVICE DELIVERY

Sebastian (aged 36 years) has recently moved from living at home with his parents into a group home. Sebastian has a moderate–severe intellectual disability with limited expressive and receptive communication. His elderly mother has never sought speech pathology services for him before so was unaware of the possibility of developing an effective system to communicate with other people. Sebastian has been provided funding for six hours of speech pathology to set up a communication system so he can participate in activities of daily living. The manager of the home contacts Jerome, a speech pathologist with significant experience and expertise in augmentative and alternative communication (AAC) and in developing communication skills using a variety of AAC formats and devices. Jerome is extremely concerned that the funded time will not be sufficient for the assessment and intervention required, including the need for staff training to support Sebastian. Jerome speaks with the manager about accessing more funds to increase the time allocated. The manager says that the organisation is unable to fund any more time and tells Jerome to just use what is allocated and to 'do what can be done in the time' and that anything extra is 'not the responsibility of the organisation'.

What Are the Legal/Ethical Issues That Arise From This Case?

- Jerome has an ethical obligation to provide evidence-based interventions that deliver benefits to clients.

- The evidence shows that six hours of speech pathology is insufficient to provide benefit to a client in this context.
- The demand being placed on the speech pathologist to provide insufficient intervention could potentially be considered a breach of duty of care for Sebastian.

What Could Be the Personal Reaction to This Case?

Jerome may feel concerned that the external funding limitation may place him in a position of not providing evidence-based practice or 'best practice' care. (From a legal perspective, apart from Jerome's ethical obligation, a breach of that duty of care could potentially be considered negligence, as described in Chapter 6.)

Jerome may be worried that little benefit can be achieved for Sebastian within the funded time and that a 'poor' result may influence access to further appropriate levels of funding. Further, he may be aware that an ineffective use of AAC may impact on Sebastian, his family and the group home staff's understanding of the possible benefit of AAC and engagement with AAC and speech pathology in the future.

Flowing on from this may be feelings of frustration that professional knowledge is not recognised and respected.

What Facts May Be Relevant Regarding This Situation?

- Sebastian has recently moved into a group home.
- He has a moderate–severe intellectual disability with limited expressive and receptive communication. The residents and care staff are all new to him and he will have difficulty communicating with them. He has no current AAC support to assist effective communication.
- Sebastian would benefit from the opportunity to have access to AAC so he can participate more in activities of daily living.
- Funding is only available for six hours to identify an appropriate mode of AAC and to set up and implement a system and training for others to support Sebastian to use the AAC.
- Six hours is not considered adequate to assess, prescribe, set up and implement an AAC system and to provide training for carers.

- The manager has said there is no more funding and has directed Jerome to do what he can in six hours.

What Values May Be at Stake?

This scenario challenges the values of integrity, professionalism, respect and care as well as quality standards and continuing competence for the speech pathologist.

Jerome is seeking to balance beneficence and non-maleficence for Sebastian while providing a service that is considered at an appropriate level for the duty of care he has to Sebastian.

Service provision is an element included in Speech Pathology Australia's *Competency based Occupational Standards* (2011), specifically: 'Element 4.2 Implement an evidence-based speech pathology intervention according to the information obtained from speech pathology assessment, interpretation and planning'.

The Speech Pathology Australia *Code of Ethics* (2010) also contains professional obligations regarding duty of care in Principle 2.3 Fairness (Justice): 'We provide accurate information. We strive to provide clients with access to services consistent with their need'.

What Are the Options in This Case?

Jerome could:

- go ahead and do the best he can in six hours
- refuse to prescribe any AAC system because six hours will not achieve benefit and may be detrimental to future engagement with AAC
- attempt to find alternative sources of funding
- meet with the manager to argue the case for why extra funding should be sought to allow time to achieve a significant improvement in Sebastian's ability to communicate, which will benefit him as well as staff
- meet with Sebastian's elderly mother to inform her about AAC and the benefits for her son
- use the six hours to assess Sebastian and prepare a report for the funding agency. The report could identify how adequate funding would allow an appropriate AAC method to be selected and pay for training for carers to support Sebastian to use it so he can achieve his participation goals.

What Should Have Occurred in This Case?

Jerome has a duty of care to provide evidence-based practice for clients. A casuistry approach to ethical reasoning involves drawing on the knowledge and experience gained from previous cases to inform decisions.[35] Jerome can use his experience to inform the selection of appropriate AAC.

Jerome also has an obligation to advocate for an appropriate level of funding for this client.

Jerome should use the current allocated funding to begin the assessment to select an appropriate AAC method and to prepare a report to support allocating further funding at a level to allow for a service that will provide benefit to Sebastian.

Could the Problem Have Been Prevented?

Community capacity building to develop an understanding of the value and cost-benefit of AAC is an important advocacy role for a speech pathologist. Education of the public and funding agencies could have averted the inappropriately small allocation of funds in the first instance.

Jerome may be able to develop an ongoing professional relationship with the manager to improve the manager's understanding of appropriate access to services and actions that satisfy duty of care.

CASE 2: CONSENT, PRIVACY AND CONFIDENTIALITY – DIAGNOSIS

Jill, a speech pathologist, told the parents of Chloe, aged five, that she thought their child's communication problems were related to autism. While both parents respected the speech pathologist and had been quite pleased with her services to date, they were shocked and disputed the diagnosis. Neither parent had noticed any unusual behaviour and said that Chloe had recently started to see a pediatrician, who had not mentioned anything about autism. They told Jill that it was not her role to make such a diagnosis. They were extremely distressed when their daughter started kindergarten to find that the speech pathologist had contacted the kindergarten in relation to their child's communication problems. In the conversation with the kindergarten director, the speech pathologist had raised the notion of autism. The parents feel that the kindergarten, having heard this information from a professional, is treating their child differently – for example, by labelling behaviours that the parents consider to be normal as 'autistic'. They are concerned that this inappropriate 'label' will now stick with their child even though, in their opinion, it is not an accurate diagnosis.

What Are the Legal/Ethical Issues That Arise From This Case?

This case raises issues regarding consent, privacy and confidentiality. It is not clear that the speech pathologist has consent to share information regarding her client with others. The issue is complicated by the fact that the diagnosis is disputed by the parents but does not mitigate the fact that a practitioner should have informed consent to share information.

Confidentiality is important in establishing and maintaining trust between a practitioner and their clients. There is also a legal obligation not to breach the privacy or confidentiality of patient information.

What Could Be the Personal Reaction to This Case?

It appears that Jill spoke about the child without the parents' permission, relaying information that was not even confirmed, and breaching confidence.

It seems as if Jill has taken an 'expert knows best' view and has not considered the feelings and wishes of the family. Jill has either not felt that she needed to obtain permission or has decided it is in the best interests of the child for her to let the kindergarten know about her view. It may be that Jill works with a few other children at the same kindergarten and does not want the teacher to think she knew Chloe had difficulties but had not told her. It may also be that Jill was worried that Chloe needed extra support at kindergarten; therefore felt she had an obligation to tell the teacher her concerns.

What Facts May Be Relevant Regarding This Situation?

- A diagnosis has not been made by an interdisciplinary team.
- The speech pathologist does not appear to have spoken to the paediatrician or followed up the discussion with the family.
- Consent does not appear to have been sought nor provided to disclose information.

What Values May Be at Stake?

This case raises issues around the values of integrity, professionalism, respect and care and autonomy. It also raises issues of consent and confidentiality.

Taking a narrative approach to ethical reasoning, we do not know the back stories of those involved.[36]

Why does the speech pathologist feel confident to make a diagnosis without discussing it with the paediatrician and given the parents' concerns? Why are the parents shocked about the possible diagnosis, and why do they not feel that autism is a possibility? It would be important to consider their voices in this scenario and try to understand their perspectives.

Confidentiality is a standard included in Speech Pathology Australia's *Code of Ethics* (2010):

> *3.1.4 Confidentiality: We treat as confidential all information we handle in the course of our professional services. We do not disclose information about our clients, or the confidences they share with us, unless: our clients consent to this; the law requires us to disclose it; or there are compelling moral and ethical reasons for us to disclose it.*

The value of professionalism also states: 'we provide professional services irrespective of our personal interests, aims and opinions'.

As mentioned in Chapter 5, it is important to remember that health professionals are under a strict ethical and legal duty to keep patient information confidential ('secret') unless the law permits disclosure.

What Are the Options in This Case?

The speech pathologist could arrange a meeting with the parents to acknowledge their concerns regarding confidentiality and to discuss her assessment findings and identify an appropriate plan of services that the parents agree with.

A case conference could be arranged with all stakeholders – the parents, the speech pathologist, the paediatrician and the kindergarten teacher – for all to present their perspectives and reflect on the implications for this child.

The parents might consider making a complaint about the speech pathologist to her professional association for sharing information without their consent.

What Should Occur in This Case?

Respectful communication with the parents is an imperative for managing this situation. A meeting with the parents would allow them to air their concerns regarding confidentiality and discuss the impact they foresee on their daughter's future. The discussion could allow the speech pathologist to demonstrate respect for their position and acknowledge their perspective.

The speech pathologist could provide information to support her professional opinion and present the benefits of a case conference with all stakeholders. This would provide an opportunity for all to present their perspectives and reflect on the implications for this child and would allow them to create a future story that will provide the best-case scenario for Chloe.

The speech pathologist needs to review her understanding of privacy and confidentiality and should develop a clear protocol for obtaining consent to share information.

Could the Problem Have Been Prevented?

As outlined in Chapter 5, it is clear that the speech pathologist must ensure consent is obtained to release any client-related information and maintain confidentiality. Confidentiality relates to nondisclosure of all information that comes to a speech pathologist during their relationship with a client, who has control over their information.

- Sharing information without consent falls below the expected standard of care and breaches the code of ethics.
- The speech pathologist must comply with the Speech Pathology Australia *Code of Ethics* and is obliged to follow federal laws. She should therefore be familiar with privacy legislation including the Commonwealth *Privacy Act 1988* and the Australian Privacy Principles.
- It is also an ethical obligation for speech pathologists to not be influenced by personal interests in their professional work.
- The speech pathologist must be mindful of acting in a professional manner in all situations and be aware where personal interests may potentially influence actions.
- Having an understanding of her professional obligations and a clear protocol for obtaining consent during intake procedures would act to prevent this scenario taking place.

CASE 3: POOR RECORD KEEPING

Gemma sends an email to an advisor at her professional association:

'I'm the manager of a private practice where we employed a part-time speech pathologist who only stayed with us for six months and has now moved overseas for work. A mother asked me for the report from her child's assessment with this speech pathologist, which took place four months ago, because she is moving to another city and needs it to apply for support at school. When I looked in the child's file I couldn't find all the information that should have been there. There are only about six file note entries for therapy sessions, but our system shows this child attended at least 20 sessions. I then conducted a quick audit of most of her case load files and I've discovered there are a lot of gaps in most of them – progress notes are missing, for example. I made sure I used the Speech Pathology Australia proforma to develop our *Policy and procedures manual*, and our clinic has all the right forms. I'm sure I went through all this with the speech pathologist when she started.

'What do I tell this mother?'

What Are the Legal/Ethical Issues That Arise From This Case?

This case raises a number of ethical and legal issues:

- The speech pathologist has not complied with her record-keeping responsibilities.
- The speech pathologist has not complied with her responsibilities to the client.
- The practice manager, Gemma, is concerned that her clinic has not maintained accurate patient records.
- The family needs an accurate and up-to-date report to apply for support for the child, who may lose access to services in the short (and even long) term without this information.

As described in Chapter 5, records serve to facilitate optimal patient outcomes provided they are accurate and up to date. The lack of records in this case undermines confidence in the professional services provided.

What Could Be the Personal Reaction to This Case?

Gemma is very angry and feels let down by the speech pathologist. She feels she did the right thing by developing policy documents and forms for the practice to support compliance with ethical and legal obligations,

and by alerting the employee to these. However, she is concerned that she should have done more to ensure compliance with the policy. She is very worried about what to tell the parents and the implications for them and her practice.

What Facts May Be Relevant Regarding This Situation?

- The manager was asked to provide a copy of a report for a child by the mother.
- The report is not in the file, and neither are many case notes.
- Upon further checking, case notes are missing from many of this speech pathologist's client files.
- The family requires a copy of the report because they are moving interstate and it is required for an application for support at school and to inform a new clinician.
- The speech pathologist who saw the child has left the practice and is now working overseas.

What Values May Be at Stake?

This case raises issues around the values of integrity, professionalism, respect and care as well as quality standards and continuing competence.

Assessment reporting is an element described in Speech Pathology Australia's *Competency based Occupational Standards* (2011), specifically: Element 2.4 'Report on analysis and interpretation', Element 2.5 'Provide feedback on results of interpreted speech pathology assessments to the client and/or significant others and referral sources, and discuss management', and Element 5.2 'Use and maintain an efficient information management system'.

The performance criteria that apply to these elements include:

- 'Maintain efficient systems of records, consistent with organisational requirements, for the purposes of service delivery, planning, accountability, monitoring client status and ensuring a high quality of service.
- Consistently apply quality management and continuous improvement principles.
- Show ability to comply with workplace requirements for electronic record keeping, data collection and video conferencing.

- Demonstrate a capacity to use or learn other relevant programs as required. Information management system education must be provided by the employer in a timely manner to ensure ethical delivery of services'.

The Speech Pathology Australia *Code of Ethics* (2010) describes the relevant ethical obligation in standard 3.1.2 Accurate and Timely Information: 'We make sure that our clients and the community receive accurate and current information in a timely manner. This includes information relating to: clinical assessment and research results and the implications of these'.

As outlined in Chapter 5, documentation of patient information should be contemporaneous with the event. Preparing a record at a much later date may not be seen as an appropriate professional record.

What Are the Options in This Case?

The manager could:

- tell the family that nothing can be done (she could also offer to fund an assessment by a new speech pathologist once the family has moved)
- offer a free review assessment and report as soon as possible
- attempt to create a report using the notes that exist.

In addition, the manager could:

- attempt to contact the speech pathologist
- consider making a complaint regarding unprofessional conduct of the speech pathologist to the Speech Pathology Australia ethics board.

What Should Occur in This Case?

Gemma should be honest with the family about the missing information and offer a free review assessment with another speech pathologist in the practice and a new report as soon as possible. This would allow the family to apply for funding to support the child.

In addition, she should put a plan in place to review clinic procedures, including documentation and training for new staff, regular audits of clinic files and exit procedures when staff leave the practice.

Could the Problem Have Been Prevented?

Taking a proactive approach would involve more than simply developing and having policies and procedures for practice staff. It would involve clear training, a clear understanding of obligations, regular audits and compliance checks, creating a culture of appropriate management of healthcare information.

Adopting a proactive approach will minimise the risk of similar issues arising in the future through improved governance and develop the professionalism of the workplace culture.

CASE 4: WORSENING DYSPHAGIA, REFUSAL OF FOOD MODIFICATIONS

Emma is a speech pathologist who works with a client, Maria, living with advanced multiple sclerosis (MS). Maria lives in a residential aged care facility. She has significant dysphagia, which is getting progressively worse. Emma has recommended modifications to the texture of food and fluids due to Maria's swallowing difficulties and has prescribed level 2 mildly thick fluids and level 5 minced and moist foods. Maria regularly refuses this diet and demands that she be given regular foods and drink. The carers are worried for her safety because she coughs and splutters with thin drinks when she is tired, so they do not want to provide them for her. Maria has had two bouts of aspiration pneumonia in the past eight months, which significantly affect her general level of function and distress her greatly.

What Are the Legal/Ethical Issues That Arise From This Case?

- Maria has MS resulting in worsening dysphagia.
- Maria has regularly refused the speech pathologist's 'treatment' in terms of the diet and fluid texture modifications recommended for her.
- Maria is currently able to make her own decisions and is choosing to exercise her autonomy, understands her prognosis and believes she knows what is best for her.
- The carers are put in a difficult situation when Maria demands unmodified drinks because she has obvious difficulty when drinking them.

What Could Be the Personal Reaction to This Case?

Emma is aware that, for Maria, an occasional drink of thin fluids (including a glass of wine) gives her pleasure.

She understands that Maria is in the advanced stages of MS and is nearing the end of her life and wishes to respect Maria's autonomy in making decisions about what she eats and drinks for her quality of life. This is balanced with concern about choking and the strong possibility of Maria developing aspiration pneumonia with subsequent detriment to her function and wellbeing.

Emma knows that choking is the second highest cause of death in residential aged care and is anxious that if Maria has an adverse event due to her swallowing difficulty, she may end up being blamed.

Emma is also very aware that the carers are distressed when they see Maria choking and share Emma's concern about choking. Emma is taking a narrative approach to ethical reasoning to consider the perspectives of all involved in this scenario.[37]

What Facts May Be Relevant Regarding This Situation?

- Maria is in the end stages of life.
- Maria is currently able to make her own decisions – at this stage these decisions are placing her life at increased risk.
- There is increasing conflict between Maria and carers about providing thin fluids when she asks for them.

What Values May Be at Stake?

The principle of autonomy underpins this scenario because Maria is exerting her choice and control by refusing texture-modified food and fluids; however, she may require further information to be fully informed about the risks.

This scenario challenges the values of integrity, professionalism, respect and care, which are professional obligations described in the Speech Pathology Australia *Code of Ethics* (2010).

Emma is seeking to balance her responsibilities to provide beneficence and non-maleficence for Maria while considering the risk involved and her duty of care.

What Are the Options in This Case?

- Emma could turn a blind eye and allow the situation to remain 'as is'.

- Emma could refuse to provide ongoing speech pathology services for Maria due to Maria not following her recommendations.
- Emma could organise a case conference with Maria and the staff to ensure all understand the risks involved and possible consequences, and support Maria to make an informed choice about her oral intake.
- Emma could discuss with the facility managers how to support care staff who are reluctant to provide thin fluids to Maria. The team could develop a care plan to reduce the risk of aspiration using other strategies, which would involve training for carers in using the strategies.
- Emma could also suggest that Maria prepares an advance care directive as described in Chapter 12 to detail her wishes regarding enteral feeding in the event that her swallow function deteriorates further.

What Should Occur in This Case?

Emma considers that she has a duty of care to continue to support Maria in making an informed choice and considers that the best course of action is to initiate open discussion and clear communication with Maria.

Emma should set up a case meeting to ensure that Maria understands the possible consequences of drinking thin fluids, in particular the risk of aspiration when she is tired. The discussion can result in an agreed plan on how to support Maria to eat and drink as safely as possible while still allowing for her choices relating to quality of life.

Emma is mindful that the care staff require training and support to assist Maria to reduce the risk when drinking thin fluids, which will also reduce their distress when Maria is choking.

A care plan should be developed following consultation with all stakeholders that considers Maria's choices, the role of the care staff to minimise risk as much as possible, and consideration of Maria's advance care plan for future decisions.

Could the Problem Have Been Prevented?

MS is a neurodegenerative disease. If a person living with MS experiences dysphagia as a consequence of the disease, it is common that deterioration in swallow function may occur. Emma could have had a discussion at the beginning of her professional relationship with Maria regarding possible prognosis and her wishes in the event that her swallow function did deteriorate. This would allow better planning, and staff training could have been provided before the situation reached this point.

Emma also could have ensured that the facility managers were aware of the potential for Maria's swallow function to deteriorate so that resources and training to minimise the risk of aspiration were available for staff from the start.

It would have been appropriate for a discussion to be held with Maria early after coming to live in the facility regarding her wish to continue to drink thin fluids against the advice of the speech pathologist so that Maria's autonomy could be upheld from the outset.

CASE 5: RIGHT TO COMMUNICATION; PHYSICAL AND PSYCHOLOGICAL ABUSE

Liz has worked in the disability sector with clients with a range of conditions for most of her 30-year career as a speech pathologist. She has recently begun to work with Adele, aged 16, who has a diagnosis of intellectual disability and severe language disorder. Adele has emerging verbal communication that is not yet sufficient for all of her communication needs and uses a high-tech AAC device to support her communication. Adele will begin working in a supported workplace next year so Liz is asked to help her to prepare to leave the education system. Adele is very excited to have a work placement trial organised and Liz goes with her to provide training for the other staff in how to support Adele to use her AAC device.

A few months go by and Adele's family contact Liz. Adele is now attending the supported workplace twice a week in a transition program, but the family have concerns that she is becoming reluctant to go and frequently comes home upset. The family is aware that the workplace supervisor decided that Adele should be using verbal communication and makes her lock her AAC device in her locker when she gets to work and will not let her use it during the day because she 'needs to get used to talking'. Another work placement student told the family she has heard him yell at Adele that she is 'lazy' when she doesn't talk, and she has told her family that he locked her in the time-out room when she asked to use her AAC device. Adele has also come home with a bruise on her arm that looks a bit like finger marks. Liz is not sure what to do. She works in a state where speech pathologists are not listed as mandatory reporters.

What Are the Legal/Ethical Issues That Arise From This Case?

The family's phone call makes Liz question if Adele is being shown respect and care in the workplace.

- Communication is a basic human right; the family's comments indicate that Adele's rights may not be respected.
- The workplace supervisor may be using restrictive practices and there is a question of whether physical and psychological abuse are occurring.

What Could Be the Personal Reaction to This Case?

Liz feels concerned that she had just begun to develop a relationship of trust with Adele and that this experience may threaten the therapeutic alliance and Adele's confidence with future workplace experiences.

Liz is unsure of her professional obligation to get involved; however, she considers that as a speech pathologist she does have an obligation to demonstrate professionalism – to help individuals with regard to communication. She also has an ethical obligation to advocate for clients and an overarching ethical and legal obligation to report suspected child abuse.

What Facts May Be Relevant Regarding This Situation?

Adele has effective communication when using a mixture of verbal communication and her AAC device. Liz thought that the supervisor understood that Adele needed to use a mix of communication techniques at the time she provided the training. A barrier to Adele being afforded access to her AAC device appears to be the attitudes and values of the supervisor, which disempowers her in the supported workplace.

There is a suspicion of abuse (physical and psychological).

What Values May Be at Stake?

The Speech Pathology Australia *Code of Ethics* (2010) obliges a speech pathologist to demonstrate professionalism: 'We act in an objective and professional manner to help individuals, groups and communities, particularly with regard to communication and swallowing' and respect and care, 'We respect the rights and dignity of our clients and we respect the context in which they live' at all times. Principle 2.5 describes the responsibility 'We comply with federal and state laws'; therefore, Liz has an obligation to report the suspected abuse. Standard 3.1.7 Safety and Welfare states: 'We take every precaution to ensure client safety'.

Chapter 16 of this book describes the state, territory and federal laws relating to reporting of child abuse, which Liz has a professional and ethical obligation to comply with.

What Are the Options in This Case?

Considering this scenario with an ethics of care approach,[38] Liz is aware that she has an obligation to advocate for Adele to have access to a method of communication that has been found to be effective for her.

As described in Chapter 16, Liz also has an obligation to report suspected physical or psychological abuse.

Liz could approach the supervisor directly and discuss the effect of the use of restrictive practices on someone with a significant communication impairment. She could seek to help him understand what restrictive practices are and the implications for Adele.

Liz could discuss with the workplace management team the effect of the use of restrictive practices on someone with a significant communication impairment and achieve changes in their policies. She could seek to help them understand what restrictive practices are, to introduce the use of behaviour support plans, and assist the workplace to explore developing their knowledge and skills in that area with other professional support.

What Should Occur in This Case?

Liz should demonstrate her respect and care as an advocate for Adele and organise to meet with the supervisor and the management team at the supported workplace to ascertain their understanding of severe communication impairment. She should provide education regarding the use of AAC to support communication and why Adele needs to be allowed to exercise her rights to communication through all the modalities that are appropriate for her.

Liz could ask to bring a psychologist to the meeting to discuss restrictive practices and positive behaviour support. This could inform development of appropriate policies and procedures for this workplace.

Liz could also contact the appropriate state agency to discuss the suspected physical and psychological abuse. The agency can provide information and resources to assist her to monitor the situation.

Following these actions, Liz could meet with the family (and Adele if appropriate) to talk about changes that will support Adele into the future. This would ensure that Adele and her family are able to have a voice in the process.

Could the Problem Have Been Prevented?

Liz was concerned that her initial education may not have been sufficiently detailed for Adele's supervisor to understand Adele's communication support needs from the beginning of the placement. To prevent this happening in the future she could revise her educational materials and presentation. She could add more detail regarding communication as a basic human right and how people must be supported in using modalities that provide effective communication for them individually.

CONCLUSION

Physical, mental and social health and wellbeing are of primary importance to patients and practitioners. In Australia the health system aims to provide high-quality care in a timely manner, reducing the morbidity and mortality associated with many diseases. Principles of ethics and law support such a system and its success, and Australian laws and policies work to support and prevent disease and early death.

In this book we have seen that health law is broad and complex. Health practitioners do not need to be legal experts, but they must understand legal concepts that relate to the framework for the health system within which they work and that govern their practice. It is important for health practitioners to be aware of the numerous 'core' areas of law (such as tort, contract and criminal laws), fundamental legal concepts (such as privacy, confidentiality and consent) and their obligations relevant to specific areas of health practice and concerns. It is also important to recognise that identifying the law does not suffice. While everyday practice is governed by the law, it is also essential to understand that different situations may raise ethical or legal dilemmas, or both. Being able to critically evaluate the situation, to acknowledge one's own morals or judgments, and to move forward in a particular case by adopting a reasoned decision-making approach is essential to delivering good health services.

This book has therefore provided discussion and analysis of the health system and ethical and legal concepts relevant to healthcare delivery across the life span. It has also provided information regarding working with legal professionals. In this final chapter, the case studies have provided the opportunity for practical application and analysis of the ethical and legal concepts discussed throughout this book. They draw together the fundamental principles that guide healthcare services and demonstrate situations in which health practitioners must meet legal and ethical standards when providing health treatment and promoting good health. The book is not a substitute for ethical or legal consultation or advice, which should be sought when required. However, it has presented the foundation for health practitioners to move forward with a good critical understanding of the health system in which they work, their ethical and legal obligations and ways to uphold them.

FURTHER READING

Australian College of Midwives. *National Midwifery Guidelines for Consultation and Referral*. 3rd ed. Issue 2 (reprinted 2017). Canberra, ACT: Australian College of Midwives; 2014.

Australian Health Practitioner Regulation Agency. *For Registered Health Practitioners: Social Media Policy*. Melbourne, VIC: AHPRA; 2014.

Benetoli A, Chen TF, Schaefer M, Chaar B, Aslani P. Pharmacists' perceptions of professionalism on social networking sites. *Res Social Adm Pharm*. 2017; 13(3):575–588.

Boyce P, Buist A. Management of bipolar disorder over the perinatal period. *Aust Fam Physician*. 2016; 45(12):890–893.

Chaar B. Ethical dilemmas: Are you across the EHC guidelines? *Aust Pharm*. 2016; 35(11):72.

Collins JC, Schneider CR, Moles RJ. Emergency contraception supply in Australian pharmacies after the introduction of ulipristal acetate: a mystery shopping mixed-methods study. *Contraception*. 2018; 98(3):243–246.

Douglas K. Social media. *ANMJ*. 2014; 22(1):24–28.

Ekor M. The growing use of herbal medicines: issues relating to adverse reactions and challenges in monitoring safety. *Front Pharmacol*. 2014;4:177.

International Confederation of Midwives. *Code of ethics for midwives*. The Hague: ICM; 2014.

International Council of Nurses. *ICN Code of Ethics for Nurses*. Geneva: ICN; 2012.

Iyer P, McFarland R, La Caze A. Expectations and responsibilities regarding the sale of complementary medicines in pharmacies: perspectives of consumers and pharmacy support staff. *J Pharm Pract*. 2017; 25(4):292–300.

Jones S-A. Ethically questionable situations. *ANMJ*. 2016; 24(2):48.

Leitão S, Bradd P, McAllister L, Russell A, Block S, Kenny B, Smith H et al. *Ethics Education Package*. Melbourne, VIC: The Speech Pathology Association of Australia Ltd; 2014.

New South Wales Health. *Medication Handling in NSW Public Health Facilities*. Sydney, NSW: NSW Government; 2013.

Nursing and Midwifery Board of Australia. *Code of Conduct for Midwives*. Melbourne, VIC: NMBA; 2018.

Nursing and Midwifery Board of Australia. *The Midwife Standards for Practice*. Melbourne, VIC: NMBA; 2018.

Oliver J, McLennan B. Pharmacy and privacy laws: Privacy law reforms and you. *Aust J Pharm*, 2013; 94(1122):56.

Speech Pathology Australia. *Code of Ethics*. Melbourne, VIC: The Speech Pathology Association of Australia Ltd; 2010.

Speech Pathology Australia. *Competency-Based Occupational Standards (CBOS) for Speech Pathologists*. Melbourne, VIC: The Speech Pathology Association of Australia Ltd; 2011.

Zuscak SJ, Peisah C, Ferguson A. A collaborative approach to supporting communication in the assessment of decision-making capacity. *Disabil Rehabil*. 2016; 38(11):1107–1114.

ENDNOTES

1. Nursing and Midwifery Board (NMBA). Position Statement on Nurses, Midwives and Vaccination. https://www.nursingmidwifery board.gov.au/codes-guidelines-statements/position-statements/vaccination.aspx. Accessed 22 April 2019.
2. Australian Health Practitioner Regulation Agency. *For Registered Health Practitioners: Social Media Policy*. Melbourne, VIC: AHPRA; 2014.
3. Nursing and Midwifery Board (NMBA). Position Statement on Nurses, Midwives and Vaccination. https://www.nursingmidwifery board.gov.au/codes-guidelines-statements/position-statements/vaccination.aspx. Accessed 22 April 2019.
4. Power A. Is Facebook an appropriate platform for professional discourse? *British Journal of Midwifery*. 2015 Feb; 23(2):140–2.
5. Australian Health Practitioner Regulation Agency. *For Registered Health Practitioners: Social Media Policy*. Melbourne, VIC: AHPRA; 2014.
6. Australian College of Midwives. *National Midwifery Guidelines for Consultation and Referral*. 3rd ed. Issue 2 (reprinted 2017). Canberra, ACT: Australian College of Midwives; 2014.
7. Ibid.
8. Nursing and Midwifery Board of Australia. *Code of Conduct for Midwives*. Melbourne, VIC: NMBA; 2018.
9. Nursing and Midwifery Board of Australia. *The Midwife Standards for Practice*. Melbourne, VIC: NMBA; 2018.
10. International Confederation of Midwives. *Code of Conduct for Midwives*. The Hague: ICM; 2014.
11. Australian College of Midwives. *National Midwifery Guidelines for Consultation and Referral*. 3rd ed. Issue 2 (reprinted 2017). Canberra, ACT: Australian College of Midwives; 2014.
12. Ibid.
13. Ibid.
14. See the Australian College of Midwives website: https://www.midwives.org.au/position-statements.
15. Jones S-A. Ethically questionable situations. *ANMJ*. 2016; 24(2): 48.

16. Boyce P, Buist A. Management of bipolar disorder over the perinatal period. *Aust Fam Physician*. 2016; 45(12):890–893.

17. Jones S, Jones I, Jones SC. Pharmacological management of bipolar disorder in pregnancy. *CNS Drugs*. 2017;31(9):737–745.

18. Ibid.

19. Nursing and Midwifery Board of Australia. *The Midwife Standards for Practice*. Melbourne, VIC: NMBA; 2018.

20. Royal Australian and New Zealand College of Obstetricians and Gynaecologists. *Prenatal Assessment of Fetal Structural Conditions*. East Melbourne, VIC: RANZCOG; 2016. From: https://www.ranzcog.edu.au/RANZCOG_SITE/media/RANZCOG-MEDIA/Women's%20Health/Statement%20and%20guidelines/Clinical-Obstetrics/Prenatal-assessment-of-fetal-structural-conditions-(C-Obs-60)-Amended-May-2016_1.pdf?ext=.pdf. Accessed 22 April 2019.

21. Ibid.

22. Nursing and Midwifery Board of Australia. *The Midwife Standards for Practice*. Melbourne, VIC: NMBA; 2018, p. 11.

23. Ibid.

24. Ibid.

25. See the NSW Health website: https://www1.health.nsw.gov.au/pds/ActivePDSDocuments/PD2013_043.pdf.

26. Paramedicine Board of Australia. Code of Conduct. https://www.paramedicineboard.gov.au/Professional-standards/Codes-guidelines-and-policies/Code-of-conduct.aspx. Accessed 22 April 2019.

27. Ibid.

28. '[T]he assent of belief is given on more slender evidence than proof. Belief is an inclination of the mind towards assenting to, rather than rejecting, a proposition': *George v Rockett* (1990) 170 CLR 104, at [14].

29. See the *Code of Ethics for Australian Pharmacists*: https://www.psa.org.au/wp-content/uploads/2018/07/PSA-Code-of-Ethics-2017.

30. Pharmaceutical Society of Australia. Code of Ethics for Pharmacists: p. 12. https://www.psa.org.au/membership/ethics/. Accessed 22 April 2019.

31. Dowdy C. Dealing with reality: Oral emergency contraception in community pharmacy – what you need to know. *Aust J Pharm*. 2017;98(1166):84.

32. Pharmaceutical Society of Australia. Professional Practice Standards. https://www.psa.org.au/practice-support-industry/professional-practice-standards/. Accessed 22 April 2019.

33. Pharmacy Board of Australia. Code of Conduct. https://www.pharmacyboard.gov.au/codes-guidelines/code-of-conduct.aspx. Accessed 22 April 2019, p. 11.

34. For examples of legislative definitions in this regard see *Guardianship Act 1987* (NSW) s 33(2); *Guardianship and Administration Act 2000* (Qld) Sch 4; *Powers of Attorney Act 1998* (Qld) Schedule 3; *Guardianship and Administration Act 1995* (Tas) s 36(2); *Guardianship and Administration Act 1986* (Vic) s 36(2).

35. Leitão S, Bradd P, McAllister L, Russell A, Block S, Kenny B, Smith H et al. *Ethics Education Package*. Melbourne, VIC: The Speech Pathology Association of Australia Ltd; 2014.

36. Ibid.

37. Ibid.

38. Ibid.

INDEX

Page numbers followed by '*f*' indicate figures, '*t*' indicate tables, and '*b*' indicate boxes.

A

Abnormal chromosome, screening of, 124
Aboriginal and Torres Strait Islander
    Health Practice Board, 36
Abortion, 116–120
  Australian position, 117–120
  early English law, 116–117
  laws in Australia relevant to, 118*t*–119*t*
Absolute privilege, 89
Accomplices, parties to offences, 95–96
Active euthanasia, 99
Actus reus, 94–95
Admissible evidence, 187
Advance Care Directives Act 2013, 134
Advance care planning, 132–143
  directives and, 132–134
    common law advance care directives,
      133
    not need to be followed, 134
    statutory advance directives, 133–134
Adversarial, defined, 9
Affidavits, 184–185
Aged care, 21–22
  home care, 21
  home support, 21
  residential care, 21–22
Aged Care Act 1997, 22, 180
'Agent', in decision making, 135
Aggravated damages, 72, 87
AHPRA. *see* Australian Health
    Practitioners Regulation Agency
Altruistic surrogacy, 129
APAC. *see* Australian Pharmaceutical
    Advisory Council
Apologies, negligence, 73, 74*t*
Appellant, 12*b*
Applied ethics, 25
APPs. *see* Australian Privacy Principles
ART. *see* Assisted reproduction
    technologies
Artificial insemination, 124–125
Assault, 79–81, 102

Assisted dying, 99–100
Assisted reproduction technologies (ART),
    124–131
  access to, 125–126
  defined, 125
  information access, by donor-conceived
    people, 126–127
  numerical limits for donation, 127
  parentage and, 126
  posthumous use of gametes, 128–129
  regulation and oversight of, 124–125
  surrogacy and, 129–130
Assisted Reproductive Treatment Act 1988,
    125, 128
Assisted Reproductive Treatment Act 2008,
    125
'Attorney', in decision making, 135
Australia
  abortion in, 117–120, 118*t*–119*t*
  death certificates in, 111
  suicide in, 99–100
Australian Capital Territory
  access to health information, 57
  birth notification requirements in, 109*t*
  child abuse, laws regarding mandatory
    reporting of, 176*t*–179*t*
  child protection legislation, principal
    Acts, 175*t*
  consequences of an apology or
    expression of regret, 74*t*
  drug and poisons legislation by
    jurisdiction, 154*t*
  Health Records (Privacy and Access) Act,
    60
  laws relevant to abortion, 118*t*–119*t*
  legislation authorising medical
    intervention for children and
    young people, 87*t*
  mental health legislation by jurisdiction,
    166*t*
  National Law, 33*t*
  statutory advance directives in, 133

substitute decision-makers, 136*t*
  appointed by a tribunal, 138*t*
  recognised by legislation, 137*t*
  in tissue removal, 148
Australian Health Practitioners Regulation
    Agency (AHPRA), 33
Australian health system, 16–23
  access to health care, evolving schemes,
    19–22
    aged care, 21–22
    issues with the current scheme, 21
    Medicare, 20
    National Disability Insurance Scheme
      (NDIS), 21
    private health insurance, 20–21
  charter of healthcare rights, 22–23
  Commonwealth responsibility for
    healthcare services, 16–17, 17*b*
  healthcare expenditure, 22
  local governments, 17–18
  shared responsibilities between the
    Commonwealth and states/
    territories, 17, 18*b*
  state powers and responsibilities
    regarding the health system, 17, 17*b*
  universal health system, history of,
    18–19
    access to medicines, Pharmaceutical
      Benefits Scheme, 18–19
    private prescriptions, 19
Australian legal system, 2–14
  Australia as federation, 2
  court hierarchy, 10–11
    courts/tribunals, 10–11
    original and appellate jurisdiction, 10
    understanding jurisdiction, 10
  distribution of power between the states
    and the Commonwealth, 2–4
  general features of, 9–10
    alternative dispute resolution, 9–10
    natural justice, 9
    presumption of innocence, 9

legislation, 4–8
  common law, 6–8, 7f
  delegated, 6
  passage of, 4–6, 5f
  separation of powers, 4, 4b
  skills relevant to understanding judicial
      decisions and legislation, 12–13
    reading judicial decisions (cases),
        12–13, 12b
    regulations, 13
    statutory interpretation, 13, 13b–14b
  types of law, 8–9
    procedural law, 8
    substantive law, 8
Australian Open Disclosure Framework,
    73–74
Australian Organ and Tissue Donation
    and Transplantation Authority
    (OTA), 150
Australian Organ and Tissue Donation and
    Transplantation Authority Act 2008,
    150
Australian Pharmaceutical Advisory
    Council (APAC), 155
Australian policies and standards, for
    mental health, 164–165
Australian position, 117–120
  conscientious objection, 117–120
Australian Privacy Principle Guidelines, 53
Australian Privacy Principles (APPs), 53
Australian Red Cross Blood Service, 147
Automatism, criminal law defence, 97
Autopsy, 113
  medicolegal, 113

B

Barristers, 188
Battery, 79, 81
Beneficence, 28
Best evidence, 190
Bioethics, 25
Birth
  registration of, 108–110
    change of sex, 110
    children born ex-nuptially, 110
    notification and, 108–111, 109t
    perinatal data collection, 109–110
  wrongful, claims regarding, 120–122
Blood
  donation of, 146–151
    ethical and legal issues in, 146–150
  transfusion of, 147
Board, person appointed by, in decision
    making, 135
Bodily harm, 102
Body, ownership of, 113

Breach of duty of care, negligence, 67–69
  assessment to be made with reference to
      the time of the breach, 69
  failure to provide warnings or
      information, 68–69
  treatment and diagnosis, defence, 68
  warnings about obvious and inherent
      risks, 69
Bulk-billing, 20
'Burden of proof', 93

C

Calculus of negligence, 68
Capacity, 82–83
  children and, to consent to healthcare
      decisions, 86
Care outside the guidelines, 201b–202b
Case studies, 196–248
  on medicine, 197–246
    death and organ donation, 199b
    mandatory reporting, 198b
    mental health and involuntary
        treatment, 197b
  on midwifery, 200–206
    care outside the guidelines,
        201b–202b
    consent to treatment of minor, 205b
    professional boundaries, 206b
    refusal of treatment, 203b
    testimonials and confidentiality, 200b
  on nursing, 207–211
    private life can affect professional life,
        210b
    sexual relationship with patient, 209b
    stealing a patient's money, 208b
    stealing and self-administration of
        Schedule 8 drugs, 207b
  on paramedicine, 211–218
    end of life and family conflict, 213b
    impairment of fellow worker, 215b
    mental health, 211b
    negligence, 217b
    privacy, 212b
  on pharmacy, 218–224
    impaired pharmacy student, 222b
    patients with dementia, 221b
    pharmacists and complementary
        medicines, 218b
    pharmacists and family, 223b
    pharmacists' personal versus
        professional views and practices,
        219b
  on physiotherapy, 224–232
    family on active physiotherapy, 224b
    patient-centred care conflicts with
        evidence-based care, 228b

    sports therapist's obligations,
        226b–227b
    standards of care and physiotherapy
        treatment, 230b
    treatment disagreement, 228b–229b
  on podiatry, 232–238
    accepting gifts, 236b
    incomplete patient notes, 232b
    issues of consent, 233b
    possible elder abuse, 237b
    social media, 235b
  on speech pathology, 238–246
    consent, privacy and confidentiality,
        240b
    inadequate funding and service
        delivery, 238b
    physical and psychological abuse,
        245b
    poor record keeping, 242b
    right to communication, 245b
    worsening dysphagia, refusal of food
        modifications, 243b
Causation, negligence, 69–70
  factual causation, 69–70
    failure to give advice, information or
        warning cases, 69–70
  new intervening acts, 70
    damages, 71–72
    defences, 70–71
    other types of damages, 72–73
    remoteness of harm, 70
    scope of liability, 70
Central register, in assisted reproduction
    technologies (ART), 126–127
'Certified' person, 147
Child abuse, 174–182, 175t
  reporting, 175–179
    mandatory, 176–179, 176t–179t
    voluntary, 175–176
Child destruction, 101–102
Child Protection Act 1999, 176, 176t–179t
Child protection legislation, 175t
Child Wellbeing and Safety Act 2005, 109
Children
  capacity to consent to healthcare
      decision, 86
  consent to healthcare treatment to,
      85–86
Children, Young Persons and Their Families
    Act 1997, 176, 176t–179t
Children, Youth and Families Act 2005, 176,
    176t–179t
Children and Community Services Act
    2004, 176t–179t
Children and Young People Act 2008, 86,
    176t–179t

Children and Young Persons (Care and Protection) Act 1998, 86, 176, 176*t*–179*t*
Children born ex-nuptially, 110
Children's Protection Act 1993, 176*t*–179*t*
Circumstantial evidence, 190
Civil cases, 188
Civil Liability Act 2002, 121
Civil Liability Act 2003, 121
'Code', 93
Code of Conduct, 80
Commercial surrogacy, 129
Common assault, 102
Common law, 6–8, 7*f*
  equitable principles, 8
Common law advance care directives, 133
Commonwealth legislation, 56–57, 137
  government agencies, 56
  private businesses, 56–57
Commonwealth Parliament, 3
Commonwealth privacy legislation, 53–54
  access to, and correction of, personal information, 54
    access, 54
    correction, 54
  collection of personal information, 53–54
    notification, 54
    solicited, 53
    unsolicited, 53–54
  dealing with personal information, 54
    adoption, use or disclosure of government-related identifiers, 54
    cross-border disclosure of personal information, 54
    direct marketing, 54
    use or disclosure of personal information, 54
  integrity of personal information, 54
    quality, 54
    security, 54
  personal information privacy, consideration of, 53
    anonymity and pseudonymity, 53
    open and transparent management of personal information, 53
Communication, right to, 245*b*
Compensation. *see* Damages
Complementary medicines, 218*b*
  regulation for, 156
Completely incapacitated, 132
Conception/birth, wrongful, 120–121
Concurrent, defined, 3
Confidentiality, 51–53
  breach of confidence, 52
  case study

    on midwifery, 200*b*
    on speech pathology, 240*b*
  common law negligence, 52
  limits of obligation of, 52–53
  professional codes of conduct and regulation, 52
  statute, 52
Conscientious objection, 117–120
Consent, 132
  defence, 82–86
  defences to action in defamation, 89
  emergency, 86
  forms of, 84–85
  to healthcare treatment in relation to children, 85–86
  implied, 84
  issues of, 233*b*
  refusal to, 83–84
  relates to specific treatment or procedures, 83
  to research, 84
  revocation of, in tissue removal, 148
  on speech pathology, 240*b*
  to treatment of minor, 205*b*
  verbal, 84–85
  voluntary, 83
  written, 85
Consent to Medical Treatment and Palliative Care Act 1995, 86
Consequentialism, 27
Constitutional law, 8
Continuing Professional Development Registration Standard, 35
Contract law, 8
Convention on the Elimination of all Forms of Discrimination against Women, 3
Convention on the Rights of Persons with Disabilities, 3–4
Convention on the Rights of the Child, 3
Coroners Court, 111–114
  finding regarding professional practice, 113–114
  functions of, 111–112
Coronial inquests, 112–113
Costs, 90
Counsel/procure crime, 95–96
Court, person appointed by, in decision making, 135
Court of Petty Sessions, 113
Courts/tribunals, 10–11
Crime
  counsel/procure, 95–96
  definition of, 92–93
  elements of, 94–95
Crimes Act 1900 (NSW), 120
Crimes Act 1958, 117, 176*t*–179*t*

Criminal Code, 96
Criminal History Registration Standard, 35–36
Criminal law, 8
  defences, 96–97
  features of, 93–94
  and issues related to health care, 92–104
    additional criminal offence, 102–104
    child destruction and feticide, 101–102
    crime, 92–93
    criminal law defences, 96–97
    criminal negligence, 95
    elements of crime, 94–95
    euthanasia, 98–101
    homicide, 97–98
    parties to offences, accomplices, 95–96
    strict liability, 95
  negligence, 95
  parties to offences, accomplices, 95–96
  sources of, 93
Criminal negligence, 95
Criminal offence
  additional, 102–104
  terminology related to, 93
Cross-examination, trial, 189
Custodial sentences, 93

D

Damages, 90
  negligence, 71–72
Death, 199*b*
  definition of, 110
  perinatal, 111
  registration of, 110–111
    definition of, 110
    notification and, 108–111
    obligation to notify, 111
    perinatal, 111
    reportable, 112
  tissue removal after, 149–150
Decision-makers
  in decision making, 135
  support or substitute, 135–137
Decision making
  for legally incompetent adults, 140, 140*t*
  by substitute decision-makers, 135–137
'Decision-making capacity', 134
Defamation, 87–89
  action, elements of, 88–89
  defences to an action in, 89
  statements, categories of, 88
Defences
  to an action in defamation, 89
  of another person, 87

criminal law, 96–97
  emergency, 86
  statutory authority, 86–87, 87*t*
  to trespass to person, 82–87
Defendant, 12*b*, 64
Dementia, patients with, 221*b*
Dental Board of Australia, 36–37
Deontology, 27–28
'Deponent', 184–185
Diminished responsibility, criminal law
    defence, 97
Direct evidence, 190
Disclosure
  of documents, 185–186
  non-party, 186
Discovery, of documents, 185–186
District Courts (County Courts), 10–11
'Do not resuscitate' order, 137–139
Documents
  discovery (disclosure) of, 185–186
  inspection of, 185–186
Donation, numerical limits for, 127
Donor-conceived people, information
    access by, 126–127
'Double effect', principle of, 100–101
Drugs, regulation of, 152–161
  administration, 157–158
  complementary medicines, 156
  customs import and export, 153
  definitions of, 156
  drug schedules for, 154, 155*t*
  federal, 152–153
  medication errors and, 159–160
  for nurse-initiated drugs, 158–159
  policy, 154–156
  prescribing and, 157
  standing orders, 159
  state and territory, 153–154, 154*t*
  storage and, 156–157
  verbal orders for, 158
Duty of care, negligence, 65–69
  breach of, 67–69
    assessment to be made with reference
      to the time of the breach, 69
    failure to provide warnings or
      information, 68–69
    treatment and diagnosis, defence, 68
    warnings about obvious and inherent
      risks, 69
  duty of care not found, 65
  duty of care not tested, 65–66
  duty to rescue, 66–67
  duty to the unborn, 66
  duty to third parties, 65
  mental harm, 67
Dysphagia, worsening, 243*b*

E
Early embryo screening, 124
Early English law, 116–117
  Australian position, 117–120
  rights of fetus and father, 120
Education (General Provisions) Act 2006,
    176*t*–179*t*
Elder abuse, 174–182, 237*b*
  disciplinary responses in, 181–182
  issues relevant to, 180
  limitations of, 181
  relevant law in, 180–181
Electroconvulsive therapy, for mental
    health, 170
Emergency, consent, 86
Emotional abuse, in child abuse, 174–175
End of life, case study on, 213*b*
'Enduring Attorney', in decision making,
    135
'Enduring Guardian', in decision making,
    135
English Language Skills Registration
    Standard, 36
Ethical decision making, 24–30
  deriving a process for, 29–30
*Ethical Guidelines on the Use of Assisted
    Reproductive Technology in Clinical
    Practice and Research* (the
    NHMRC Ethical Guidelines),
    124–125
Ethical issues
  on accepting gifts, 236
  on care outside the guidelines, 202
  on consent, privacy and confidentiality,
    240
  on consent to treatment of minor,
    205
  on death and organ donation, 199
  on end of life and family conflict,
    214
  on family on active physiotherapy,
    225
  on impaired pharmacy student, 223
  on impairment of fellow worker,
    215–216
  on inadequate funding and service
    delivery, 238–239
  on incomplete patient notes, 232
  on involuntary treatment, 197
  on issues of consent, 233–234
  on mandatory reporting, 198
  on mental health, 197, 211–212
  on negligence, 217
  on patient-centred care conflict with
    evidence-based care, 228
  on patients with dementia, 221

  on pharmacists and complementary
    medicines, 218–219
  on pharmacists and family, 224
  on pharmacists' personal *versus*
    professional views and practices,
    220
  on poor record keeping, 242
  on possible elder abuse, 237
  on privacy, 213
  on private life affecting your
    professional life, 210
  on professional boundaries, 206
  on refusal of treatment, 203–204
  on right to communication; physical
    and psychological abuse, 245
  on sexual relationship with patient, 209
  on social media, 235
  on sports therapist's obligations, 227
  on stealing and self-administration of
    Schedule 8 drugs, 207
  on stealing patient's money, 208
  on testimonials and confidentiality, 200
  on treatment disagreement, 229
  on worsening dysphagia, refusal of food
    modifications, 243
Ethics
  applied, 25
  bioethics, 25
  codes of, 26
  decision making when faced with an
    ethical dilemma, 26–28
    consequentialism, 27
    deontology, 27–28
    principles-based approach, 28
    virtue ethics, 28
  definition, 24–25
  law *vs.*, 26, 27*t*
  normative, 25
Euthanasia, 98–101
  active, 99
  homicide and, 99
Evidence, categories of
  best evidence, 190
  circumstantial evidence, 190
  direct evidence, 190
  original and hearsay evidence, 190
  perjury, 190
  secondary evidence, 190
Evidence Act 1977, 190
Evidence-based care, patient-centred care
    conflicts with, 228*b*
Evidential burden, discharging, 188
Examination-in-chief, trial, 189
Exclusive, defined, 3
Exemplary damages, 72–73, 87
Expert evidence, 191

F

Factual causation, 69–70
 failure to give advice, information or warning cases, 69–70
False imprisonment, 79, 81–82
Family
 pharmacists and, 223*b*
 on physiotherapy, 224*b*
Family conflict, case study on, 213*b*
Family Court, in tissue removal, 147–148
Family Court Act 1997, 141, 176*t*–179*t*
Family Law Act 1975, 120, 176–179
Father, rights of, 120
Federal Circuit Court, 11
Federal Court of Australia, 11
Federal regulation, for drug and poisons, 152–153
Fellow worker, impairment of, 215*b*
Felonies, 93
Female genital mutilation, 103–104
Feticide, 101–102
Fetus, rights of, 120
Fifth National Mental Health and Suicide Prevention Plan, 165
Food modification, refusal of, 243*b*
'Forensic pathology', 194
Forensic science, 193–194
Freedom of Information Act 1982, 56

G

Gabrielsen v Nurses Board of South Australia, 181
Gamete intrafallopian transfer, 124
Gametes, posthumous use of, 128–129
General damages, 72
General registration, health practitioners, 34
Gifts, accepting, 236*b*
'Gillick competent', 86
Golden rule, 13
Government policy and legislation, in child abuse, 175
Grievous bodily harm, 102
Guardian ad litem, 64
Guardianship Act 1987, 133
Guardianship and Administration Act 1990, 134
Guardianship decision, on withholding and withdrawal of treatment, 139–142

H

HCCC v Gabrielsen, 181
Health, alternative dispute mechanisms in, 194

Health care
 criminal law and issues related to, 92–104
  additional criminal offence, 102–104
  child destruction and feticide, 101–102
  crime, 92–93
  criminal law defences, 96–97
  criminal negligence, 95
  defences, 96–97
  elements of crime, 94–95
  euthanasia, 98–101
  features of, 93–94
  homicide, 97–98
  negligence, 95
  parties to offences, accomplices, 95–96
  sources of, 93
  strict liability, 95
 fraudulent consent and provision of, 103*b*
Health information, management of, 48–62
 access pursuant to the court process, 60
 access to health information, 56–59
  Commonwealth legislation, 56–57
  state and territory legislation, 57–59
 collecting health information via third party, 56
 computerised records and electronic health, 50–51
  National Strategy for Digital Health Records, 50–51
 government policy, 59–60
 healthcare records, establishing and maintaining, 48–62
 privacy and confidentiality of health information, 51–55
  confidentiality, 51–53
  exceptions to the protection of sensitive or health information, 54–55
  privacy, 53–54
  state and territory health privacy legislation, 55
 storage and disposal of healthcare records, 60–61
  destroying health information and records, 60–61
  retiring or closing a practice, 60
Health Insurance Act, 20
Health Ombudsman Act 2013, 42
Health practitioners
 child abuse and, 175
 of intentional torts, 79
 professional regulation of, 32–46

 codes of conduct, 38–39
 disciplinary issues, 39–40
 disciplinary process, 40–43
 guidelines for advertising regulated health services, 38
 health practitioners not regulated by the National Scheme, 43–45
 mental or physical incapacity or impairment, 40
 National Registration and Accreditation Scheme, 32–38
 voluntary notifications, 38
 registration of, 34–35
  general registration, 34
  limited registration, 34
  non-practising registration, 35
  provisional registration, 35
  specialist registration, 34
  student registration, 35
Health Services Act 1997, 67
Health system, Australian, 16–23
 access to health care, evolving schemes, 19–22
  aged care, 21–22
  issues with the current scheme, 21
  Medicare, 20
  National Disability Insurance Scheme (NDIS), 21
  private health insurance, 20–21
 charter of healthcare rights, 22–23
 Commonwealth responsibility for healthcare services, 16–17, 17*b*
 healthcare expenditure, 22
 local governments, 17–18
 shared responsibilities between the Commonwealth and states/territories, 17, 18*b*
 state powers and responsibilities regarding the health system, 17, 17*b*
 universal health system, history of, 18–19
  access to medicines, Pharmaceutical Benefits Scheme, 18–19
  private prescriptions, 19
Hearsay evidence, 190
High Court, 11
Home care, 21
Home support, 21
Homicide, 97–98
 euthanasia and, 99
Honest opinion (defence of fair comment at common law), 89
Human leukocyte antigen (HLA) typing, screening of, 124

Human Reproductive Technology Act 1991, 125–126, 128–129
Human Tissue And Transplant Act 1982, 128
Human tissue and transplantation, 128
Hunter and New England Area Health Service v A (2009), 133

I

Impaired pharmacy student, 222*b*
Implied consent, 84
In vitro fertilisation (IVF), 124–126
Inadequate funding, case study on, 238*b*
Incompetent adult, tissue removal from, 148–149
Incomplete patient notes, 232*b*
Indictable/summary offences, 94
Industrial (or employment) law, 8
Infant Life (Preservation) Act 1929 (UK), 116
Infanticide, 102
Information access, by donor-conceived people, 126–127
Injunctions, 193
Injunctive relief, 193
Inquisitorial approach, defined, 9
Insanity, criminal law defence, 97
Insemination, artificial, 124–125
Inspection, of documents, 185–186
Intent to assist, 96
Intentional act, 79
Intentional torts, 79–91
    apologies, 89–90
    damages and costs, 90
    defamation, 87–89
    trespass to person, 79–87, 80*f*
Interim injunction, 193
Interlocutory injunction, 193
Interlocutory steps, 188
International Covenant on Economic, Social and Cultural Rights, 3
Interrogatories, 185–186
Involuntary admission, mental health and, 166–167
Involuntary euthanasia, 99
Involuntary manslaughter, 98
Involuntary treatment, case study on, 197*b*
IVF. *see* In vitro fertilisation

J

Judge-made or common law, 4*b*
Jurisdiction, 10
Justice, 28
Justice of the Peace, 185
Justification/truth, defences to action in defamation, 89

K

'Known donor', 126

L

Law
    ethics *vs.*, 26, 27*t*
    ignorance of, 94
Law Reform Act 1995, 67
Lawyer, 188
Legal and ethical principles, 196–248
Legal documents
    affidavits as, 184–185
    Justices of the Peace, 185
Legal issues
    on accepting gifts, 236
    on care outside the guidelines, 202
    on consent, privacy and confidentiality, 240
    on consent to treatment of minor, 205
    on death and organ donation, 199
    on end of life and family conflict, 213–214
    on family on active physiotherapy, 224–225
    on impaired pharmacy student, 222–223
    on impairment of fellow worker, 215
    on inadequate funding and service delivery, 238–239
    on involuntary treatment, 197
    on issues of consent, 233–234
    on mandatory reporting, 198
    on mental health, 197, 211
    on negligence, 217
    on patient-centred care conflict with evidence-based care, 228
    on patients with dementia, 221
    on pharmacists and complementary medicines, 218
    on pharmacists and family, 224
    on pharmacists' personal *versus* professional views and practices, 220
    on poor record keeping, 242
    on possible elder abuse, 237
    on privacy, 212
    on private life affecting your professional life, 210
    on professional boundaries, 206
    on refusal of treatment, 203–204
    on right to communication; physical and psychological abuse, 245
    on sexual relationship with patient, 209
    on social media, 235
    on sports therapist's obligations, 227
    on standards of care and physiotherapy treatment, 230–231
    on stealing and self-administration of Schedule 8 drugs, 207
    on stealing patient's money, 208
    on testimonials and confidentiality, 200
    on treatment disagreement, 229
    on worsening dysphagia, refusal of food modifications, 243
Legal practitioner, 188
Legal recognition, 120
Legal representatives, 184–195
    discovery (disclosure) and inspection of documents, 185–186
    interrogatories, 186
    notice of non-party disclosure, 186
    rules of evidence and standards of proof, 187–188
    statutory declarations as, 184
    subpoenas, 186–187
Legal system, Australian, 2–14
    Australia as federation, 2
    court hierarchy, 10–11
        courts/tribunals, 10–11
        original and appellate jurisdiction, 10
        understanding jurisdiction, 10
    distribution of power between the states and the Commonwealth, 2–4
    general features of, 9–10
        alternative dispute resolution, 9–10
        natural justice, 9
        presumption of innocence, 9
    legislation, 4–8
        common law, 6–8, 7*f*
        delegated, 6
        passage of, 4–6, 5*f*
    separation of powers, 4, 4*b*
    skills relevant to understanding judicial decisions and legislation, 12–13
        reading judicial decisions (cases), 12–13, 12*b*
        regulations, 13
        statutory interpretation, 13, 13*b*–14*b*
    types of law, 8–9
        procedural law, 8
        substantive law, 8
Legally incompetent adults, decision making for, 140, 140*t*
Legislation
    for mental health, 162–173
        Australian policies and standards for, 164–165
        Fifth National Mental Health and Suicide Prevention Plan, 165
        international law and policy for, 162–164

mental health statement of rights and responsibilities, 165
national mental health policy, 164
national recovery-oriented mental health practice framework, 165
national standards for mental health services, 164
state and territory legislation, 165, 166t
or statutory law, 4b
LHC. see Lifetime Health Cover
Liability, 93–94
strict, 95
Life, wrongful, 121–122
claims regarding, 120–122
Life-sustaining measure, 133–134
Lifetime Health Cover (LHC), 20–21
Limited registration, health practitioners, 34
area of need, 34
postgraduate training or supervised practice, 34
public interest, 34
teaching or research, 34
Literal rule, 13
'Living will', 132
Local Court, 113

M

Magistrates' Courts (Local Courts), 10
Mandatory injunction, 193
Mandatory reporting, 198b
of child abuse, 176–179, 176t–179t
Manslaughter, homicide, 98
Material risks, 68–69
Medibank, 20
Medical abortions, 116
'Medical decision-maker', in decision making, 135
Medical malpractice, 63b
Medical negligence, 63b
Medical Practice Regulations 2003, 60
Medical Practitioner's Act 1958, 66–67
Medical professionals, South Australia, 117
'Medical treatment decision', 134
Medical Treatment Planning and Decisions Act 2016, 134
Medicare, 20
Medicare levy, 20
Medication error, 159–160
Medicine, case studies on, 197–246
death and organ donation, 199b
mandatory reporting, 198b
mental health and involuntary treatment, 197b
Medicolegal autopsy, 113

'Menhennitt ruling', 117
Mens rea, 95
Mental health
case studies
on medicine, 197b
on paramedicine, 211b
definitions of, 165–166
electroconvulsive therapy for, 170
hospital and care orders, 166–167
restraint and, 169
restricted treatment for, 169–170
review boards/ tribunals, 170–171
seclusion with, 169
and treatment without the patient's consent, 167–169
Mental health legislation, 162–173
Australian policies and standards for, 164–165
Fifth National Mental Health and Suicide Prevention Plan, 165
international law and policy for, 162–164
mental health statement of rights and responsibilities, 165
National Mental Health Policy, 164
national recovery-oriented mental health practice framework, 165
National Standards for Mental Health Services, 164
state and territory legislation, 165, 166t
Mental health statement of rights and responsibilities, 165
Metaethics, 25
Midwifery, case studies on, 200–206
care outside the guidelines, 201b–202b
consent to treatment of minor, 205b
professional boundaries, 206b
refusal of treatment, 203b
testimonials and confidentiality, 200b
Minors
consent to treatment of, 205b
withholding and withdrawal of treatment for, 140–142
'Miscarriage', 116
Miscarriage of Women Act 1803 (UK), 116
'M'Naghten rule', 97
Murder, 97–98

N

Narcotic Drug Act 1967, 153
Narcotic drugs, regulations for, 153
National Boards, 33–34
National Code of Conduct, 44
National Disability Insurance Agency (NDIA), 21

National Disability Insurance Scheme (NDIS), 21
National Drugs and Poisons Schedule Committee, 153
National Electronic Health Transitional Authority (NEHTA), 50–51
National Framework for Protecting Australia's Children 2009-2020, 175
National Health Act 1953, 157
National Health and Medical Research Council Guidelines, 150
National Health Scheme, 19–20
National Health Service Act, 19
National Law, 32–34, 33t
National Mental Health Policy, 164
National Perinatal Data Collection, 109
National recovery-oriented mental health practice framework, 165
National Registration and Accreditation Scheme, 32–38
fifteen health professions: APRHA and the National Boards, 32–34
Australian Health Practitioners Regulation Agency (AHPRA), 33
National Boards, 33–34
registration of health practitioners, 34–35
general registration, 34
limited registration, 34
non-practising registration, 35
provisional registration, 35
specialist registration, 34
student registration, 35
registration standards, 35–38
additional standards, 36–37
Continuing Professional Development Registration Standard, 35
Criminal History Registration Standard, 35–36
English Language Skills Registration Standard, 36
guidelines, codes and policies, 37
guidelines and requirements for mandatory reporting, 37–38
Professional Indemnity Insurance Arrangements Registration Standard, 36
Recency of Practice Registration Standard, 36
National Standards for Mental Health Services, 164
Natural justice, 9
NDIA. see National Disability Insurance Agency

NDIS. *see* National Disability Insurance Scheme
Neglect
  in child abuse, 175
  mental illness and, 170
Negligence, 63–78, 63*b*, 120, 217*b*
  alternative actions, 76
    complaints and professional regulation, 76
    consumer protection, 76
  apologies, 73, 74*t*
  Australian Open Disclosure Framework, 73–74
  criminal, 95
  elements, 64–73
    causation, 69–70
    damage, 69
    duty of care, 65–69
  non-delegable duty of care, 75–76
  parties, 64
  proof, 64
  vicarious liability, 74–75
  wrongful death, 73
Negligent manslaughter, 98
NEHTA. *see* National Electronic Health Transitional Authority
Neurosurgery for mental illness (NMI), 170
New South Wales, 41–42, 118*t*–119*t*
  access to health information, 57–58
  birth notification requirements in, 109*t*
  child abuse, laws regarding mandatory reporting of, 176*t*–179*t*
  child protection legislation, principal Acts, 175*t*
  consequences of an apology or expression of regret, 74*t*
  drug and poisons legislation by jurisdiction, 154*t*
  Health Records and Information Privacy Act, 60
  legislation authorising medical intervention for children and young people, 87*t*
  mental health legislation by jurisdiction, 166*t*
  National Law, 33*t*
  substitute decision-makers, 136*t*
    appointed by a tribunal, 138*t*
    recognised by legislation, 137*t*
Next friend, 64
NMI. *see* Neurosurgery for mental illness
Non-custodial sentences, 93
Non-maleficence, 28
Non-party disclosure, 186

Non-practising registration, health practitioners, 35
Non-regenerative tissue, removal of, 148
Non-voluntary euthanasia, 99
Normal fortitude, 67
Normative ethics, 25
Northern Territory
  access to health information, 58
  birth notification requirements in, 109*t*
  child abuse, laws regarding mandatory reporting of, 176*t*–179*t*
  child protection legislation, principal Acts, 175*t*
  conscientious objection, 117
  consequences of an apology or expression of regret, 74*t*
  drug and poisons legislation by jurisdiction, 154*t*
  laws relevant to abortion, 118*t*–119*t*
  legislation authorising medical intervention for children and young people, 87*t*
  mental health legislation by jurisdiction, 166*t*
  National Law, 33*t*
  statutory advance directives in, 133
  substitute decision-makers, 136*t*
    appointed by a tribunal, 138*t*
    recognised by legislation, 137*t*
'Not for resuscitation' order, 137–139
Nurse-initiated drugs, regulations for, 158–159
Nursing, case studies on, 207–211
  private life can affect professional life, 210*b*
  sexual relationship with patient, 209*b*
  stealing a patient's money, 208*b*
  stealing and self-administration of Schedule 8 drugs, 207*b*
Nursing and Midwifery Board of Australia v Millikan, 182

O
Obvious risks, 69
Offences, 95
  charge for, cannot be retrospective, 94
Older persons and the law, 180
Omission to act, 96
Optometry Board of Australia, 37
'Ordinary costs', 121
Organ donation, 199*b*
Organs, donation of, 146–151
  ethical and legal issues in, 146–150
Original evidence, 190

P
Panel, person appointed by, in decision making, 135
Paramedicine, case studies on, 211–218
  end of life and family conflict, 213*b*
  impairment of fellow worker, 215*b*
  mental health, 211*b*
  negligence, 217*b*
  privacy, 212*b*
Parens patriae power, 149
'Parent', in tissue removal, 147
Parentage, 126
Parental decision-making authority, 85
Partner abuse, exposure to intimate, 175
Passive euthanasia, 99
Patient-centred care, conflicts with evidence-based care, 228*b*
Patient notes, incomplete, 232*b*
Perinatal data collection, for notification of birth, 109–110
Perinatal death, 111
Perjury, 190
Perpetual injunction, 193
Person appointed, in decision making, 135, 136*t*
Person recognised/assigned by legislation, in decision making, 135, 137*t*
Person responsible
  in decision making, 135
  for notification of birth, 108–109
Personal reaction
  on accepting gifts, 236
  on care outside the guidelines, 202
  on consent, privacy and confidentiality, 240
  on consent to treatment of minor, 205
  on death and organ donation, 199
  on end of life and family conflict, 214
  on family on active physiotherapy, 225
  on impairment of fellow worker, 216
  on inadequate funding and service delivery, 239
  on incomplete patient notes, 232
  on involuntary treatment, 197
  on issues of consent, 234
  on mandatory reporting, 198
  on mental health, 197, 212
  on negligence, 217–218
  on pharmacists' personal *versus* professional views and practices, 220
  on poor record keeping, 242
  on possible elder abuse, 237
  on privacy, 213
  on private life affecting your professional life, 210

on professional boundaries, 206
on refusal of treatment, 204
on right to communication; physical
    and psychological abuse, 245
on sexual relationship with patient, 209
on social media, 235
on sports therapist's obligations, 227
on stealing and self-administration of
    Schedule 8 drugs, 207
on stealing patient's money, 208
on testimonials and confidentiality,
    200
on treatment disagreement, 229
on worsening dysphagia, refusal of food
    modifications, 243–244
Pharmaceutical Benefits Scheme, 153
Pharmacists, 218b
    and family, 223b
    versus professional views and practices,
        219b
Pharmacy, case studies on, 218–224
    impaired pharmacy student, 222b
    patients with dementia, 221b
    pharmacists and complementary
        medicines, 218b
    pharmacists and family, 223b
    pharmacists' personal versus
        professional views and practices,
        219b
Physical abuse
    case study on, 245b
    in child abuse, 174
Physiotherapy, case studies on, 224–232
    family on active physiotherapy, 224b
    patient-centred care conflicts with
        evidence-based care, 228b
    sports therapist's obligations,
        226b–227b
    standards of care and physiotherapy
        treatment, 230b
    treatment disagreement, 228b–229b
Plaintiff, 12b, 64
Planning, advance care, 132–143
    directives and, 132–134
        common law advance care directives,
            133
        not need to be followed, 134
        statutory advance directives,
            133–134
Pleadings, 188
Podiatry, case studies on, 232–238
    accepting gifts, 236b
    incomplete patient notes, 232b
    issues of consent, 233b
    possible elder abuse, 237b
    social media, 235b

Poisons, regulations of, 152–161
    customs import and export, 153
    drug schedules for, 154, 155t
    federal, 152–153
    policy, 154–156
    state and territory, 153–154, 154t
Posthumous use, of gametes, 128–129
Postmortem/autopsy, 113
'Postmortem examination', 113
Powers of Attorney Act 1998, 133–134
Pregnancy
    active termination of, 116
    termination of, 116
Prenatal injury, 122
    claims regarding, 120–122
Prescribing, regulation of drugs and, 157
Presumption of innocence, 9
Privacy, 53–54
    case study
        on paramedicine, 212b
        on speech pathology, 240b
    Commonwealth privacy legislation,
        53–54
Privacy Act, 53
Private health insurance, 20–21
Private life, affect professional life, 210b
Privilege, 192–193
Procedural law, 8
Professional boundaries, 206b
Professional Indemnity Insurance
    Arrangements Registration
    Standard, 36
Professional issues
    on impaired pharmacy student, 223
    on patients with dementia, 221
Professional life, private life affect, 210b
Professional practice, Coroners Court
    finding regarding, 113–114
Professional regulation, of health
    practitioners, 32–46
    codes of conduct, 38–39
    disciplinary issues, 39–40
    disciplinary process, 40–43
        decisions by responsible tribunals,
            41–43
        disciplinary tribunal processes, 43
    guidelines for advertising regulated
        health services, 38
    health practitioners not regulated by
        the National Scheme, 43–45
    codes of conduct, 43–44
    self regulation, 43
    who does the National Code of
        Conduct apply to?, 44–45
    mental or physical incapacity or
        impairment, 40

National Registration and Accreditation
    Scheme, 32–38
    fifteen health professions: APRHA
        and the National Boards, 32–34
    registration of health practitioners,
        34–35
    voluntary notifications, 38
Prosecution, 93
Provision of information, 83
Provisional registration, health
    practitioners, 35
Provocation, defence of, 96
Psychological abuse
    case study on, 245b
    in child abuse, 174–175
Psychology Board of Australia, 37
Psychosurgery, 170
Punitive damages. see Exemplary damages
Pure mental harm, 67
Purpose rule, 13

Q

Qualified privilege, 89
Quality of Care Principles 2014, 181
Queensland, 42–43, 118t–119t
    access to health information, 58
    birth notification requirements in, 109t
    child abuse, laws regarding mandatory
        reporting of, 176t–179t
    child protection legislation, principal
        Acts, 175t
    consequences of an apology or
        expression of regret, 74t
    drug and poisons legislation by
        jurisdiction, 154t
    legislation authorising medical
        intervention for children and
        young people, 87t
    mental health legislation by jurisdiction,
        166t
    National Law, 33t
    statutory advance directives in, 133–134
    substitute decision-makers, 136t
        appointed by a tribunal, 138t
        recognised by legislation, 137t

R

R v Byrne, 97
Rape, 102–103
    current categories of, 103
Reasonable creature, victim, 98
Recency of Practice Registration Standard,
    36
Record keeping, poor, 242b
Re-examination, trial, 189–190
Refusal of treatment, 203b

Regenerative tissue, removal of, 146–148
Registration
    of birth, 108–110
        change of sex, 110
        children born ex-nuptially, 110
        notification and, 108–111, 109t
        perinatal data collection, 109–110
    of death, 110–111
        definition of, 110
        notification and, 108–111
        obligation to notify, 111
        perinatal, 111
    of health practitioners, 34–35
        general registration, 34
        limited registration, 34
        non-practising registration, 35
        provisional registration, 35
        specialist registration, 34
        student registration, 35
    standards, 35–38
        additional standards, 36–37
        Continuing Professional
            Development Registration
            Standard, 35
        Criminal History Registration
            Standard, 35–36
        English Language Skills Registration
            Standard, 36
        guidelines, codes and policies,
            37
        guidelines and requirements for
            mandatory reporting, 37–38
        Professional Indemnity Insurance
            Arrangements Registration
            Standard, 36
        Recency of Practice Registration
            Standard, 36
Regulations of drugs, 152–161
    administration, 157–158
    complementary medicines, 156
    customs import and export, 153
    definitions of, 156
    drug schedules for, 154, 155t
    federal, 152–153
    medication errors and, 159–160
    for nurse-initiated drugs, 158–159
    policy, 154–156
    prescribing and, 157
    standing orders, 159
    state and territory, 153–154, 154t
    storage and, 156–157
    verbal orders for, 158
Reportable deaths, 112
Reporting, of child abuse, 175–179
    mandatory, 176–179, 176t–179t
    voluntary, 175–176

Reproductive Technology Accreditation
    Council (RTAC), 124–125
    code, 127
Res ipsa loquitur, 64
Research, consent to, 84
Residential care, 21–22
Residual, defined, 3
Respect for autonomy, 28
Respondent, 12b
Restraint, 169
Restricted treatment, for mental health,
    169–170
Restrictive injunction, 193
Review boards, mental health, 170–171
Role of the courts, 85–86
RTAC. see Reproductive Technology
    Accreditation Council
Rules of evidence, 187–188

S
Satisfactory conduct, 39
Science, forensic, 193–194
Seclusion, 169
Secondary evidence, 190
Self-administration, of Schedule 8 drugs,
    207b
Self-defence, 87
    criminal law defence, 96
Service delivery, case study on, 238b
Sex, change of, 110
Sex Discrimination Act 1984, 126
Sexual abuse, in child abuse, 175
Sexual relationship, with patient, 209b
'Sibling', in tissue removal, 147
Single Convention on Narcotic Drugs
    (1961), 153
Social media, 235b
Solicitors, 188
Sound memory and age, criminal law, 98
South Australia, 118t–119t
    access to health information, 58
    birth notification requirements in, 109t
    child abuse, laws regarding mandatory
        reporting of, 176t–179t
    child protection legislation, principal
        Acts, 175t
    consequences of an apology or
        expression of regret, 74t
    drug and poisons legislation by
        jurisdiction, 154t
    legislation authorising medical
        intervention for children and
        young people, 87t
    medical professionals, 117
    mental health legislation by jurisdiction,
        166t

National Law, 33t
statutory advance directives in, 134
substitute decision-makers, 136t
    appointed by a tribunal, 138t
    recognised by legislation, 137t
South Australian Act, in assisted
    reproduction technologies (ART),
    125
Special medical procedure, 85
Specialist registration, health practitioners,
    34
Specialist titles, 34
Specific/special damages, 72
Speech pathology, case studies on,
    238–246
    consent, privacy, and confidentiality,
        240b
    inadequate funding and service delivery,
        238b
    physical and psychological abuse, 245b
    poor record keeping, 242b
    right to communication, 245b
    worsening dysphagia, refusal of food
        modifications, 243b
Sports therapist, 226b–227b
Standard for the Uniform Scheduling of
    Medicines and Poisons (SUSMP),
    154, 155t
Standards of care, in physiotherapy, 230b
Standing orders, 159
State and territory legislation, for mental
    health, 165, 166t
State and territory regulation, for drug
    and poisons, 153–154, 154t
State parliaments, 3
Statutory advance directives, advance care
    planning in, 133–134
Statutory authority, defence, 86–87, 87t
Statutory declarations, 184
'Statutory health attorney', in decision
    making, 135
Statutory interpretation, 13, 13b–14b
    golden rule, 13
    literal rule, 13
    purpose rule, 13
Stealing
    of patient's money, 208b
    of Schedule 8 drugs, 207b
Stillbirth, 109
Strict liability, 95
Student registration, health practitioners,
    35
Subpoenas, 186–187
Substantive law, 8
    constitutional law, 8
    contract law, 8

criminal law, 8
industrial (or employment) law, 8
tort law, 8
Substitute decision-makers, decision
    making by, 135–137
Substitute decisions, 83
Summons, 187
Support or substitute decision-makers,
    135–137
'Support person', in decision making, 135
Supported decisions, 83
Supreme Courts, 11
Surrogacy, 129–130
    altruistic, 129
Surrogacy Act, 126
SUSMP. *see* Standard for the Uniform
    Scheduling of Medicines and
    Poisons

T
Tasmania
    access to health information, 58–59
    birth notification requirements in, 109*t*
    child abuse, laws regarding mandatory
        reporting of, 176*t*–179*t*
    child protection legislation, principal
        Acts, 175*t*
    consequences of an apology or
        expression of regret, 74*t*
    drug and poisons legislation by
        jurisdiction, 154*t*
    laws relevant to abortion, 118*t*–119*t*
    legislation authorising medical
        intervention for children and
        young people, 87*t*
    mental health legislation by jurisdiction,
        166*t*
    National Law, 33*t*
    substitute decision-makers, 136*t*
        appointed by a tribunal, 138*t*
        recognised by legislation, 137*t*
'Termination of pregnancy', 116
Testimonials, 200*b*
*The Care and Protection of Children Act
    2007*, 176*t*–179*t*
The presumption of innocence, 93
The standard of proof, 93
Therapeutic Goods Act 1989, 152–153
Therapeutic privilege, 68–69
Tissue, removal and donation of, 146–151
    after death, 149–150
    Australian Organ and Tissue Donation
        and Transplantation Authority
        (OTA), 150
    clinical guidelines for, 150
    consent revocation in, 148

ethical and legal issues in, 146–150
    from incompetent adult, 148–149
    *National Health and Medical Research
        Council Guidelines*, 150
    non-regenerative tissue, 148
    regenerative tissue, 146–148
To aid, abet, 95–96
Tort law, 8
Treatment
    Commonwealth legislation, 137
    'not for resuscitation' or 'do not
        resuscitate' orders, 137–139
    revocation and limits of decision in,
        134–135
    support or substitute decision-makers,
        135–137
    withholding and withdrawal of,
        132–143
        guardianship decision on, 139–142
        for minors, 140–142
Trespass to person, 79–87, 80*f*
    assault, 80–81
    battery, 81
    damages for, 87
    defences to, 82–87
    false imprisonment, 81–82
Trial, sequence of, 188–190
    cross-examination, 189
    examination-in-chief, 189
    re-examination, 189–190
Trial process, 188
Tribunals, 11
    person appointed by, in decision
        making, 135, 138*t*
Triviality, defence of, 89

U
Universal Declaration of Human Rights, 3
Unlawfully kills, homicide, 98
Unprofessional conduct, 39–40
Unsatisfactory professional performance,
    39
Users Rights Principles 2014, 181

V
Values
    on accepting gifts, 236
    on care outside the guidelines, 202
    on consent, privacy and confidentiality,
        240–241
    on consent to treatment of minor, 205
    on end of life and family conflict, 215
    on family on active physiotherapy, 226
    on impairment of fellow worker, 216
    on inadequate funding and service
        delivery, 239

on incomplete patient notes, 232
    on involuntary treatment, 198
    on issues of consent, 234
    on mandatory reporting, 198
    on mental health, 198, 212
    on negligence, 218
    on patient-centred care conflict with
        evidence-based care, 228
    on poor record keeping, 242–243
    on possible elder abuse, 238
    on privacy, 213
    on private life affecting your
        professional life, 210
    on professional boundaries, 206
    on refusal of treatment, 204
    on right to communication; physical
        and psychological abuse, 245–246
    on sexual relationship with patient, 209
    on social media, 235
    on sports therapist's obligations, 227
    on stealing and self-administration of
        Schedule 8 drugs, 207–208
    on stealing patient's money, 208
    on testimonials and confidentiality, 200
    on treatment disagreement, 230
    on worsening dysphagia, refusal of food
        modifications, 244
Verbal consent, 84–85
Verbal orders, for drugs, 158
Vicarious liability, 74–75
Victoria
    access to health information, 59
    birth notification requirements in, 109*t*
    child abuse, laws regarding mandatory
        reporting of, 176*t*–179*t*
    child protection legislation, principal
        Acts, 175*t*
    consequences of an apology or
        expression of regret, 74*t*
    drug and poisons legislation by
        jurisdiction, 154*t*
    laws relevant to abortion, 118*t*–119*t*
    legislation authorising medical
        intervention for children and
        young people, 87*t*
    mental health legislation by jurisdiction,
        166*t*
    National Law, 33*t*
    statutory advance directives in, 134
    substitute decision-makers, 136*t*
        appointed by a tribunal, 138*t*
        recognised by legislation, 137*t*
Victorian Health Records Act, 60
Victoria's *Abortion Law Reform Act 2008*,
    119
Virtue ethics, 28

Voluntary admission, mental health and, 166
Voluntary euthanasia, 99
Voluntary manslaughter, 98
'Voluntary register', 127
Voluntary reporting, of child abuse, 175–176

W

Western Australia
    access to health information, 59
    birth notification requirements in, 109*t*
    child abuse, laws regarding mandatory reporting of, 176*t*–179*t*
    child protection legislation, principal Acts, 175*t*

consequences of an apology or expression of regret, 74*t*
drug and poisons legislation by jurisdiction, 154*t*
Health Act 1911, 119–120
laws relevant to abortion, 118*t*–119*t*
legislation authorising medical intervention for children and young people, 87*t*
mental health legislation by jurisdiction, 166*t*
National Law, 33*t*
statutory advance directives in, 134
substitute decision-makers, 136*t*
    appointed by a tribunal, 138*t*
    recognised by legislation, 137*t*
Williams, Glanville, 92

Withholding and withdrawal, of treatment, 132–143
    guardianship decision on, 139–142
    for minors, 140–142
Witness, 191–192
Witnesses, professional expertise, 191–194
Written consent, 85
Wrongful birth, claims regarding, 120–122
Wrongful conception/birth, 120–121
Wrongful death, 73
Wrongful life, 121–122
    claims regarding, 120–122

Y

Young Persons and their Families Act 1997, 86